Complications in
Facial Plastic Surgery

Thieme

Complications in Facial Plastic Surgery

Randolph B. Capone, MD, FACS
Director, The Baltimore Center for Facial Plastic Surgery
Assistant Professor of Otolaryngology/Head and Neck Surgery
Division of Facial Plastic and Reconstructive Surgery
The Johns Hopkins University School of Medicine
Baltimore, Maryland

Jonathan M. Sykes, MD, FACS
Immediate Past President, AAFPRS
Professor of Otolaryngology/Head and Neck Surgery
Director, Facial Plastic and Reconstructive Surgery
University of California–Davis Medical Center
Sacramento, California

2012

Thieme
New York · Stuttgart

Thieme Medical Publishers, Inc.
333 Seventh Ave.
New York, NY 10001

Executive Editor: Timothy Hiscock
Managing Editor: J. Owen Zurhellen IV
Editorial Assistant: Elizabeth Berg
Editorial Director, Clinical Reference: Michael Wachinger
Production Editor: Kenneth L. Chumbley
International Production Director: Andreas Schabert
Senior Vice President, International Marketing and Sales: Cornelia Schulze
Vice President, Finance and Accounts: Sarah Vanderbilt
President: Brian D. Scanlan
Illustrator: Robert J. Brown
Compositor: Prairie Papers Inc.
Cover Illustration: *Shipwreck* (1854) by Ivan K. Aivazovsky. Image courtesy of the State Russian Museum, Saint
    Petersburg, Russia, whose collection includes this painting.
Printer: Leo Paper Group

Library of Congress Cataloging-in-Publication Data

Complications in facial plastic surgery / [edited by] Randolph B. Capone, Jonathan M. Sykes.
    p. ; cm.
Includes bibliographical references.
ISBN 978-1-60406-026-3 (hardback)
I. Capone, Randolph B. II. Sykes, Jonathan M.
[DNLM: 1. Cosmetic Techniques—adverse effects. 2. Face—surgery. 3. Medical Errors—prevention & control.
4. Reconstructive Surgical Procedures—adverse effects. WE 705]

617.5'20592—dc23

2011052040

Important note: Medical knowledge is ever-changing. As new research and clinical experience broaden our knowledge, changes in treatment and drug therapy may be required. The authors and editors of the material herein have consulted sources believed to be reliable in their efforts to provide information that is complete and in accord with the standards accepted at the time of publication. However, in view of the possibility of human error by the authors, editors, or publisher of the work herein or changes in medical knowledge, neither the authors, editors, nor publisher, nor any other party who has been involved in the preparation of this work, warrants that the information contained herein is in every respect accurate or complete, and they are not responsible for any errors or omissions or for the results obtained from use of such information. Readers are encouraged to confirm the information contained herein with other sources. For example, readers are advised to check the product information sheet included in the package of each drug they plan to administer to be certain that the information contained in this publication is accurate and that changes have not been made in the recommended dose or in the contraindications for administration. This recommendation is of particular importance in connection with new or infrequently used drugs.

Some of the product names, patents, and registered designs referred to in this book are in fact registered trademarks or proprietary names even though specific reference to this fact is not always made in the text. Therefore, the appearance of a name without designation as proprietary is not to be construed as a representation by the publisher that it is in the public domain.

Printed in China

5 4 3 2 1

ISBN 978-1-60406-026-3
eISBN 978-1-60406-027-0

Complications are inescapable. This text is therefore dedicated to all who practice plastic surgery of the face, regardless of experience or expertise. Special emphasis, however, is placed on individuals early in practice so that they might learn from the adversity of others. While untoward outcomes are experienced as fellows, residents, and medical students, these doctors will now encounter them singularly as the patient's surgeon. Although their preparation has been thorough, they will acquire additional experience in the more challenging, yet more rewarding, school of experience.

Randolph B. Capone, MD, FACS
Jonathan M. Sykes, MD, FACS

Contents

Foreword

Randolph B. Capone and Jonathan M. Sykes have given us a wise and important book, *Complications in Facial Plastic Surgery*. Complications—and especially their prevention—are far too infrequent a focus in our scientific literature. The importance of preventing complications rose to national prominence with the publication in 1999 of the Institute of Medicine (IOM) report, *To Err Is Human: Building a Safer Health Care System*. The IOM report stated that "medical errors can be defined as the failure of a planned action to be completed as intended or the use of a wrong plan to achieve an aim." Its strong conclusion that "health care in the United States is not as safe as it should be—and can be" became a stimulus for the now widely accepted quality movement in American medicine.

Dr. Capone's own first chapter is humanistic and emphasizes the unique nature of aesthetic surgery. This book appropriately expands the usual definition of complications as "an unfavorable outcome" to now include "patient dissatisfaction." All those who work in the exciting, creative, and sometimes frustrating specialty of facial plastic surgery recognize that patient satisfaction is a key outcome measure. Dr. Sykes provides thoughtful advice in his chapter "Management of the Dissatisfied Patient." Their general recommendation—that surgeons swiftly acknowledge and address complications—has become almost universally recognized but is appropriately emphasized here.

This book is well organized, with recognized experts discussing the major areas of facial plastic surgery. Tables provide a good summary of the cause, prevention, and treatments of specific complications. Complex subjects such as facial implants are explored with a thorough review of the data and presented honestly without oversimplification. The pearls of wisdom in each chapter highlight the authors' experience and judgment and provide an easily accessible summary for each topic. The major topics, from minimally invasive procedures to reconstruction surgery to aesthetic surgery, will be of interest to all facial plastic surgeons.

Drs. Capone and Sykes are to be congratulated for a work that will doubtless be widely read and improve outcomes for our patients. I hope to see many future editions of this fine book.

Wayne F. Larrabee Jr., MD
Clinical Professor
Department of Otolaryngology–
Head and Neck Surgery
University of Washington
Editor in Chief
The Archives of Facial Plastic Surgery
Seattle, Washington

Preface

No one yearns to be associated with a complications text, nor wants notoriety as an expert in adverse outcomes. Yet complications occur and are a fact of surgical practice. As the colloquial definition goes, an expert is one who is well versed in failure, and this certainly applies to the art and practice of surgery. Surgeons often learn more from the sting of a misstep than the satisfaction of a triumph.

A text that is never far from reach in the resident call room is a surgical complications book, and the information contained within has helped countless surgeons on the wards, in the operating room, and at weekly morbidity conferences.[1] Such books provided motivation, in part, for the present work.

Facial plastic surgeons perform a surprising breadth of procedures in a variety of venues, including the office, the hospital operating room, the outpatient surgical center, and in some instances, the commercial medspa. The editors have attempted, therefore, to include chapters by seasoned authors that cover all aspects of contemporary facial plastic surgery. Even so, it is difficult to successfully describe the management of all complications in all scenarios, and the editors make no claims that this work is by any means exhaustive. There are undoubtedly numerous complications that occur but are absent from this text.

Another aspect of this work that should be anticipated is that statistics on this topic are often significantly lacking in the literature, or if present, are determined from only a small sample. Therefore, universally accepted incidences for the complications discussed hereafter are typically unknown. Much of the data is either estimated, anecdotal, or simply absent. However, physicians in general, and surgeons in particular, learn from their individual observations. The use of anecdotal experience to mold knowledge and influence decision making is common practice in medicine. So even though the evidence in this book often does not rise above the level of the observations of experts, this knowledge can be used to improve others' level of care and improve patient outcomes.

Upon completion of training, surgeons cross a stark divide where one day there is ample supervision, and the next day there is none. It is hoped that a work of this sort can serve in some small way as a surrogate supervisor or companion to help provide guidance. The editors have tried to create such a text for those who practice plastic surgery of the face, and are indebted to its contributors. It is our hope that with continued, careful review of all outcomes good and bad, such a work will help encourage open and frank dialogue between all colleagues of plastic surgery, and especially with our patients.

> "Success is going from failure to failure without losing confidence."
> —*Abraham Lincoln*

Reference

1. Eisele DW, Johns ME. Complications in Head & Neck Surgery. First Edition. Mosby–Year Book, 1993.

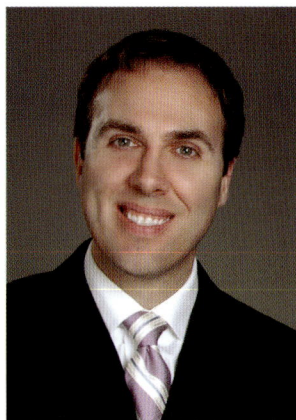

Randolph B. Capone, MD, FACS   *Jonathan M. Sykes, MD, FACS*

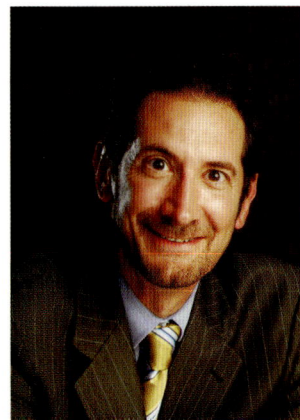

Contributors

Sydney C. Butts, MD
Assistant Professor and Chief
Division of Facial Plastic and Reconstructive Surgery
Department of Otolaryngology
SUNY Downstate Medical Center
Brooklyn, New York

Patrick J. Byrne, MD
Director
Division of Facial Plastic and Reconstructive Surgery
Associate Professor
The Johns Hopkins University School of Medicine
Baltimore, Maryland

Randolph B. Capone, MD
Director, The Baltimore Center for Facial Plastic Surgery
Assistant Professor of Otolaryngology/Head and Neck
    Surgery
Division of Facial Plastic and Reconstructive Surgery
The Johns Hopkins University School of Medicine
Baltimore, Maryland

Christopher R. Cote, MD
Faces First Cosmetic Surgery
Denver, Colorado

Jaimie DeRosa, MD, MS, FACS
Assistant Professor
Harvard Medical School
Facial Plastic and Reconstructive Surgeon
Department of Otology and Laryngology
Massachusetts Eye and Ear Infirmary
Boston, Massachusetts

John H. Eichhorn, MD
Professor of Anesthesiology
College of Medicine
Provost's Distinguished Service Professor
University of Kentucky
Department of Anesthesiology
University of Kentucky Medical Center
Lexington, Kentucky

John E. Frank, MD, FACS
Founder, Anapelli Hair Clinic
Assistant Professor of Clinical Otolaryngology
Columbia University College of Physicians and Surgeons
New York, New York

Robert A. Goldberg, MD
Karen and Frank Dabby Professor of Opthalmology
Chief, Orbital and Ophthalmic Plastic Surgery Division
Director, Orbital Disease Center
Co-Director, Aesthetic Center
Jules Stein Eye Institute
Los Angeles, California

Daniel T. Goulson, MD
Vice President for Medical Affairs
Our Lady of Bellefonte Hospital
Ashland, Kentucky

Ryan M. Greene, MD, PhD
Voluntary Assistant Professor
Division of Facial Plastic and Reconstructive Surgery
Department of Otolaryngology–Head and Neck Surgery
University of Miami Miller School of Medicine
Miami, Florida
Private Practice
Fort Lauderdale, Florida

Robert M. Kellman, MD, FACS
Professor and Chair
Department of Otolaryngology and Communication Sciences
SUNY Upstate Medical University
Syracuse, New York

Ji-Eon Kim
Fellow
Facial Plastic and Reconstructive Surgery
University of California–Davis School of Medicine
Sacramento, California

Srinivasan Krishna, MD, MPH
Director
Facial Plastic and Reconstructive Surgery
Bronx Lebanon Hospital Center
Bronx, New York

Corey S. Maas, MD, FACS
Founder and Director
The Maas Clinic
Associate Clinical Professor
University of California–San Francisco
Director
Facial Plastic Surgery Fellowship Training Program
American Academy of Facial Plastic and Reconstructive
  Surgery
San Francisco, California

Gary D. Monheit, MD
Total Skin and Beauty Dermatology Center, P.C.
Associate Clinical Professor
Departments of Dermatology and Ophthalmology
University of Alabama at Birmingham
Birmingham, Alabama

Ira D. Papel, MD
Associate Professor
Division of Facial Plastic Surgery
Department of Otolaryngology–Head and Neck Surgery
The Johns Hopkins University
Baltimore, Maryland

Shepherd G. Pryor V, MD, FACS
Founding Director
Valley Facial Plastic Surgery
Private Practice
Scottsdale, Arizona

Nicholas W. Rotas, DDS
Assistant Clinical Professor
Department of Otolaryngology
University of California–Davis School of Medicine
Sacramento, California

David A. Sherris, MD
Professor and Chairman
Department of Otolaryngology
University at Buffalo
Buffalo, New York

Sven-Olrik Streubel, MD, MBA
Pediatric Otolaryngology and Craniomaxillofacial Surgery
Assistant Professor
Department of Otolaryngology
Children's Hospital Colorado
University of Colorado School of Medicine
Aurora, Colorado

Jonathan M. Sykes, MD, FACS
Immediate Past President, AAFPRS
Professor of Otolaryngology/Head and Neck Surgery
Director
Facial Plastic and Reconstructive Surgery
University of California–Davis Medical Center
Sacramento, California

Sherard Austin Tatum III, MD, FAAP, FACS
Professor of Otolaryngology
Pediatrics Medical Director
Cleft and Craniofacial Center
SUNY Upstate Medical University
Syracuse, New York

Travis T. Tollefson, MD, MPH, FACS
Associate Professor
Department of Facial Plastic and Reconstructive Surgery/
  Cleft and Craniofacial Program/Otolaryngology–Head
  and Neck Surgery
University of California–Davis
Sacramento, California

Dean M. Toriumi, MD
Professor
Department of Otolaryngology–Head and Neck Surgery
University of Illinois–Chicago
Chicago, Illinois

Tom D. Wang, MD
Professor
Facial Plastic and Reconstructive Surgery
Oregon Health and Science University
Portland, Oregon

Edwin F. Williams III, MD
Medical Director
Williams Plastic Surgery Specialists
Latham, New York
Clinical Professor of Surgery
Albany Medical College
Albany, New York

Andrew A. Winkler, MD
Assistant Professor
Department of Otolaryngology
University of Colorado School of Medicine
Denver, Colorado

Paul R. Young, MD
Resident
Department of Otolaryngology
University at Buffalo
Buffalo, New York

1

Facial Plastic Surgery Complications: An Overview

Randolph B. Capone

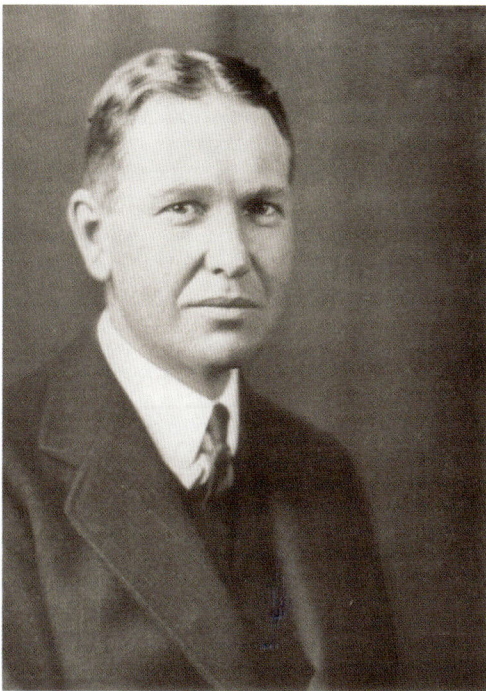

Fig. 1.1 Francis Weld Peabody. Used with permission from J Clin Invest. 1927 December; 5(1): 1.b1–6.

While lecturing at the Harvard Medical School in the fall of 1925, Frances Weld Peabody first made his memorable remark that "the secret of the care of the patient is in caring for the patient."[1] At the time, there was growing concern that rapid increases in scientific knowledge and emphasis on the pathophysiology of disease were consuming the attention of those studying medicine. Peabody felt the pendulum had swung too far toward medicine as a science than as an art, and his assertion that physicians should spend as much time caring for patients as attempting to understand what ails them secured Peabody a spot in American medical education history. Two years later, his remarks were published in JAMA:

> What is spoken of as a 'clinical picture' is not just a photograph of a sick man in bed; it is an impressionistic painting of the patient surrounded by his home, his work, his relations, his friends, his joys, sorrows, hopes, and fears.[1]
>
> *Peabody, 1927*

Although such a philosophy should be asserted by physicians daily in modern medical practice, empathy alone will unfortunately not protect our patients from undesirable healthcare events or untoward surgical outcomes. The surgeon cannot control predictably and reliably the multitude of variables involved in the care of a surgical patient. Surgical complications inevitably occur and do so in many varieties and with differing degrees of severity. Untoward outcomes stem from events that occur intraoperatively or postoperatively and can occur because of an undesirable patient characteristic (e.g., tobacco abuse, diabetes, malnutrition, or willful neglect), or because of an undesirable surgeon characteristic (e.g., technical error or poor judgment).

Unlike the airline industry, in which a successful flight can be defined as one that takes off and lands uneventfully without loss of life or limb, surgical complications occur along a greater spectrum of possible outcomes. This is especially true in plastic surgery, where the success of the outcome is not simply a matter of whether the flap lives or dies or whether the wound heals or does not; rather, it is a complex interplay of actual results, intended results, and expected results. At no time is this more important than when the surgeon's subject is the human face, for an undesirable outcome from an operation on the face is difficult to conceal in contemporary society and harbors unique significance:

> In civilized man, the face alone remains unclothed and exposed. An injury resulting in distortion of the features thus sets the unfortunate individual apart in a highly organized society where a premium is placed upon beauty and facial symmetry. Because disfigurement of the face becomes a serious social handicap, the surgical treatment of facial injuries is of special significance, as it serves to restore the inner feelings of happiness and well-being in addition to the outer appearance and function.[2]
>
> *Varstad Kazanjian and John Converse, 1949*

This text was conceived and crafted to help surgeons help their patients, so it is devoted to the prevention, identification, and management of unfavorable outcomes in contemporary facial plastic surgery.

◆ What Is a Complication?

Plastic surgeons and patients often interpret surgical results differently, and an undesirable result can be real or perceived. What the surgeon sees as a technical victory, the patient can easily view as unsightly. To complicate matters further, an undesirable outcome for one patient might be overlooked by another or even lauded by yet another. Despite such variability, there is a consistent emotion associated with poor surgical outcomes that all surgeons will inevitably experience during their careers: the sinking feeling that always accompanies the appearance of an undesirable result, the associated loss of patient confidence, and the uncomfortable torque that ensues on the patient-doctor relationship.

For the purposes of this text, it is necessary to understand the definition of a complication in facial plastic surgery. Because of the aesthetic nature of the specialty, the familiar definition has been expanded to include patient dissatisfaction as a complication. Therefore, a complication can be defined as an undesirable outcome that occurs because of the presence of one or more of four conditions: (1) inappropriate surgical technique, (2) inappropriate surgical judgment, (3) inappropriate recovery, and (4) inappropriate patient expectations. Inappropriate technique includes both equipment failure and doing the advisable procedure but performing it incorrectly. Inappropriate judgment includes both poor patient selection and doing an ill-advised procedure but performing it correctly. Inappropriate surgical recovery includes any aberration in wound healing or other complication that arises in the recovery period, and inappropriate patient expectations occur when the surgical result falls significantly short of the outcome the patient desired. Because this latter condition is extremely

important in aesthetic surgery, it is therefore included with the more traditional types of surgical complications, because *any* outcome whereby the patient is truly not happy is an undesirable outcome.

Complications in facial plastic surgery are not uniformly the result of errors by the surgeon, although it has been estimated that 60–82% of adverse events in healthcare might be attributed to human error.[3,4] Therefore, avoidance of the terms "error" or "mistake" in the previous descriptions is purposeful, so as not to imply fault. While consulting the chapters of this book, readers should keep this framework in mind and are encouraged to develop familiarity with these four forms of causation. Surgeons can then hope to identify deftly, manage adeptly, and reconstruct appropriately the cause of their patient's unfortunate result, for both the benefit of the patient and the prevention of future problems.

◆ How Are Complications Avoided?

PATIENT VIGNETTE: A patient desiring revision rhinoplasty displays columellar malposition with accompanying nostril asymmetry. She desires symmetric nostrils. Her request during consultation is straightforward, and she instructs the surgeon emphatically, "Just please make them equal, doctor." After careful examination, the surgeon indicates that if given the opportunity, he would do everything he could to repair her columella and improve her nostril symmetry, but that revision rhinoplasty is a challenging operation devoid of guarantees. Although he shows her photos of previous patients he has helped with a similar problem, he emphasizes that many factors affect the position of the skin bridge between the nostrils and that he cannot know with certainty why she healed this way or what the prior surgeon did that might have affected this area. During the discussion, he indicates that his surgical fee is for the attempt, not the result, and he emphasizes the importance of this distinction. This dialogue helps modify the expectations of the patient, so that when after the operation her columellar position and nostril symmetry appear improved but not perfect, she is still pleased. If the surgeon had not communicated with the patient effectively, she could easily have been significantly disturbed by the lack of perfection that she thought she was paying for.

As illustrated, communication between patient and plastic surgeon is a powerfully helpful tool to avert the untoward outcome of patient dissatisfaction with the surgery. Adequately trained and empathic surgeons who are most adept at the skills of communication will fare better than others in preventing poor outcomes and mitigating their resultant sequela. Thorough discussion and repetitive counseling before scheduling surgery will give surgeons additional opportunities to judge the patient's goals and expectations and also to temper them. It is the responsibility of the surgeon to make patients understand firmly that the goal of facial plastic surgery procedures is improvement, not perfection. If a patient has inappropriate or unrealistic motivations or expectations for surgery, it is ultimately better to refuse to perform the surgery or to alter strategy than to proceed. This is critically important, because typically patients with the most realistic expectations at the outset are the ones most enamored with their surgical experience. Eugene Kern sagely advises that preoperative patient preparation be taken even a step further and encourages surgeons to prepare their patients for a second operation before performing the first.[5] Such realistic forecasting brings to mind the saying that one should strive to underpromise but overdeliver.

Problems in recovery are mitigated by prudent patient selection, elimination of high-risk individuals, and meticulous postoperative care, while solid surgical experience and careful preparation will help eliminate problems in judgment and technique. Surgeons are frequently encouraged to perform their procedures three times to help with preparation and reflection for future improvement: once mentally before the case, once physically during the actual procedure, and once again mentally after completion of the case. Other techniques for avoiding adverse outcomes are outlined in **Table 1.1**; although decidedly incomplete, the table attempts to organize further this complex topic by showing how undesirable outcomes in facial plastic surgery might be avoided.

◆ What Should Be Done When a Complication Is Identified?

Complications are onerous to surgeons as well as their patients, and it is a natural coping mechanism for surgeons to rationalize, conceal, or deny their presence. Surgeons typically will want to avoid unhappy patients altogether, seeing them in the office or visiting them in the hospital less frequently. Even with weekly morbidity and mortality (M&M) conferences at nearly all institutions, it is rare for a plastic surgeon to present electively the patients who did not like their facelifts or felt their noses were still too big. Understandably, M&M is reserved for presentation and discussion of "true" morbidities, and topics concerning questionable morbidities are not usually discussed. But in spite of this, surgeons should do just the opposite and pay increased attention to their unhappy patients, listening avidly and repeatedly to their concerns and being ever present for their benefit. Mindful of the saying that recommends "holding your friends close and your adversaries closer," surgeons should seek out their patients who experience complications. In some cases, they should offer daily visits. Listen intently, without trying to explain continually what might have gone wrong. Never presuppose what impact a facial plastic surgery complication has on a patient. Who can say that a facial tic after rhytidectomy is worse than xerophthalmia after blepharoplasty, or that new nasal obstruction after cosmetic rhinoplasty

Table 1.1

Techniques to Help Avoid Adverse Outcomes	
Complication Category	**Avoidance Techniques**
Inappropriate surgical judgment Inappropriate surgical technique	Solid surgical training Maintenance of certification Continuing medical education Familiarity with current literature Regular attendance at M&M conferences and journal clubs Avoid practicing in a vacuum—attend professional meetings Careful surgeon preparation Know whom you can help and whom you can't Test equipment prior to surgery Surgical time outs Surgical site markings
Inappropriate recovery	Meticulous patient selection Elimination of high-risk individuals Thorough postoperative patient and caretaker education Careful performance of postoperative care
Inappropriate patient expectations	Superlative patient communication Thorough informed consent process Realistic preoperative imaging display Review of prior patient photos and outcomes with prospective patients Encouragement of prospective patients to speak with prior surgical patients

is worse than malocclusion after facial fracture repair? Only patients can judge this impact.

Careful reflection on the course of events and critical review while driving or in the quiet moments before sleep can help discover and illuminate any missteps, bad judgments, technical errors, or insufficient preoperative discussions. Surgeons should confer with trusted colleagues, either in private or in a collegial meeting format such as M&M conference. Other surgeons have likely had similar experiences and can offer counsel, helping to convey what should or should not be done.

◆ Conclusion

As Francis Peabody suggested to his medical students nearly 90 years ago, surgeons must sit with and listen to patients after a complication and be ever empathetic, for most often this is what patients primarily want from their surgeons after an undesirable outcome. They want to know that the surgeon comprehends the gravity of what they are going through and is there emotionally to help them bear the burden of an adverse recovery. Other actions, such as issuing apologies, giving refunds, and notifying a medical liability carrier, are outside the scope of this text but might be beneficial. Consideration of all such factors involved with undesirable surgical outcomes will help surgeons better understand the medical, social, and psychological interplay of the variables, and such an understanding will lead to improvements in outcome. Plastic surgery, after all, is not simply performing the complex or innovative steps that define a particular procedure; rather it involves taking a patient with a facial deformity or undesirable trait and striving to improve form, function, and self-image simultaneously. This is a weighty yet rewarding task.

PEARLS OF WISDOM

The secret of the care of the patient is caring for the patient.[1]

Complication prevention is always the best practice.

Prepare patients for revision surgery before performing the primary operation.[5]

Perform each case three times: twice mentally and once physically.

Swift acknowledgment of a complication is paramount.

Be present emotionally and physically for your patients with untoward results. See them frequently and listen actively.

Patients with the most appropriate expectations are often the most enamored with their surgical result.

References

1. Peabody FW. The care of the patient. JAMA 1927;88(12):877–882
2. Kazanjian VH, Converse JM. The Surgical Treatment of Facial Injuries. Baltimore: Williams and Wilkins; 1949
3. Kohn LT, Corrigan JM, Donaldson MS, Eds. To Err Is Human: Building a Safer Health System. The Institute of Medicine; 2000
4. Cooper JB, Newbower RS, Long CD, McPeek B. Preventable anesthesia mishaps: A study of human factors. Anesthesiology 1978;49(6):399–406
5. Kern EB. The preoperative discussion as a prelude to managing a complication. Arch Otolaryngol Head Neck Surg Nov 2003;129:1163–1165

2

Management of the Dissatisfied Patient

Jonathan M. Sykes

The goals and expectations of patients seeking plastic surgery are complex. For most patients, the overt desire is to change their physical appearance or function. However, patients have unspoken desires, which may include improving their self-esteem and overall quality of life. Although unstated, these desires to improve overall quality of life clearly affect an individual patient's eventual satisfaction with his or her surgical outcome.

The goal of the facial plastic surgeon is to achieve the best possible aesthetic and functional surgical outcome. However, improved function and aesthetic appearance are clearly matters of the individual's perception. An individual patient's perception of their surgery is a product of many factors that include not only the physical result but also the less objective characteristics of self-esteem and ego strength.

This chapter focuses on diagnosis and treatment of the psychological aspects of the plastic surgery patient. This includes preoperative identification of the well-adjusted patient, who is likely to appreciate the benefits of well-performed surgery. The preoperative consultation should also identify potentially problematic patients. This chapter outlines a systematic approach to evaluate patients who are likely to be dissatisfied with plastic surgery and provides an algorithm for dealing with these patients. A detailed outline of how to communicate with all patients is included. Although the plastic surgeon receives minimal training in dealing with the psychological concerns of the plastic surgery patient, attention to this subject is mandatory for a successful plastic surgery practice.

◆ Preoperative Considerations

The Consultation

The initial consultation between the facial plastic surgeon and a prospective patient is a complex interaction that involves two-way diagnosis and decision making. While evaluating the medical history and physical suitability of the patient, the surgeon is also beginning a process of deciding whether or not the patient is a good psychological candidate for surgery. Simultaneously, the patient is evaluating the surgeon and deciding whether to be operated on by the surgeon.

Most patients seeking a plastic surgery consultation have already considered the process of making a decision about surgery. Unlike non-cosmetic surgery patients, who often hope that surgeons will recommend not having surgery, plastic surgery patients desire change and usually request surgery. For this reason, careful communication during the consultation is essential in establishing a healthy and open surgeon-patient relationship. It is important that the surgeon identify characteristics that may predispose the patient toward postoperative dissatisfaction with the surgical result.

The personality characteristics of both the patient and the surgeon are noticeable during the initial consultation. The overt goals of the patient are to evaluate the competence and expertise of the surgeon; that is, to answer the question "Will the surgeon be able to improve the function and appearance of my face?" The less frequently stated goals of whether or not the surgeon can care for and comfort the patient during the healing process are at least as important as surgical competence is to the patient. Thus, the decision to choose a given surgeon is a complex one based on reputation, perceived competence, empathy, and comfort during the consultation.

The surgeon also must make an important evaluation of the patient's psychological profile during the consultation. This begins with the surgeon trying to understand the patient's position, perspective, and (most importantly) motivation for having surgery. If the surgeon feels that the patient has a poor self-image and is generally unhappy, the motivation for surgery may be to create personal happiness. If such patients are disappointed with the surgical results, their resulting dissatisfaction is accentuated. Furthermore, if patients have poor self-image, it is more likely that surgery will not meet their expectations. The failure to meet patient's expectation usually results from a patient's initial unhealthy motivation for having surgery. All of these factors mandate that the surgeon be aware of the patient's psychological profile and communicate any potential issues with the patient preoperatively.

Selecting Patients

The first step to obtaining a successful outcome in facial plastic surgery is to select the patient carefully. This requires the surgeon to delve beneath the surface and to determine the patient's inner strength and ability to deal with the postoperative healing process. Surgeons are taught how and when to operate, but the skill of knowing when not to operate requires experience and good judgment. At the end of their careers, surgeons will rarely be disappointed that they did not operate on a particular patient; however, operating on the wrong patient (one with a poor psychological profile) often creates anger and frustration for both the patient and surgeon. To exclude or discourage certain facial plastic surgery patients from having surgery, the surgeon must be aware of patient profiles that are problematic. **Table 2.1** lists the traits of patients who are predisposed to unhappiness or dissatisfaction.

The Demanding Patient

Patients who exhibit the need for special treatment from either the doctor or staff are difficult to please and will tend to be dissatisfied with their surgical results. These patients will often request special treatment, including special timing for their appointments. They will often seem annoyed by or irritated with the manner in which they are treated. Physicians should listen carefully to staff warnings regarding these patients, as demanding patients will often mask these characteristics from their physicians.

The Perfectionist Patient

Patients who need to control every detail relating to surgery are also potential problems. These patients ask many detail-oriented questions and often bring in many photographs depicting their desired results. Perfectionist patients often do not understand the limitations of surgery. In addition, these patients will often be preoccupied with minimal aesthetic problems or deformities. These patients require a significant time commitment from the surgeon to explain surgical limitations and to set appropriate and realistic expectations. If appropriate surgical expectations are set and limitations of surgery are outlined in advance, perfectionist patients can be very pleased with postoperative results.

Patients Critical of Other Surgeons

A patient who is dissatisfied with prior aesthetic surgery and is vocally critical of past medical care is a dangerous patient to treat. The facial plastic surgeon should listen carefully to how the criticism is spoken. If a patient explains a prior surgery with an underlying tone of anger, this patient should be avoided. If the surgeon operates on the patient before the anger issues are dealt with, the anger will likely resurface during the postoperative period after the revision surgery.

Surgeons often feel that their surgical skill is enough to overcome the results of prior surgery that led to patient dissatisfaction. This idea is reinforced by the patient who states: "Doctor, I know you are the best! You can fix me." The surgeon should not be trapped by the histrionic patient who appeals to the surgeon's ego while criticizing prior care. Surgeons should realize that such a patient will be quick to criticize them later when the surgical result falls short of expectations.

The Depressed Patient

Many members of society have periods of depression. These periods are often helped by mood-elevating prescription medications. However, some people have more deep-seated endogenous depression that often is not helped by medication. It is important for the facial plastic surgeon to identify how severe a patient's depression is and whether or not the condition is treatable. If the depression is treatable, many patients will do very well with proper preoperative teaching and postoperative empathetic care. If the depression is not well controlled and the patient has more deeply rooted neuroses, plastic surgery will usually expose and may even accentuate these problems. It is appropriate for the surgeon to discuss these issues directly and to schedule multiple visits or have the patient seek psychiatric consultation prior to scheduling any surgery.

Body Dysmorphic Disorder (BDD)

Patients with body dysmorphic disorder (BDD) represent an increasingly growing percentage in the aesthetic surgeon's practice. BDD is listed in the DSM-IV under somatization disorders, but clinically it seems to have

Table 2.1

Behaviors Associated with Body Dysmorphic Disorder[2]
• Frequent glancing in reflective surfaces
• Avoidance of mirrors
• Skin picking
• Repeatedly measuring or palpating the defect
• Repeated requests for reassurance about the defect
• Elaborate grooming rituals
• Camouflaging some aspect of the patient's appearance with a hand, a hat, or makeup
• Avoiding social situations where others might see the defect
• Social anxiety
• Depressed mood and suicidal ideation

similarities to obsessive-compulsive disorder (OCD).[1] These patients universally are dissatisfied with themselves and want significant changes in their appearance. They generally have a poor self-image, fixate on small aesthetic issues, and allow these issues to become important and even overwhelming problems.

Their significant distortions in self-image make it very difficult to satisfy patients with BDD. They often desire changes in multiple body parts yet often hide these wants from the surgeon. Although patients with BDD desire multiple changes, they are embarrassed by their wants, because they have some insight into their narcissistic desires. An example of this behavior is the patient with anorexia nervosa, who feels too fat but does not want to share this feeling with others. Patients with BDD are dangerous for the aesthetic surgeon and therefore warrant early identification. The other behaviors commonly associated with BDD that can be useful in detecting the condition are outlined in **Table 2.1**.

These patients usually cannot be satisfied, as their underlying problem is poor self-image, and not a desire to change a single body part or feature. These patients rarely comprehend the limitations of the plastic surgery and almost always desire multiple procedures. A patient with BDD commonly asks the question, "When can we schedule my next procedure?" It is important for the surgeon to see through the patient's poor self-image and to advise them not to have too much surgery. In a sense, the surgeon must protect patients with BDD from themselves.

Patients with Poor Self-Image

The self-esteem and self-image of patients vary significantly. The personality characteristics of patients range from those who are totally secure with their status and image to those who feel inadequate and want to change themselves totally. Ironically, people with the best self-image are the best psychological candidates for cosmetic surgery, but they often do not request surgical change.

Cosmetic surgery results in some change in self-image. This is often evidenced by patients who have rhinoplasty and then change their hairstyles and makeup postoperatively. If the patient has a positive change in self-image after the cosmetic surgery change, the patient will be very happy with the results. However, when patients have a negative change in self-image, they are rarely satisfied postoperatively with the surgical result.

Because the patients' ultimate evaluations of their surgical results are based on their preoperative self-image, it behooves the surgeon to evaluate each patient's sense of self preoperatively. It is their strength of self-image that will allow the patients to accept their physical changes postoperatively, as swelling and bruising occur and eventually give way to a changed appearance. A patient's self-esteem also allows the patient to accept the postoperative reactions of family members, friends, and coworkers.

For all of these reasons, the surgeon should assess the patient's self-image and ego strength during all preoperative consultations. This assessment should include the manner in which the patients discuss their own cosmetic issues. If patients discuss a minor problem as a major deformity and are self-berating, they are likely to exaggerate postoperative issues such as swelling, bruising, or minor cosmetic healing irregularities. These patients will often become very upset postoperatively with minor criticisms from family and friends. Patients with poor self-esteem are also likely to judge postoperative results too quickly and with too much volatility; for example, they are often happy on one visit and upset at the next. The surgeon should ask questions at the initial consultation that help to evaluate the patient's overall sense of self.

◆ The Surgeon's Relationship with the Cosmetic Surgery Patient

Surgeons are taught to diagnose and treat patients. Plastic surgeons are taught surgical techniques to improve the function and appearance of their patients. However, most surgeons are not taught techniques for communicating effectively with their patients. Effective communication is the key to all successful physician-patient interaction. Communication is the basis of trust and understanding.

Communication allows the surgeon to understand the patient's motivations for and expectations of surgery. The surgeon should ask questions such as, "When did you first consider changing your appearance?" and "Why do you want to change your nose?" The answers to such questions will give the surgeon insight into the patient's goals and motivations. More importantly, the manner in which the patient answers these and similar questions will give the surgeon a sense of the patient's self-image and the patient's ability to withstand the physical and emotional stresses of surgery.

Effective communication is especially important in the postoperative period, when the plastic surgery patient often feels vulnerable and insecure about the surgical results. It is particularly important that the patient experiences "being heard" by the surgeon. If the patient has a postoperative concern, the surgeon should avoid the tendency to diagnose and treat the problem immediately. The patient usually does not require immediate treatment (in fact, the surgeon cannot provide this anyway) but instead needs a listening, caring provider. The surgeon should use reflective listening, which includes repeating or paraphrasing the speaker's intents. This technique includes phrases such as, "So it sounds like you're saying…," or "What I hear you saying is…" This form of listening allows the patients to feel that they are being heard. The use of these communication skills will allow the surgeon to avoid the frustration and anger that often accompany the dissatisfied postoperative patient.

◆ The Four Es of Effective Communication

The clinician can use a systematic approach to improving communication with patients. The four Es of communication—engage, empathize, educate, and enlist—give the provider a model to use in any patient interaction. These communication skills are useful during both preoperative consultations and postoperative visits. The four Es are especially effective in dealing with difficult, demanding, or dissatisfied patients.

Engagement is the initial connection with the patient. This includes orienting the patient to the process of the visit or the care to be given. It is important that the practitioner elicit statements about the patient's goals and expectations and identify all complaints. The physician should be curious about the person prior to examining the patient. The person is engaged with statements such as, "Before we begin, tell me something about yourself." The agenda is engaged with statements such as, "What were you hoping to accomplish today?"

The ability to empathize with patients is very important in all fields of medicine but is particularly crucial in plastic surgery. Empathy allows the surgeon to accept the patients' perspectives and to understand their motivations for surgery. To empathize with the patient, the surgeon must be a caring listener. The patient should experience being heard and accepted. The surgeon can use reflective listening to allow the patient to experience being heard. Reflective listening involves repeating what the speaker says to guarantee that the speaker's words and meaning are understood. The surgeon should use short summaries to reflect what they hear. The surgeon can use stems such as, "So, you are saying that…" or "You are wondering if…," or "I hear you saying.…" The technique of reflective listening should be used in all patient interactions, beginning with the consultation and continuing through all postoperative care.

Education of patients is fundamental to all successful communication with patients. The patient should feel as though there is shared knowledge in diagnosis and in treatment options. The surgeon should ask patients about their understanding of the condition, why it is occurring, and what they know about possible treatments. This will allow the patient to better accept the surgeon's viewpoint and better assess the treatment options presented. This is particularly important with cosmetic surgery patients, who may be inundated with multiple surgical options from the media and Internet. If patients feel as though they have made educated decisions preoperatively regarding their surgical choices,

they are less likely to be angry or frustrated postoperatively. It is important for the physician to ensure that the patient understands the diagnosis and treatment options. This understanding is essential to successful patient education.

The last E in successful physician-patient communication is enlistment. Enlistment is defined as an invitation from the clinician to the patient to collaborate in making the decisions regarding the goals and plans for treatment. The surgeon should offer options, explore the pros and cons of each option, and agree with the patient on the best option. The patient should be allowed to weigh all treatment options. This is extremely important in elective cosmetic surgery, which is not a need but a want of the patient. If the patient understands that the surgery is something that they desire but do not need, there is less chance for postoperative dissatisfaction. By engaging patients in the process and enlisting them in the decision-making, the surgeon converts patients into partners.

◆ Managing the Dissatisfied Patient

Dissatisfaction after cosmetic surgery produces distress in both the patient and the surgeon. Even though only a relatively small percentage of cosmetic surgery patients are truly dissatisfied with their result, these few patients usually occupy a large amount of the surgeon's time and energy. Learning to deal with patient dissatisfaction after cosmetic surgery requires the surgeon to gain significant psychological skills.

The key to dealing with postoperative patient dissatisfaction is communication. As noted in the section above, successful communication requires empathy and compassionate listening. This will allow the surgeon to identify the specific reason(s) for the patient's dissatisfaction. It is important for the surgeon to avoid the impulse to immediately suggest a solution for the problem; rather, the surgeon should listen carefully and express compassion for the patient. The surgeon should approach the patient with postoperative issues in the same manner that is used during the initial consultation; i.e., the surgeon should use a systematic communication style that employs all four Es. This will allow the surgeon to display empathy and compassion to the patient and will usually prevent anger and frustration by the patient.

The usual cause of patient dissatisfaction after aesthetic surgery is unmet expectations. Patient often expect that cosmetic surgery improve their self-image and self-confidence. In most patients, this is the case. However, for some patients who have significant preoperative issues with their self-image, the surgery actually causes an erosion of self-esteem. Naturally, such patients then transfer their feelings of loss of confidence and self-image onto the surgical result. These patients will become extremely sensitive to the reactions and comments of family members and friends. In addition, such patients will often become overly concerned with normal postoperative swelling and bruising and will become impatient with normal healing times. It is very important that the surgeon recognize the patient's insecurity over the postoperative healing and surgical results. It is more important to show these patients compassion and empathy than it is to try assuring them that their healing is "normal."

As discussed in the "Selecting Patients" section, the best method for obtaining a successful outcome in plastic surgery is to select patients carefully. If a patient has significant postoperative dissatisfaction and communication between the patient and the surgeon erodes, the surgeon should use other means to communicate with the patient. This includes using friends and family of the patient to assist communication. Often, a friend or family member may add reason and may help the patient articulate his or her concerns and dissatisfaction. The surgeon should also use a caring staff member to attend all postoperative visits. The presence of other people (staff members and family members) during the visit will foster communication and help avoid anger and frustration. It is very important to document all visits carefully and to have staff members document their impressions of the visit separately.

In rare cases, the erosion of communication results in increased patient frustration and increased surgeon distress. The patient will occasionally ask for a financial refund. The surgeon should then consult risk management specialists and their insurance carrier. In these instances, a refund or partial refund of the surgeon's fee may be given, but it should be given only after the patient signs a full liability release. The refund of fees should terminate the relationship between the surgeon and patient.

◆ Conclusion

In training for facial plastic surgeons, the emphasis is on learning surgical technique. Very little time and education are devoted to improving surgeon-patient communi-

nication and to learning psychological skills. Although it is important for all surgeons to maximize their surgical skills, the success of any cosmetic surgeon's practice is related to the surgeon's ability to interact with patients. Careful selection and screening are crucial to patient satisfaction. Use of a systematic method—the four Es—gives the surgeon a consistent template for communication. If communication is used effectively, facial plastic surgery can be rewarding for both the patient and the surgeon.

PEARLS OF WISDOM

It is important that the surgeon determine the patient's motivations for, and expectations of, surgery.

Patient selection in plastic surgery is as important as surgical execution.

Certain personality types predispose the patient to postoperative unhappiness or dissatisfaction. These include the demanding, the perfectionist, and the depressed patient.

Patients with body dysmorphic disorder (BDD) frequently request aesthetic surgery. These patients have significant distortion in self-image and are difficult to satisfy surgically.

The four Es of effective communication—engage, empathize, educate, and enlist—allow the provider a model to use in any patient interaction.

The surgeon should use reflective listening when interacting with the patient. This will allow the patient to feel understood and accepted.

Successful methods for dealing with postoperative patient dissatisfaction include listening and understanding the patient.

References

1. Jakubietz M, Jakubietz RJ, Kloss DF, Gruenert JJ. Body dysmorphic disorder: diagnosis and approach. Plast Reconstr Surg 2007;119(6):1924–1930
2. Phillips KA. The Broken Mirror: Understanding and Treating Body Dysmorphic Disorder. New York: Oxford University Press; 1996:391

3

Complications in the Cosmetic Office Setting

Corey S. Maas

Intradermal and hypodermal injections have become a multimillion dollar industry in contemporary cosmetic medicine. Minimally invasive facial rejuvenation techniques, such as soft-tissue augmentation with dermal fillers and rhytid effacement with botulinum neurotoxin type A (BT-A), have exponentially increased in popularity. This increase in popularity and demand is due to a combination of fast results with minimal recovery time as well as excellent product safety records. As more patients seek cosmetic and aesthetic improvement without surgery, a review of the potential complications that can occur from these minimally invasive techniques can be advantageous. By reviewing complications associated with the most often used injectables, both the physician and the patient will become better informed of both potential complications and expected results. This chapter will discuss BT-A, review its associated complications, outline the most commonly used injectable fillers, and briefly discuss the potential complications associated with each product: collagens, hyaluronic acids, Radiesse, Sculptra, and synthetic injectables.

◆ Botulinum Toxin

Botulinum toxins have been used successfully to manage facial aging by effacing rhytides and hyperkinetic lines of the face and neck. Although seven different serotypes of botulinum toxin are found in nature (A through G), serotype A is the most commonly used [Botox and Botox Cosmetic (Onabotulinum toxin A), Allergan, Inc., Irvine CA. Dysport (Abobotulinum toxin A), Medicis Aesthetics, Inc., Scottsdale, AZ. Xeomin (Incobotulinum toxin A), Merz Aesthetics, Inc., San Mateo, CA]. Each of the serotypes is defined by its specific biologic action, specifically the cleaving of different proteins involved in active transport of acetylcholine into the neurosynaptic cleft responsible for muscle contraction. Relaxing the muscle leads to effacement of rhytides, causing an improved cosmetic appearance. Although extensive research and

data have been collected to support the safety of BT-A in therapeutic doses, it is important to note that complications can occur. Complications related to BT-A are usually minimal, short-lived, and reversible. The majority of complications can be prevented with proper injection techniques, correct dosing, and a thorough knowledge of facial anatomy.

Potential Complications with BT-A Injections

Bruising, Pain, and Edema

Bruising, pain, and edema can occur from BT-A injections; however, it should be noted that they are usually associated with the injection itself and are not complications of the neurotoxin. Mild bruising has been reported in as many as 11% to 25% of patients who received Botox injections.[4] Bruising is increased in patients taking nonsteroidal anti-inflammatory drugs, aspirin, anticoagulant medications, vitamin E, or large doses of ginseng, garlic, and ginkgo. Patients should be advised to discontinue taking these products 7 to 10 days before treatment if medically possible.

Injection site pain is an adverse event associated with any injection, but it can be minimized with the use of a topical lidocaine (Topicaine, ESBA Laboratories, Mountain View, CA) and benzocaine, lidocaine, tetracaine (BLT, TLC Pharmacy, Hermosa Beach, CA). Both pain and edema can each be minimized by applying ice to the injection sites directly after injection. The use of 32-gauge needles will also help to minimize bruising and discomfort.

Immunogenicity

Immune responses to BT-A have occurred in patients receiving local injections of botulinum toxin (BTX). Development of antibodies and T lymphocytes primed to epitopes on the heavy chain of the toxin has been reported.[4] Loss of action can occur in patients who have received one or more previous BTX injections; upon a subsequent injection, the patient does not respond to treatment. Although BT-A resistance occurs in only 5% of patients, it is an important factor to consider.[1] This immunogenicity is presumed to be caused by the formation of serum antibodies.[4] The antibodies formed against BT-A can block the activity of the neurotoxin by blocking the presynaptic terminals, thereby allowing the release of acetylcholine and leaving the patients as nonresponders. Resistance can be measured using the Frontalis Type A Antibody Test (FTAT), where patients are injected with 15–20 units of BT-A in the frontalis muscle. The patient is considered a nonresponder or resistant if the eyebrows can be raised after two weeks.[2]

The immunogenicity of BT-A is thought to be dependent on the amount used, the duration between injections, and the amount of protein surrounding the toxin. It has been noted that repeat treatments with large doses may increase the likelihood of developing antibodies.[3] Immune response can be minimized by using the smallest effective dose and by increasing the amount of time between injections. BT-A has a large therapeutic window, which increases the possibility of overtreatment. As a simple rule, the minimal effective dose should be used to give maximum efficacy with a lower risk of developing immunogenicity. Because the protein content may be proportional to antigenicity, Botox has released recent batches with lower protein content in the hope of decreasing immunogenicity.[3] Dysport, another serotype A toxin, was recently approved by the FDA and has a lower protein load.[4]

In patients who have demonstrated nonresponsiveness, different serotypes of the botulinum neurotoxin may result in different antibody responses, thus serotype B (Myobloc) may be an option for these patients.

Brow Ptosis

BT-A is commonly injected into the frontalis muscle to reduce transverse forehead rhytides. However, overtreatment of the frontalis muscle can produce brow ptosis, a complication resulting in a drop of the brow below the supraorbital rim. Brow ptosis can be easily avoided by reviewing facial anatomy and using correct injection techniques, as well as adhering to patient selection criteria. The frontalis muscle lies beneath a thick layer of sebaceous skin and subcutaneous tissue. The muscle originates on the galea aponeurotic layer superiorly and interdigitates with the procerus, corrugator and orbicularis oculi muscles that overlie the brow region. Successful rejuvenation of the rhytides requires some relaxation of the frontalis muscles, but not enough to cause subsequent brow ptosis through the unopposed drepressor activity of the procerus, corrugator and orbicularis oculi muscles. Deep injections into the muscle are performed in a staggered distribution, with ~1 cm distance between injections positioned at least 1.5 cm to 2.0 cm above the brow margin. If injections stay above the brow, subsequent ptosis and brow asymmetry are avoided.

Correct patient selection is also an important consideration to avoid brow ptosis. Patients with heavy, thick brows should be avoided, as well as patients who had brow ptosis before receiving botulinum toxin.

Blepharoptosis (Figs. 3.1, 3.2)

Bepharaptosis (eyelid) ptosis is defined as inferior malposition of the upper eyelids; it can occur from the use of BT-A and most commonly occurs when BT-A is injected into the orbicularis oculi, corrugator supercilii and procerus muscles[5] (**Fig. 3.1**). Eyelid ptosis usually occurs from either incorrect placement of BT-A or diffusion of the toxin through the orbital septum to the levator palpebrae superioris muscle. The onset of ptosis can range from 48 hours up to 14 days after the injection and can last for two to four weeks. Blepharoptosis is usually subtle; however it can become exaggerated at the end of the day or when patients feel tired. Ptosis can very easily be avoided by advising patients to avoid manipulation and to remain in the upright position for 3 to 4 hours after the injection. Injections to reduce glabellar rhytides should not be performed lateral to the midpupillary line.

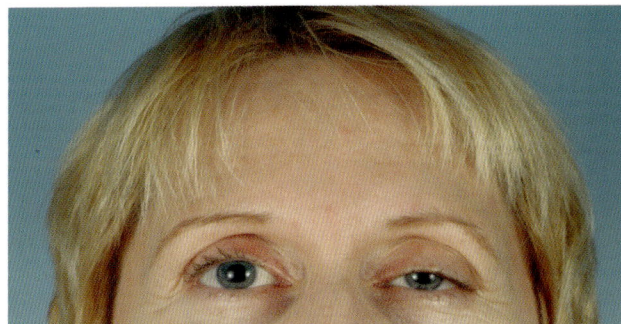

Fig. 3.1 Patient with eyelid ptosis of left lid.

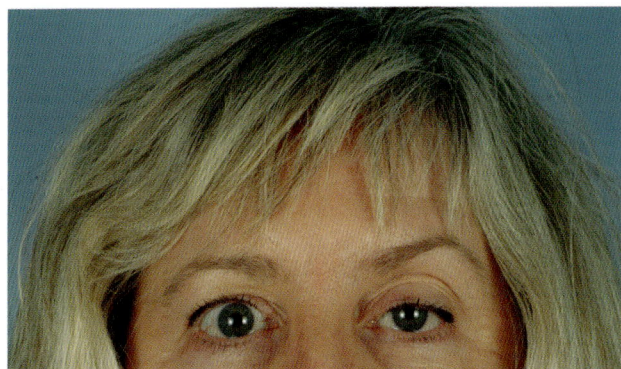

Fig. 3.2 Patient with eyelid ptosis of left lid. Note attempted frontalis compensation (elevated left eyebrow).

If ptosis occurs, the use of apraclonidine eye drops, 0.5% (Iopidine, Alcon Laboratories, Forth Worth, TX) can be an effective therapy.[6] Apraclonidine is an α2-adrenergic agonist, causing contraction of the Müller muscles and a resulting elevation of the eyelid. One or two drops should be applied three times daily until ptosis resolves. It is important to note that contact dermatitis has been noted as a potential complication with use of apraclonidine.[7]

Systemic Complications of BT-A

Systemic complications are not an issue when botulinum toxin is used in small quantities with standard preparations. There are, however, reports that botulinum toxin has been detected in the hypothalamus after intradermal injection, which would indicate it travels systemically and even crosses the blood-brain barrier. There have also been misadventures with treated individuals contracting systemic toxicity (botulism) after injections of botulinum toxin when non-standard preparations and large doses were used. It is imperative, therefore, that physicians who treat patients with botulinum toxin use only the recommended doses of FDA-approved toxins. Whatever the actual mechanism, the lack of deleterious systemic effects with these simple guidelines implies that while research into BT-A mechanisms continues, physicians can safely use BTX for therapy.[8]

◆ Dermal Fillers

Throughout the aging process, elasticity and collagen levels decrease, creating wrinkles in a fairly predictable manner. As a corrective measure, dermal fillers offer a successful method for soft-tissue augmentation and facial rejuvenation without the risks associated with surgery. Thus, as these products gain popularity and more products emerge, it becomes increasingly important to discuss the differences between the products and the complications involved with each. For all dermal fillers, the potential complications can be divided into either early or late complications. Early complications, which can be seen with all fillers, include bruising, erythema, and edema. Late complications are usually due to an immunological response or an incorrect injection technique. The following sections thoroughly discuss the potential complications associated with each filler and review strategies to avoid and treat adverse events, so complications can be minimized and hopefully avoided.

Nasolabial folds, perioral lines and lips are the most commonly treated areas; however, dermal fillers can also be used for many other corrections, such as glabellar lines, marionette lines, scarring, cheek augmentation, chin and jaw line contouring, and lipoatrophy. The list of dermal fillers and areas of use are constantly growing, making it increasingly important to discuss the proper usage and potential complications associated with each product. Some commonly used FDA-approved fillers are outlined below.

◆ Bovine, Porcine, and Human Collagen

Collagen has been used as a soft-tissue filler since the 1980s, and its popularity peaked in the 1990s. Although no longer in significant use, it is included in this discussion largely for historical purposes. The most abundant protein in the body, collagen acts as a successful, nonpermanent biocompatible treatment for soft-tissue deficiencies. Cells from animals, including cows and pigs, are a useful source of collagens (Evolence, Ortho-McNeil-Janssen-Pharmaceuticals, Inc., Los Angeles, CA). The first bovine collagen approved for soft tissue augmentation was Zyderm (Palo Alto, CA). Bovine collagen comes in three types, produced by Inamed Aesthetics (Santa Barbara, CA). Zyderm I received its FDA approval in 1981 and became the first non-autologous agent approved in the United States for use in soft-tissue augmentation.[9] The approval of Zyderm II and Zyplast quickly followed. Zyderm is a preparation of bovine collagen that has been purified, digested with pepsin, and suspended in phosphate-buffered saline with 0.3% lidocaine.[10] Zyderm II has a higher concentration of collagen (6.5% compared with 3.5% in Zyderm I). Zyplast is collagen cross-linked with glutaraldehyde, leading to longer durability with a decrease in antigenicity.[11] The effects of bovine collagen treatments last between 3 and 6 months.

Cosmoderm and Cosmoplast, approved by the FDA for cosmetic use in 2003, are bioengineered human collagens used to correct facial rhytides. These products contain purified collagen derived from cell cultures of human fibroblasts. The cell lines are screened for viruses, tumorigenicity, and other potential pathogens; the collagen produced is devoid of antigenic determinants, which makes the product nonimmunogenic and thus eliminates the need for a skin test.

◆ Hyaluronic Acid

Hyaluronic acid (HA) is a naturally occurring polysaccharide found in all living organisms that has virtually supplanted the use of collagens for cosmetic purposes. HA fillers are nonimmunogenic and therefore bypass the need for skin testing. HA fillers are also strongly hydrophilic, which serves to hydrate and plump the skin. A rapidly developing area, there are eight formulations currently approved by the FDA at the time of this writing: Restylane, Perlane (Medicis Aesthetics, Inc., Scottsdale, AZ), Prevelle Silk (Mentor Corporation, Santa Barbara, CA), Captique (Inamed Aesthetics, Santa Barbara CA), Hylaform, HylaformPlus (Biomatrix, Ridgefield, NJ), Juvederm Ultra, and Juvederm Ultra Plus (Allergan, Inc. Irvine, CA). All are nonanimal stabilized hyaluronic acids (NASHAs), except Hylaform and Hylaform Plus, which are a cross-linked variety derived from rooster combs. Restylane, Perlane, Juvederm Ultra, and Juvederm Ultra Plus are cross-linked and are derived from bacterial fermentation.[12] This process causes Restylane and Juvederm to contain up to four times as much protein as Hylaform for the same volume. Both products are safe, but since Restylane and Juvederm are not derived from an animal source, there is a lower risk of an allergic skin reaction [13]

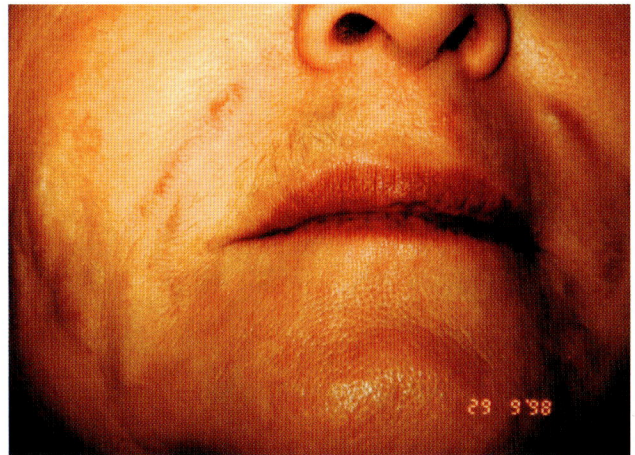

Fig. 3.3 Patient with polymethylmethacrylate granulomata in the nasolabial folds.

◆ Calcium Hydroxylapatite

Radiesse (Merz Aesthetics, Inc., San Mateo, CA) is a non-immunogenic synthetic material composed of microscopic calcium hydroxylapatite particles ranging in size from 25 to 40 μm and suspended in a carboxymethylcellulose gel. As the polysaccharide gel degrades, new tissue infiltrates and surrounds the hydroxylapatite particles. Thus it acts as a framework for new tissue ingrowth. These effects last from 12 to 24 months.

◆ Poly-L-Lactic Acid

Sculptra (Sanofi Aventis Inc., Bridgewater, NJ) is a synthetic, nontoxic, nonimmunogenic injectable form of poly-L-lactic acid, a biocompatible and biodegradable compound that has been used in absorbable suture material for over 40 years. Sculptra is composed of crystalline microparticles of poly-L-lactic acid. It is packaged as a sterile, freeze-dried powder, which must be reconstituted with sterile water, typically with lidocaine.

Proper reconstitution and massage have proven to be very important in decreasing the possibility of nodule formation. The original reconstitution volume, which used 2 cc of saline, was problematic. It was noted that using a larger amount of diluent (5 to 10 cc of saline) with longer reconstitution time (a minimum of 12 hours) decreased the risk of nodule formation.[14] The addition of lidocaine to the product just prior to injection has led to enhanced patient comfort.

Polymethylmethacrylate (Fig. 3.3)

ArteFill (Suneva Medical, San Diego, CA) is an injectable filler used for long-lasting aesthetic results. Consisting of homogeneous polymethylmethacrylate (PMMA) microspheres ranging from 32 to 40 microns in size, it is evenly suspended in a solution of partly denatured bovine collagen and therefore requires a skin test prior to use. It is considered a permanent filler, because the microspheres are not biodegradable.

Silikon (Fig. 3.4)

Silikon 1000 (purified polydimethylsiloxane) is a highly purified long-chain polydimethylsiloxane trimethylsiloxy terminated silicone oil. It is sterile, not pyrogenic, clear, and colorless, and it has a viscosity of 1000 cs. Silikon 1000 has been approved by the FDA for prolonged retinal tamponade since 1998. Silikon is also considered a permanent filler.

◆ Potential Complications with Dermal Fillers

Although some complications are unique to specific fillers, many complications can be seen with all of the fill-

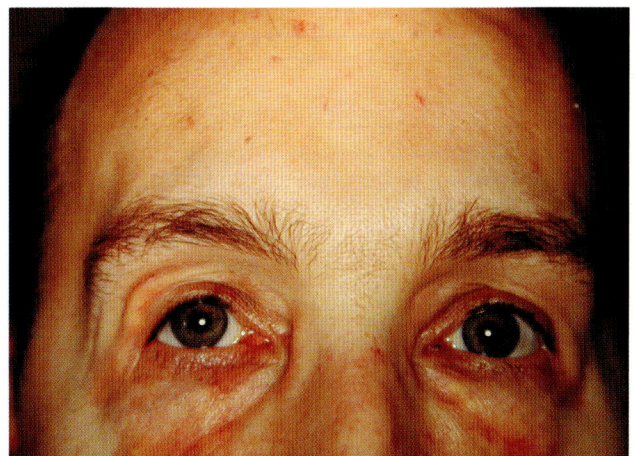

Fig. 3.4 Patient with periocular granulomata from silicone injections.

ers outlined above. Complications common to all fillers will be discussed below, as well as filler-specific adverse effects.

Bruising, Pain, Erythema, and Edema

Bruising, pain, erythema, and edema can occur directly after treatment with any filler. These complications are usually caused by the injection itself and should not necessarily be attributed to the product. However, certain precautions can be taken to minimize these events. Bruising can be minimized by advising patients who are taking aspirin, vitamin E, and NSAIDs to stop using these products 7 to 10 days before treatment, if medically advisable. Pain can be decreased by using local nerve block anesthesia in combination with topical anesthetics, such as Topicaine or BLT, and with ice. Erythema and edema can be minimized by advising patients to use ice packs after the injection.

Vascular Occlusion

Direct injection of any filler into the lumen of a vessel can cause vascular occlusion, leading to ischemia or (more significantly) irreversible tissue necrosis. Injections of fillers into the glabellar region have a higher risk of vascular occlusion than those into the nasolabial folds. Vascular occlusion is very rare (estimated at less than 0.001%), and its occurrence can be reduced with appropriate technique and correct placement. Bolus injections with overlying skin tumescence should be avoided, and injections into areas at increased risk must be done with elevated caution. Knowledge of vascular anatomy is important, and injections should be oriented orthogonal to the lumen of known vessels to limit intraluminal injections. Checking for bloody flashback before injection is helpful. Recent developments in needle design, with emphasis on blunt cannula delivery, might prove helpful for reducing the incidence of intravascular injections.

Suspected necrosis or arterial occlusion subsequent to dermal filler injection should be treated aggressively. Immediate cessation of the injection, vigorous massage, warm compresses, 2% nitroglycerin paste, and hyperbaric oxygen therapy have been used with benefit.[15] An additional protocol for the treatment of impending necrosis after dermal filler injection has been published[16] but its efficacy has yet to be shown definitively (**Table 3.1**).

Hypersensitivity

While a hypersensitivity reaction can theoretically occur with any filler, this complication is much more common with fillers derived from animal products. In fact, the major drawback to using bovine collagen is the risk

of an allergic reaction. When bovine collagen (Zyderm) is used, a skin test is necessary and extremely important to determine if the patient experiences any allergic response to the product. Usually, a skin test of 0.1 mL is placed intradermally in the volar forearm area. Upon exposure, a positive skin test is indicated by the development of a wheal characterized by edema, erythema, pain, and itching. A positive skin test is seen in 3.0% to 3.5% of patients. More importantly, there is a 1.3% to 6.2% false-negative rate in skin testing.[17] For this reason, a second skin test is recommended two weeks after the initial test. Treatments can begin two to four weeks after a second negative skin test. Hypersensitivity reactions are indicated by erythema, edema, pain, and tenderness. When hypersensitivity occurs, it can be treated with hydrocortisone cream. Abscess formation is a rare occurrence, but it is thought to be related to hypersensitivity.[18] Severe hypersensitivity is very rare; however, there have been reports of anaphylactic shock.[19]

Most of the hyaluronic acid fillers are of nonanimal origin and therefore have a very low risk of hypersensitivity reactions. Rare cases of hypersensitivity to hyaluronic acid are thought to be due to impurities of bacterial fermentation or potentially from biofilm formation. Hypersensitivity reactions comprised 0.02% of all injections.[20] These consisted of swelling, erythema, and induration at the implant site, with a median duration of 15 days.[21]

Tyndall Effect

The Tyndall effect is caused by the fact that different wavelengths of light scatter differently, depending on

Table 3.1

Vascular Occlusion: Treatment Options
1. Inject hyaluronidase (Vitrase, ISTA Pharmaceuticals, Inc., Irvine, CA), 10–30 units diluted 1:1 with saline, at the first recognition of vascular compromise.
2. Nitropaste (nitroglycerin ointment, 2%) applied to the affected watershed area of compromise.
3. Aspirin, 325 mg each day.
4. Warm compresses and massage.
5. Topical Dermacyte (Oxygen Biotherapeutics, Inc., Durham, NC), an oxygen cosmeceutical, applied to the area of concern q.i.d.
6. See the patient daily. If there is no improvement, repeat regimen and add a Medrol dose pack.

the size of particles they encounter. Because blue and violet light have the shortest wavelengths in the visible spectrum, they are more easily scattered than any other color. This physical phenomenon is related to the appearance of skin and veins. A vein appears blue, in part, because longer wavelengths of light (e.g., red) travel deeply enough into the skin to be absorbed and shorter wavelengths are scattered, giving the vein a bluish hue.[22]

Subdermal injection of any clear filler can lead to the Tyndall effect. An inexperienced injector may inject too superficially, leaving a bluish discoloration at the injection sites. Therefore, HAs should be injected in the mid to lower dermis to avoid this complication. If this complication arises, it is fortunately reversible with filler degradation using hyaluronidase, with aspiration of the product or with the use of selective photothermolysis. Hyaluronidase, an enzyme not requiring ATP, catabolizes HAs. The use of a small amount of hyaluronidase (10 to 30 units) can dissolve the HA filler and correct the problem. The QS 1064 nm laser has also been used as an effective therapy.[22]

Nodules

Nodules are a relatively common complication that can be seen with any soft-tissue filler. Most nonerythematous nodules result from uneven distribution of product and are not due to an allergenic response. The size of a nodule tends to remain constant until it is absorbed or removed. If nodules or lumps result from superficial injection of product, they can be unroofed and excised using a 19-gauge needle. Despite its efficacy in other parts of the face, Radiesse has a higher incidence of nodule formation in the lips and is therefore not recommended in this area. It is thought that with excessive lip motion, the hydroxylapatite becomes clumped together to form nodules.

Nodules can theoretically result from an immune response to fillers. These nodules may or may not be painful and can manifest in the dermis or subcutaneously. There have been reports of painful erythematous nodules evolving into abscesses.[23,24] The important thing to note is the time of onset of the nodules. If they occur within the first few weeks of treatment, they are usually simply due to uneven distribution of the product. However, when a delayed reaction is seen, it is more likely caused by an allergic response.

Granulomata

Foreign body reactions can occur from the injection of certain dermal fillers and may result in the formation of granulomata. These occur at a rate 0.01% to 1.0%, depending on the filler.[1] A granuloma forms as a result of a foreign body that causes an immune response lead-ing to inflammation and the build-up of various epithelioid cells and lymphocytes. Clinically, granulomata are characterized by erythema and edema. They often will enlarge if left untreated. Granulomata lack a well-defined border, making excision difficult. Hence, local steroid therapy is the suggested treatment protocol. Kenalog (1mg/cc) injections every four to six weeks can be beneficial in reducing the size and appearance of a granuloma.

With the large number of dermal fillers on the market, it is important to remember that thorough product knowledge and correct injection technique play major roles in minimizing the potential adverse events associated with injectable fillers. There are three basic techniques used with injectable fillers to deliver material to the deep dermis or subcutaneous level: linear threading, droplet, and serial puncture. Linear threading refers to delivering the product in a uniform, retrograde fashion while the needle is slowly withdrawn from the tissue. Linear threading is a useful technique that is very effective for lip augmentation along the mucocutaneous border as well as for augmentation of the nasolabial fold. The development of blunt cannulas for injections has made the linear threading technique most popular, and it purportedly reduces the incidence of bruising and intravascular injection. The droplet technique is used in a manner similar to that in linear threading, except that instead of an even distribution of filler as the needle is withdrawn, microdroplets of filler are delivered into the tissue by gentle pumping on the syringe as the needle is withdrawn. This technique has been advocated for injecting silicone. Finally, the serial puncture technique involves the delivery of small aliquots of filler at multiple spots, with the goal of an even distribution over a two-dimensional area. Using the proper technique for each filler can help minimize complications.

◆ Conclusion

The use of botulinum toxin and dermal filler injections slows the appearance of facial aging. The loss of facial volume can be mitigated with fillers, and botulinum proteins relax unwanted hyperkinetic lines. The results that have been obtained from these products have caused an overwhelming surge of products to the market, and more are in the midst of clinical trials. With the success of such injectables, limited restrictions on physician specialty use, and the rise of nonphysician injectors, more complicated outcomes have followed. The complications discussed can be minimized with thorough product knowledge, use of correct injection techniques, intimate knowledge of facial anatomy, and adherence to safe practices.

PEARLS OF WISDOM

Injection of botulinum toxin inferior to the eyebrows or lateral to the midpupillary line risks blepharoptosis.

Injection of the lateral frontalis muscles risks brow ptosis, with resultant decompensation and aggravation of underlying blepharoptosis.

Use the smallest possible dose of botulinum toxin that will achieve the desired result to impede the development of immunogenicity.

Apraclonidine eyedrops are useful in the event of botulinum toxin-related blepharoptosis.

Use a graduated approach to dermal fillers—consider starting patients with shorter-duration fillers and advance to longer-duration fillers once appropriate patient satisfaction has been acknowledged.

Permanent fillers can lead to permanent problems.

References

1. Ludlow CL, Hallett M, Rhew K, et al. Therapeutic use of type F botulinum toxin. N Engl J Med 1992;326(5):349–350

2. Panicker JN, Muthane UB. Botulinum toxin: pharmacology and its current therapeutic evidence for use. Neurol India 2003;51(4):455–460

3. Klein AW. Contraindications and complications with the use of botulinum toxin. Clin Dermatol 2004;22(1):66–75

4. Pickett AM, O'Keeffe R, Panjwani N. The protein load of therapeutic botulinum toxins. Eur J Neurol 2007;14(4):e11

5. Vartanian AJ, Dayan SH. Complications of botulinum toxin use in facial rejuvenation. Facial Plast Surg Clin North Am 2003;11:483–492

6. Scheinfeld N. The use of apraclonidine eyedrops to treat ptosis after the administration of botulinum toxin to the upper face. Dermatol Online J 2005;11(1):9

7. Silvestre JF, Carnero L, Ramón R, Albares MP, Botella R. Allergic contact dermatitis from apraclonidine in eyedrops. Contact Dermat 2001;45(4):251

8. Currà A, Berardelli A. Do the unintended actions of botulinum toxin at distant sites have clinical implications? Neurology 2009;72(12):1095–1099

9. Monhian N, Greene D, Maas CS. The role of soft-tissue implants in scar revision. Facial Plast Surg Clin North Am 1998;6: 183–190

10. Knapp TR, Kaplan EN, Daniels JR. Injectable collagen for soft tissue augmentation. Plast Reconstr Surg 1977;60(3): 398–405

11. Ramirez AL, Monhian N, Maas CS. Current concepts in soft tissue augmentation. Facial Plast Surg Clin North Am 2000;8: 235–251

12. Krauss MC. Recent advances in soft tissue augmentation. Semin Cutan Med Surg 1999;18(2):119–128

13. Lowe NJ, Maxwell CA, Lowe P, Duick MG, Shah K. Hyaluronic acid skin fillers: adverse reactions and skin testing. J Am Acad Dermatol 2001;45(6):930–933

14. Lam SM, Azizzadeh B, Garvier M. Injectible poly-L-lactic acid (Sculptra): Technical considerations in soft-tissue contouring. Plast Reconstr Surg 2006; 118(3, Suppl):55–63

15. Narins RS, Jewell M, Rubin M, Cohen J, Strobos J. Clinical Conference: Management of rare events following dermal fillers—focal necrosis and angry red bumps. Derm Surgery 2006; 32(3):426–434

16. Dyan SH. Merge September/October 2010: 22–23

17. Klein AW, Rish DC. Injectable collagen update. J Dermatol Surg Oncol 1984;10(7):519–522

18. Hanke CW, Higley HR, Jolivette DM, Swanson NA, Stegman SJ. Abscess formation and local necrosis after treatment with Zyderm or Zyplast collagen implant. J Am Acad Dermatol 1991;25(2 Pt 1):319–326

19. Mullins RJ, Richards C, Walker T. Allergic reactions to oral, surgical and topical bovine collagen. Anaphylactic risk for surgeons. Aust N Z J Ophthalmol 1996;24(3):257–260

20. Matarasso SL, Carruthers JD, Jewell ML. Consensus recommendations of soft-tissue augmentation with nonanimal stabilized hyaluronic acid (Restylane). Plast Reconstr Surg 2006; 117(3, Suppl):3–34

21. Friedman PM, Mafong EA, Kauvar AN, Geronemus RG. Safety data of injectable nonanimal stabilized hyaluronic acid gel for soft tissue augmentation. Dermatol Surg 2002;28(6): 491–494

22. Hirsch RJ, Narurkar V, Carruthers J. Management of injected hyaluronic acid induced Tyndall effects. Lasers Surg Med 2006;38(3):202–204

23. Hönig JF, Brink U, Korabiowska M. Severe granulomatous allergic tissue reaction after hyaluronic acid injection in the treatment of facial lines and its surgical correction. J Craniofac Surg 2003;14(2):197–200

24. Schanz S, Schippert W, Ulmer A, Rassner G, Fierlbeck G. Arterial embolization caused by injection of hyaluronic acid (Restylane). Br J Dermatol 2002;146(5):928–929

4

Anesthesia Complications in Facial Plastic Surgery

John H. Eichhorn and Daniel T. Goulson

Surgery and anesthesia are uniquely interdependent. Each discipline cannot exist without the other. Improvements by each interact for the benefit of the patient, while the potential complications of each can negatively impact the patient. Surgeons and anesthesia professionals must cooperate and communicate to maximize patient safety through minimizing the likelihood of complications.

In hospital settings, anesthesia is administered by personnel trained in anesthesia: a physician anesthesiologist, a nurse anesthetist, an anesthesia assistant, or a team of an anesthesiologist with either of the other two. However, this is not always the case in the setting of sedation and analgesia, particularly outside traditional hospital operating rooms. The surgeon will then have a role in supervising the care given by the individual administering the sedation. In some states, the surgeon will also supervise the nurse anesthetist if an anesthesiologist is not involved in the case. Regardless of the array of practitioners, proper avoidance and management of complications requires input from all participants. Understanding, appreciation, and anticipation of risks help to prevent untoward outcomes.

◆ Outcome of Anesthesia Care

Anesthesia complications are any adverse, undesired outcomes related to anesthesia care. As with all complications of medical care, the primary focus should be on prevention. Sometimes these outcomes cause direct morbidity or mortality to the patient. At other times, they affect the patient indirectly by impeding the surgical procedure, such as intraoperative hypertension that leads to excessive bleeding or inadequate relaxation leading to patient movement at a critical delicate point in the operation.

Over all, anesthesia care is remarkably safe. Due to the lack of centralized statistics and consistent definitions, it is very difficult to determine an exact mortality rate

related solely to anesthesia. However, the risk of anesthesia catastrophe (death, permanent brain damage, or intraoperative cardiac arrest) in healthy patients is vanishingly small, in the range of 1:150,000 to 1:300,000.[1] When these catastrophes do occur, they usually involve the coincidence of two or more deviations from normal circumstances at the same time and often include unrecognized inadequate ventilation (from any of several causes—including simple inattention), failures of the oxygen supply, or, rarely, other equipment failures. This is not to say that other critical incidents (such as disconnection of the breathing circuit) are rare. These still occur with some frequency, but they usually do not cause adverse outcomes because the behaviors of the anesthesia professional, augmented by the alarms and warning signals from the safety monitoring equipment, catch such developments very early in the evolution of an event, allowing correct diagnosis and treatment long before there is any real danger to the patient.

Insight about adverse outcomes unique to anesthesiology can be found from the American Society of Anesthesiologists Closed Claims Project. Starting in 1984, many medical malpractice insurance companies were persuaded to open their closed files and allow confidential examination of the litigation records. All these cases, by definition, involved adverse anesthesia outcomes. They were examined for patterns of causes and effects regarding untoward clinical events, which were usually severe and involved at least perceived damage that led to lawsuits against anesthesiologists. A summary of the positive impact of the project during its first 17 years[2] reveals the extensive breadth of the findings.

One important initial finding was that "respiratory system adverse events" accounted for a significant fraction of the claims, particularly lawsuits involving death or brain damage.[3] The main focus of the study was not on the concept of preoperative predictors of adverse anesthesia outcome as much as it was on the causation of the adverse events. It was determined that failure to monitor adequately was the main reason for the adverse outcomes and that 93% of the preventable mishaps would have been avoided by the correct application of capnography and pulse oximetry together to help ensure appropriate ventilation and oxygenation.[4]

Traditional potential adverse outcomes that are caused largely by anesthesia care and manifest within 24 to 48 hours of surgery are listed in **Table 4.1**. Some authors might add severe bronchospasm, or airway burns, to this list of anesthesia complications.

◆ Complications of Anesthetic Medications

The practice of anesthesiology intimately involves the use of medications. An unfortunate reality is that most medications have some degree of side effect, adverse reactions, and unwanted interaction with other medications. One significant implication is that it is very important to understand and fully evaluate the patient's chronic medications because of the possibility of interactions with anesthetic medications.

Table 4.1

Traditional Potential Adverse Outcomes of Anesthesia Care
Broken teeth from laryngoscopy
Corneal abrasion
Allergy to anesthetic medications
Unintended awareness during general anesthesia
Unplanned admission to the hospital following outpatient surgery
Unplanned postoperative admission to an intensive care unit
Pneumonitis from aspiration of acid stomach contents
Emergency reintubation in the immediate postop period
Peripheral nerve injury
Neuraxial nerve injury, including stroke, with deficit
Unanticipated pulmonary edema
Malignant hyperthermia
Hypoxic brain injury
Myocardial infarction
Cardiac arrest
Death

Premedication Prior to Surgery

Most premedications given today are anxiolytics, analgesics, antiemetics, or medicines for prophylaxis against aspiration of stomach contents. Anxiolytics (such as midazolam) and especially narcotics (such as fentanyl) may lead to depression of consciousness or ventilation, which can lead to patient harm if it is not anticipated and recognized quickly. Monitoring of hemoglobin saturation with oxygen using pulse oximetry may help to detect problems, but hemoglobin desaturation is a late development in the downward spiral from excessive depressant medication, so direct visual monitoring by personnel trained to detect hypoventilation (whether from airway obstruction, CNS depression, or both) is likely to be more helpful. Patients are at higher risk for ventilatory depression if they take either anxiolytics or narcotics chronically at home, because there can be an additive effect with similar medications that may be given on the day of surgery. Extreme caution and hypervigilance should be exercised in this situation.

Metoclopramide is sometimes given for both antiemesis and (because it is a pro-motility agent intended to help empty the stomach) aspiration prophylaxis. Because it blocks post-synaptic dopaminergic receptors, dystonic and other extrapyramidal reactions can be seen, though occurring in less than 1% of patients.[5] Patients may also experience feelings of anxiety and agitation, which occur more often when the drug is administered as a rapid IV bolus as opposed to the recommended slow infusion. Such adverse reactions can typically be treated with diphenhydramine (25 or 50 mg, IV) or benztropine. Other agents that have found some success in reducing postoperative nausea and vomiting (PONV) include ondansetron, aprepitant, and Decadron.

Aspiration of acid stomach contents can be one of the most serious complications of anesthesia care. A true acid aspiration pneumonitis carries significant morbidity and an appreciable mortality. Accordingly, it is critical that patients observe the prescribed pre-op NPO regime, the recommended precise details of which are debated and are evolving.[6,7] Many efforts can be made to help minimize aspiration risks. Patients with known gastroesophageal reflux disease (GERD) and/or hiatus hernia, or even with a tendency to frequent "heartburn," may benefit from an attempt at reduced preoperative stomach acid production with either an H-2 blocker (such as famotidine) or a proton pump inhibitor (such as omeprazole), metoclopramide as noted to promote gastric emptying, and PO sodium citrate (Bicitra) to neutralize any remaining stomach acid. Such a regime may apply equally or even more so to patients scheduled for sedation and analgesia who will not have a secured airway but who may become relaxed or nauseated enough to regurgitate residual stomach contents. The gravity of the potential complications is so great that this question must be considered for every patient.

Local Anesthetic Toxicity and Allergy

Local anesthetics are drugs that produce reversible blockade of the conduction of impulses along central and peripheral nerve pathways by inhibiting passage of sodium ions through ion-selective sodium channels in nerve membranes. Removal of the local anesthetic by redistribution or metabolism is followed by spontaneous and complete return of nerve conduction with no evidence of structural damage to nerve fibers.[8] Thus, wary patients may be reassured that local anesthetics do not cause permanent dysesthesia.

Systemic toxicity from a local anesthetic occurs when there is an excess plasma concentration of the drug that may manifest in the central nervous system or cardiovascular system. Accidental direct intravascular injection is the most common mechanism for producing such an excess plasma concentration. Less often, excess plasma concentration results from absorption of significant amounts of the local anesthetic from the injection site.

Central Nervous System Toxicity

Nervous system toxicity manifests in a continuum, depending on the plasma concentration of local anesthetic. The initial symptoms of local anesthetic toxicity usually include numbness of the tongue and circumoral tissues. As the plasma concentration increases, restlessness, vertigo, and tinnitus may result from the local anesthetic crossing the blood-brain barrier. Very high plasma concentrations produce tonic-clonic seizures.

Treatment of local anesthetic-induced seizures consists of ventilation with supplemental oxygen and, if indicated, IV benzodiazepines (midazolam or diazepam). Hyperventilation lowers the P_aCO_2, which decreases cerebral blood flow, thus resulting in a decreased delivery of drug to the brain. This maneuver may be helpful in reducing the plasma concentration in the face of a seizure. Refractory seizures may require induction of general anesthesia with a barbiturate.

Cardiovascular Toxicity

The reversible blockade of sodium channels from local anesthetics can also block sodium channels in the heart, which can lead to cardiac toxicity. Myocardial conduction and automaticity may become depressed when enough of these channels become blocked. Increases in local anesthetic blood levels may lead to varying degrees of heart block, the appearance of multi-focal ectopic beats, re-entrant arrhythmias, tachycardia, and, ultimately, ventricular fibrillation. Treatment is supportive and includes oxygen, vasopressors, inotropes, and anti-dysrhythmics if needed.[9] Evidence is building that infusing a 20% lipid emulsion may be helpful when there is cardiac arrest due to bupivacaine toxicity.[10]

Among local anesthetics, there appears to be a difference in their propensity to cause cardiac toxicity. Experience has shown that bupivicaine (Marcaine) toxicity is the most likely to lead to cardiovascular collapse, which is particularly difficult to treat. This finding led to the search for a safer long-acting local anesthetic.[11] Analysis of laboratory data suggests that cardiac toxicity is associated with the dextro (R-) enantiomer of bupivacaine and that the S-enantiomer is less troublesome. Ropivacaine, which was released for use in 1996, is a pure S-isomer that has less cardiotoxicity than bupivacaine. It is more expensive than bupivacaine, but when large volumes of local anesthetic are used with a high likelihood of intravascular injection or significant absorption, its greater safety justifies the increased cost.[12]

Maximum Dose of Local Anesthetics

Even when local anesthetics are administered by infiltration into soft tissues, some is absorbed into the bloodstream, and this absorption can, in excess quantity, be toxic. **Table 4.2** shows maximum recommended infiltration doses of various local anesthetics.[13]

Local Anesthetic Allergy

Patients occasionally report "allergy" to local anesthetic agents, but true allergy to local anesthetics is quite rare. Ester local anesthetics, which produce metabolites related to para-aminobenzoic acid (PABA), are significantly more likely to lead to allergic reactions than amide local anesthetics, which do not produce these metabolites.[8]

Table 4.2

Clinical Properties of Local Anesthetic Agents

Local Anesthetic Agent	Duration of Action (h)	Maximum Safe Dosage (mg/kg)
Lidocaine (plain)	1.5–2	4
Lidocaine (with epinephrine)	2–2.5	7
Bupivacaine (plain)	3–6	1–2
Bupivacaine (with epinephrine)	6–10	2–3
Mepivacaine	2.5–3	7
Ropivacaine	6–10	1–2.5
Tetracaine	1–3	1–2
Cocaine	0.75–3	3–4

Adapted from Ahlstrom KK, Frodel JL. Local Anesthetics for Facial Plastic Procedures. Otolaryngologic Clinics of North America; 2002;35(1):29–53.

Table 4.3 shows the ester and amide classification of local anesthetics, as well as other items of comparative pharmacology. Because PABA is usually the culprit in true allergy, there is often cross-sensitivity within the ester classification. (For example, a patient allergic to tetracaine will also likely have an allergic reaction to procaine.)

Sometimes, allergies that are attributed to local anesthetics are actually caused by preservatives, such as methylparaben, used in the preparation of local anesthetic agents. These compounds are structurally related to PABA. Patients with allergies to preservatives can safely receive preservative-free local anesthetics.

Another common reason for "allergy" to local anesthetics is a normal response to epinephrine. Epinephrine is often added to local anesthetics to provide vasoconstriction, which slows the systemic absorption of the local anesthetic and therefore prolongs the action of the drug. Intravascular absorption of epinephrine can lead to tachycardia, palpitations, flushing, and hypertension, all of which the patient may incorrectly interpret as an allergic reaction, usually during dental work. Therefore, when a patient reports a drug allergy, it is important to obtain a detailed history in an attempt to determine exactly what took place during the incident and guide subsequent therapy accordingly. It is extremely unlikely that a patient is truly allergic to an amide local anesthetic. If the reaction did not include any rash, hives, swelling, or bronchospasm but does describe a typical response to epinephrine, it may be reasonable simply to proceed slowly with an amide local anesthetic (knowing that appropriate anaphylaxis treatment is available, as it always must be for every case). On the other hand, if there is genuine doubt, it is reasonable to postpone any use of local anesthetic and refer the patient to an allergist for testing.

Intravenous Sedation

Sedation is typically produced through the use of any number of intravenous medications, either alone or in combination. The classic combination is a benzodiazepine, such as midazolam, and a narcotic, such as fentanyl (which has replaced meperidine in many practices because repeated doses of meperidine are associated with the potential for seizures). Though midazolam is used commonly as the benzodiazepine of choice, several different narcotics are often used, including the ultra-potent synthetic narcotics fentanyl and remifentanil. In the past 20 years, the hypnotic drug propofol has been introduced into practice, either alone or in combination with other medications. Ketamine, a dissociative hypnotic drug, has also been used as a non-narcotic sedative.

The desired effect of IV sedation varies with the particular situation, and this drives the choice of drugs. Benzodiazepines produce anxiolysis and amnesia, but

Table 4.3

Comparative Pharmacology of Local Anesthetics

Classification	Potency	Onset	Duration after infiltration (mins)
Esters			
Procaine	1	Slow	45–60
Chloroprocaine	4	Rapid	30–45
Tetracaine	16	Slow	60–180
Amides			
Lidocaine	1	Rapid	60–120
Etidocaine	4	Slow	240–480
Prilocaine	1	Slow	60–120
Mepivacaine	1	Slow	90–180
Bupivacaine	4	Slow	240–480
Ropivacaine	4	Slow	240–480

Adapted from Stoelting RK. Pharmacology and Physiology in Anesthetic Practice. 3rd ed. Philadelphia: Lippincott-Raven;1999.

no analgesia and relatively little ventilatory or cardiovascular depression in truly conservative doses. Narcotics are analgesics that cause respiratory and cardiovascular depression, but only small amounts of anxiolysis and no appreciable amnesia. Propofol has very little analgesic effect, but produces anxiolysis and unconsciousness. Therefore, if the patient is having a procedure where excellent analgesia can reliably be achieved with local anesthesia but the patient is anxious, then sedation with only a benzodiazepine would be adequate and a narcotic would be unnecessary.

The definition of therapeutic index is the ratio between the toxic dose and the effective therapeutic dose of a drug, and it is used as a measure of the relative safety of the drug. Drugs with a small, or narrow, therapeutic index have a very little difference between the plasma concentrations that produce the desired effect and toxicity. The same concept can be applied in situations when the concern is not overt toxicity, but undesired side effects. This is the case with medications used for IV sedation. Many of these drugs, most notably propofol and remifentanil, have a very narrow therapeutic index related to ventilatory depression. This requires that these specific medications be titrated very carefully and that patients are monitored very closely for adequate ventilation and oxygenation.

Making the use of IV sedation even more difficult is the remarkable synergy that exists among many of these drugs. A dose of midazolam that produces perfect anxiolysis alone can lead to respiratory depression if a small analgesic dose of narcotic is added. Again, titration and monitoring are of utmost importance. When a patient moves or moans near the end of a facial plastic surgery case being done under IV sedation, the almost-reflex response of administering one last dose of 0.5 mg midazolam, 25 micrograms of fentanyl, or 12.5 mg meperidine could be enough to cause dangerous ventilatory insufficiency (central depression and/or airway obstruction from relaxation).

Propofol is an extreme example of this quandary because the same drug can produce both excellent conscious sedation and deep general anesthesia with an electrically silent EEG, just by varying the dose. The availability and use of this drug by non-anesthesiologists was one of the primary motivators for the American Society of Anesthesiologists to produce practice guidelines for sedation and analgesia for non-anesthesiologists.[14] This document reviews the continuum between minimal sedation, moderate sedation, deep sedation, and general anesthesia and provides definitions. Recommendations in the guidelines include items related to patient preparation, patient monitoring, training of personnel, availability of emergency equipment, use of supplemental oxygen, titration of medications, and recovery care. Facial plastic surgeons directing the administration of propofol for sedation should review and actively apply these guidelines.

Because of the narrow therapeutic index of many of the medications that are used for IV sedation, it is extremely difficult to achieve a level of "conscious" sedation, where the patient has analgesia and sedation, but is still able to respond to commands (a central definition of "conscious" sedation). When patients accidentally are put in deeper levels of sedation, it is critical that practitioners either be able to provide life support, reverse the sedation, or both. There have been many instances of failure to rescue patients from deep sedation, which often results in patient harm.[15]

Because there have been incidences of major morbidity and mortality that have been publicized, concerns about proper sedation care have appeared in the lay press. Patients are becoming more aware of potential pitfalls of sedation for procedures and are demanding that guidelines for properly trained personnel and equipment are followed.[16]

General Anesthesia

General anesthesia refers to a state of unconsciousness, amnesia, analgesia, and relaxation that permits calm surgery. This state is often produced by the administration of several different drugs to the patient by the anesthesia professional, each of which focuses on a different component of the anesthetic. As with all drugs, many of these anesthetic agents have important side effects. In adults, anesthesia is typically induced by either propofol or (rarely) sodium thiopental. Both of these induction agents are vasodilators, and sodium thiopental is a myocardial depressant as well. Some degree of hypotension is common after administration of these drugs.

After induction, anesthesia is often maintained by one of the volatile anesthetic agents. These drugs, usually desflurane and sevoflurane (or possibly isoflurane) in facial plastic surgery, can also cause vasodilation and produce hypotension. They have differing effects on the bronchial tree, with sevoflurane and isoflurane leading to bronchodilation and desflurane causing bronchoconstriction. Desflurane is often avoided in patients with reactive airway disease because of its tendency to irritate the airways.

Administration of intravenous fluids, sometimes in significant quantities, is often required to counteract the hypotension from vasodilation caused by these drugs. Routinely in healthy patients, the kidneys eventually eliminate this extra fluid, and it is of no consequence. In some patients, this fluid can lead to tissue edema. This can be significant in facial procedures, so the need for the maintenance of blood pressure must be balanced against the harm of swelling, and this is an appropriate point for preoperative discussion between the surgeon and the anesthesia professional(s).

Of the muscle relaxants in common use today, succinylcholine is the one that may potentially produce untoward side effects (beyond the expected consequence of apnea from all the muscle relaxants). Succinylcholine can cause a transient increase in plasma potassium levels, typically on the order of 0.5 mEq/l.[17] This increase may be significant in patients with already abnormally high potassium levels, such as in renal failure. In certain scenarios, such as after burns or crush injuries, the potassium increase caused by succinylcholine may be much more than 0.5 mEq/l. Succinylcholine is rapidly hydrolyzed by plasma pseudocholinesterase enzymes, and in rare cases patients have an abnormality (quantity or quality) of these enzymes, resulting in a duration of action of the drug of hours instead of minutes. Succinylcholine is also one of a handful of drugs that can trigger malignant hyperthermia (see below). However, despite its potential problems, succinylcholine is the only muscle relaxant currently available with a rapid onset and typically ultrashort duration of action, and this makes it the drug of choice in some situations, particularly facilitating intubation for short cases or with patients having potentially difficult airways.

Malignant Hyperthermia

Malignant hyperthermia (MH) is an anesthetic-related disorder of skeletal muscle metabolism.[18] It is an inherited condition that is triggered on exposure to either volatile anesthetics, succinylcholine, or both. Its importance to plastic surgeons assessing patients has been discussed.[19] When the increased metabolic state is triggered, signs include severe sudden hypercarbia, tachycardia, muscle rigidity, acidosis, and eventually hyperthermia (although this is a late development, so if there is a question, waiting to see the temperature rise allows the syndrome to advance to a very dangerous stage). The very dramatic initial sharp rise in end-tidal CO_2 with significant tachycardia should provoke a presumptive diagnosis and invoke immediate treatment.

Since MH is an inherited disease, susceptibility to it can often be predicted by taking a careful family history. If a patient is determined or suspected to be susceptible, a perioperative episode of MH can almost always be avoided by limiting exposure to triggering agents. Stated differently, if general anesthesia is necessary, then propofol, which does not trigger MH, can be used for both induction and maintenance of anesthesia by intravenous infusion.

If MH does occur, the initial treatment is straightforward: call for help and dantrolene; discontinue any possible triggering agent and hyperventilate with 100% oxygen; administer an initial dose of 2.5 mg/kg of dantrolene and also treat the confirmed blood-gas metabolic acidosis with IV bicarbonate; cool actively with iced fluids IV, in cavities, and to the skin; place a large IV and a urinary catheter. The critical component of treatment is the dantrolene, a skeletal muscle relaxant that may require repeated doses in sequence. Because of this, dantrolene must be stocked in every facility that uses any of the possible triggering medications, and a minimum of 36 vials is recommended. A patient suspected of having the disease in an office or ambulatory surgery center must be transferred to a hospital as soon as possible. Education and communication about this disorder is provided by the Malignant Hyperthermia Association of the US (MHAUS, www.mhaus.org). The MH Hotline (1–800-MHHYPER, or 1–800–644–9737) provides telephone service to medical professionals for emergency consultation.

◆ Patient and Anesthetic Technique Selection and Evaluation for Facial Plastic Surgery

Patient Factors That May Lead to Anesthetic Complications

The best way to manage complications is to avoid them. This approach helps to create an environment that promotes patient safety, which is in the forefront of medical practice today.[20] Anesthesiologists and other physicians have been interested in determining which patient-specific factors predict postoperative complications in that patient.[21]

ASA Physical Status Classification

The American Society of Anesthesiologists (ASA) Physical Status (PS) classification (**Table 4.4**) was developed in 1941 with the intent of facilitating studies of patients undergoing anesthesia and surgery. The system was enhanced in 1961 and acquired its modern form. It has provided a basis for communication among anesthesia and non-anesthesia professionals by describing the acuity and the likely anesthetic challenge of a patient and facilitates the most logical assignment of personnel and resources for a given case.

In recent years, extensive discussion of the correlation of the ASA PS classification with surgical risk factors in the database of the National Surgical Quality Improvement Program (NSQIP) has taken place. In a random sample of almost 6000 major surgical procedures, the PS classification was found to be a strong predictor of surgical outcomes. As shown in **Table 4.5**, morbidity and mortality rose with increases in the PS classification. The NSQIP database was shown to correlate with and (in some circumstances) predict surgical outcome, thus validating the ASA PS classification.[22]

Cardiovascular

Predictors of adverse surgical and anesthesia outcomes suggest that cardiac risk is the most prominent consideration. Extensive studies and recommendations have been published on this issue.[23] The greatest risks for perioperative cardiac complications include the usual suspects: recent myocardial infarction, unstable or severe angina, decompensated CHF, significant dysrhythmias, heart block, and untreated valve disease. Intraoperative risk is highest for the most invasive surgery and prolonged surgery with major fluid shifts. Many risk-scoring schemes for predicting postoperative cardiac complications exist, one being the Revised Cardiac

Table 4.4

American Society of Anesthesiologists Physical Status Classification
PS I - A normal healthy patient
PS II - A patient with mild systemic disease
PS III - A patient with severe systemic disease
PS IV - A patient with severe systemic disease that is a constant threat to life
PS V - A moribund patient who is not expected to survive with or without the operation
PS VI - A declared brain-dead patient whose organs are being removed for donor purposes

Table 4.5

Perioperative Mortality Rate and Morbidity Rate (All Causes) by ASA PS Level		
ASA PS Level	**30-Day Mortality Rate (%)**	**30-Day Morbidity Rate (%)**
I	0.0 ± 0.0	1.7 ± 0.4
II	0.2 ± 0.1	4.0 ± 0.4
III	2.2 ± 0.4	11.3 ± 0.8
IV	15.2 ± 2.4	31.7 ± 3.1
V	70.0 ± 10.5	40.0 ± 11.2

Adapted from Davenport DL, Bowe EA, Henderson WG, et al. National Surgical Quality Improvement Program (NSQIP) risk factors can be used to validate American Society of Anesthesiologists Physical Status Classification (ASA PS) levels. Ann Surg 2006;243:636–641, discussion 641–644.

Risk Index.[24] As shown in **Table 4.6**, six factors were found to predict cardiac complications. When only one of these factors is present, there is a 0.9% chance of a major cardiac complication; two increase the chance to 7% and three to 11%.

Pulmonary

The factors predicting pulmonary complications have not been studied to the same degree as cardiac risk, but the American College of Physicians has published relevant guidelines.[25] Formulated by use of systematic review techniques, these guidelines indicate that significant risk factors for postoperative pulmonary complica-

Table 4.6

Independent Correlates of Major Cardiac Complications
Revised Cardiac Risk Index
1. High-risk type of surgery
2. Ischemic heart disease
3. History of congestive heart failure
4. History of cerebrovascular disease
5. Insulin therapy for diabetes
6. Preoperative serum creatinine >2.0 mg/dL

Adapted from Lee TH, Marcantonio ER, Mangione CM, et al. Derivation and prospective validation of a simple index for prediction of cardiac risk of major noncardiac surgery. Circulation 1999;100:1043–1049.

tions are chronic obstructive pulmonary disease, age older than 60 years, ASA class of II or greater, functionally dependent, and congestive heart failure. Preexisting airway pathology, from diseased teeth to congenital or traumatic anatomic abnormalities that may prevent easy intubation, can predispose a patient to potential adverse outcomes, although patients whose airways are predicted to be easy to manage[26] may occasionally face the greatest danger due to the lack of recognition and appropriate preparation. Airway issues remain among the thorniest problems still unsolved in modern anesthesia practice,[27] and appeals for improved equipment, techniques, and management strategies persist.

Obstructive Sleep Apnea

Obstructive sleep apnea (OSA) is a specific condition with several relevant risks. Though this disease increases the risk for airway management difficulties in the immediate postoperative period, its influence on postoperative pulmonary complication rates has not been fully investigated, with only one study evaluating the risks.[28] There were nonstatistically significant trends toward higher rates of reintubation, hypercapnia, and hypoxemia for patients with obstructive sleep apnea.

The ASA has published guidelines that focus on the perioperative management of patients with OSA, who may be at increased risk for perioperative morbidity and mortality because of potential difficulty in maintaining a patent airway.[29] Further, these issues can easily be compounded in patients during or after facial plastic or reconstructive surgery. One challenge of dealing with OSA is that the vast majority of patients with this condition have not been formally diagnosed. The guidelines include risk factors for OSA, along with the recommendation that if patients are found to have a high risk, they should be treated as if they have the disease. Patients with OSA should receive extended and more intense monitoring for adverse ventilatory events both during and after facial plastic surgery.

Choice of Anesthetic Technique

Many facial plastic surgery procedures can be done with either general anesthesia (GA) or monitored anesthesia care (MAC). The surgeon often indicates a preference to the anesthesia professional(s). General anesthesia is typically produced and maintained with either intravenous or inhalational medications and usually depresses ventilation enough that some type of artificial support is necessary. That support can be provided either with an endotracheal tube or a laryngeal mask airway (LMA). From the surgeon's perspective, the advantages of GA are that the patient is completely unconscious, insensate, and still. However, several risks of GA should be considered. When combined with surgery, GA can result in physiologic stress for the patient that can upset homeostasis and result in cardiovascular or cerebrovascular complications. Since ventilation and oxygenation must be maintained artificially, GA also introduces the opportunity for complications related to management errors or simple inattention.

These potential complications and the overall degree of invasiveness have led some surgeons to attempt to avoid GA whenever possible. MAC typically involves the administration of some degree of sedation and analgesia by an anesthesiologist or nurse anesthetist, combined with local anesthesia administered by the surgeon. Because it is intended that the patient maintain spontaneous ventilation, it is tempting to think that this anesthetic technique is inherently safer. However, there are no randomized controlled trials that demonstrate a favorable difference in complication rates between general anesthesia and MAC, and there certainly have been reports of significant morbidity and mortality during and after MAC.[15,30] In the data of the closed claims project of the ASA, claims associated with MAC showed a high severity of patient injury and a liability profile similar to claims associated with general anesthesia.[31] In fact, many anesthesia professionals believe there is a greater risk with MAC than with GA for relatively extensive procedures, particularly those involving the face, head, and neck because the airway is usually not immediately accessible (as would need to be for a resuscitative jaw thrust or insertion of an oral airway device to help overcome a patient's obstructed airway following an additional dose of IV sedation medication). Therefore, it is extremely important to maintain vigilant monitoring and management of patients under MAC that is at least equal to that with GA.

Another alternative to GA is involved in tumescent liposuction. This technique includes the subcutaneous infusion of significant volumes of a solution containing lidocaine, followed by the aspiration of fat through microcannulas. It is attractive because it is reported to provide excellent anesthesia, often without the need for systemic sedation or analgesia. Though tumescent liposuction has been performed thousands of times without problems,[32,33] within the last two decades, there have been reports of morbidity and mortality after this technique was used.[34] In one study, Rao describes four deaths, three of which were probably related to lidocaine toxicity and one related to fluid overload. Guidelines now exist for dosage limits for local anesthetics and volume limits for wetting solutions;[7,35] their implementation should reduce risk but cannot eliminate it.

Qualifications of Practitioner Providing Sedation

Many different personnel models have been used at one time or another for providing sedation care to patients who are undergoing painful procedures. Though these different models have been discussed a great deal, which type of practitioner is best suited to ad-

minister the sedative or analgesic medications is unknown. On the surface, it might be proposed that an anesthesiologist is most medically qualified to do so, but this choice is also the most expensive. On the other end of the spectrum, the operating surgeon may order that the sedative medications be administered by a registered nurse, under the impression that the sedation plays only a minor role in the care of the patient and that this method serves to minimize cost and maximize convenience.

While complications during sedation have been reported when patients have been cared for by all different types of practitioners,[30] there is consensus that sedation should be provided by someone who is trained to monitor the patient adequately and who is not participating in the surgical procedure.[14] Extensive guidelines and statements by the American College of Surgeons and the American Society of Anesthesiologists on the critical issues of the depth of sedation and the appropriateness of involved personnel have been published (and undoubtedly would have medical-legal implications in the event of malpractice litigation).[36] In cases of moderate or deep sedation, the person administering sedation should also be able to rescue the patient from excess sedation, provide advanced life support skills, and establish an emergency airway. This approach helps to avoid complications by directing maximum attention specifically to the patient's sedation and analgesia, in particular the monitoring of ventilation, oxygenation, and cardiovascular function.

◆ Anesthesia Considerations and Complications Specific to Facial Plastic Surgery

Considerations Relative to the Location and Other Characteristics of the Surgery

Duration of Surgery

The duration of the procedure is one factor that has been shown to have a positive correlation with incidence of postoperative complications.[7,37] Lengthy procedures with local anesthesia and sedation or monitored anesthesia care are limited by the patient's ability to hold still on the table without requiring so much sedation as to be at risk for dangerous hypoventilation (mechanical airway obstruction, CNS depression, or both). Lengthy procedures under general anesthesia are more likely to lead to postoperative atelectasis, nausea and vomiting, and (in the setting of a planned ambulatory procedure) unplanned hospital admission. This has led some to recommend that only cases of shorter duration should be considered for an office-based procedure. The time limit for what would be considered a shorter case is subject to debate and varies among practitioners. Experience over time with a given team in a given setting often provides guidance as to a reasonable maximum.

Lengthy cases may also lead to problems with patient positioning and injuries associated with positioning issues.[38] Therefore, when a long surgical procedure is anticipated in any setting, great care should be given to position the patient so that there is no traction on nerves and minimal pressure on points of contact between the patient and the surgical environment.

Airway Management

Management of the airway is of critical importance to the patient and of utmost concern to the anesthesia professional. Several issues, such as distorted airway anatomy and intraoperative access to the airway, are relevant in both major and minor facial plastic and reconstructive cases.

In large facial reconstruction cases, the airway anatomy is often abnormal because of the pathology. When general anesthesia is induced, the abnormality may lead to the need for advanced airway techniques, such as flexible fiberoptic laryngoscopy. If MAC is being considered when the airway anatomy is abnormal, many anesthesiologists will prefer to use general anesthesia with a secured airway from the outset, rather than take the risk of losing control in the middle of the procedure if the patient develops airway obstruction. If the airway is extremely distorted or there is a high likelihood of postoperative upper airway obstruction, doing a tracheostomy before starting the planned surgical procedure should be considered.

Since in facial cases the surgical procedure is in close proximity to the airway, both the surgeon and the anesthesiologist should be aware that they must share the same space. The worst consequence of inattention to this fact occurs when (during surgical manipulation) the endotracheal tube becomes dislodged from the trachea in the middle of a case, and the problem goes unrecognized until impairment of ventilation and oxygenation raises the alarm. Then there is precious little time to restore the airway before the patient faces injury. Obviously, careful planning, open communication (before and during the case), and rigorous vigilance should help avoid such incidents.

Pitfalls of Monitored Anesthesia Care

Supplemental Oxygen and Fire

Since oxygen supports combustion, the use of monopolar electrocautery near high concentrations of oxygen can produce a risk of fire. This is the scenario in some facial cases done under sedation where there has been fire, often involving ignition of cloth or paper drapes. Supplemental oxygen administered by a nasal cannula or plastic face mask may accumulate near the surgical site if the drape configuration prevents the oxygen from dissipating into the room air. There have been sporadic reports of fire in the literature over the years.[39] There has been an increased awareness of the risk of fires, especially by accrediting bodies.[40] The American Society of Anesthesiologists has published a practice advisory providing detailed recommendations on avoiding operating room fires[41] (which, again, could have medical-legal implications); in addition, the Anesthesia Patient Safety Foundation has issued an extremely popular instructional video with illustrative scenarios (http://www.apsf.org/resources_video_watch.php).

Several strategies can be employed to reduce the risk of fire. When monopolar electrocautery is used, open delivery of supplemental oxygen should be avoided if at all possible. The reflex administration of oxygen whenever IV sedation is employed often is unnecessary and may actually be a disservice because it is likely to create a false sense of security if there is a lack of appreciation of the difference between ventilation and oxygenation. The supplemental O_2 will delay the appearance of desaturation on the pulse oximeter when extremely dangerous hypoventilation is evolving. In the rare case when supplemental oxygen is definitely required due to, for example, severe pulmonary disease and monopolar electrocautery is used near the oxygen, the oxygen flow rate delivered by either nasal cannula or mask should be reduced to the absolutely lowest level possible for that patient. The use of "open face" draping techniques or an effective venting scheme may prevent oxygen pooling. Lastly, the avoidance of alcohol-based prep solutions may eliminate one combustion fuel source. The ECRI Institute offers a large wall poster (https://www.ecri.org/Documents/Surgical_Fire_Poster(2009).pdf) on prevention of surgical fires.

Capnographic Monitoring

As noted, the ASA Closed Claims Project revealed that many malpractice claims involved adverse respiratory events (inadequate ventilation) and that a failure to monitor the patient adequately was a contributing factor in most of those cases. Facial plastic surgery, particularly without a mechanically secured airway, has among the greatest risks for intraoperative ventilatory insufficiency. The ASA standards for basic intraoperative monitoring require that capnography be employed to verify correct endotracheal tube placement and then continued throughout the general anesthetic. Further, during MAC, observation of ventilation qualitative clinical signs or capnography (which can be accomplished with certain nasal cannulae, but these may be in the surgical field) must be used.[42] The danger of hypoventilation (both CNS depression and airway obstruction) during MAC cannot be stressed enough—it is one of the greatest risks during many of the most common facial plastic surgical procedures and has appeared in the past to be frequently underappreciated by the involved surgeons.

◆ Immediate Postoperative Recovery from Facial Plastic Surgery

Patients receiving anesthesia for any type of surgery need appropriate facilities and personnel for immediate postoperative recovery. This concept was highlighted when surgical procedures began to be done commonly in an office setting, because recovery was not done in a typical postanesthesia care unit (PACU) equivalent to that found in a hospital. In offices, the anesthesia provider also is often occupied with a subsequent case or simply leaves and thus is not available to assist with postoperative problems. In the early days of office-based surgery, patients sometimes recovered in a back hallway, attended by non-clinical office staff if at all. Not surprisingly, anecdotes abound about patient deaths in such scenarios.[43]

Guidelines for office-based surgery from the American College of Surgeons and the American Society of Anesthesiologists are cited above.[36] In addition, there are three primary accrediting bodies involved with ambulatory surgery. They are the Joint Commission for Accreditation of Healthcare Organizations (JCAHO), the Accreditation Association for Ambulatory Health Care (AAAHC), and the American Association for Accreditation of Ambulatory Surgical Facilities (AAAASF). All these accrediting organizations have standards for facilities, equipment, and personnel necessary for postanesthesia recovery. All facilities where moderate sedation through general anesthesia is provided will reduce the risk of untoward complications during the recovery phase if they observe the standards of at least one of these organizations. Some plastic surgeons with operatories in their offices or office buildings have voluntarily sought formal accreditation to help maximize the safety of their patients, particularly in the immediate postoperative recovery period. Malpractice insurance carriers may offer premium discounts for plastic surgeons whose office-based facilities are formally accredited. Organizations such as the American Academy of Facial Plastic and Reconstructive Surgery and the American Society of Plastic Surgery have proactively linked their membership to the performance of surgery only in duly accredited facilities, thereby reducing the risks for their membership's patients undergoing surgery.

◆ Conclusion

The anesthesia care associated with facial plastic and reconstructive surgical cases is often underappreciated as a source of potential danger. Awareness of and attention to all of the points presented above will facilitate maximum efforts by all involved to help prevent complications and adverse anesthesia outcomes.

PEARLS OF WISDOM

The risk of overt catastrophe in healthy patients caused solely by anesthesia care is probably as low as 1:150,000 to 1:300,000, and this remarkable degree of safety is a testament to the recent improvements in anesthesia care.

Respiratory system adverse events (usually inadequate ventilation) account for a significant majority of anesthesia complications—and even more so in facial plastic surgery due to airway challenges and the significant danger of dangerous hypoventilation during monitored anesthesia care.

Many anesthesia medications have side effects that can lead to untoward events in the absence of careful planning, execution, and—above all—monitoring.

Local anesthetic toxicity can lead to CNS and cardiovascular complications. Maximum dose guidelines should be considered, particularly in tumescent liposuction.

Malignant hyperthermia, though rare, is a serious threat. Dantrolene, the antidote, should be stocked in every facility that uses general anesthesia.

The ASA guidelines for sedation and analgesia by nonanesthesiologists are extensive, valuable, and likely have medical-legal implications, and they have been referenced by many professional and accrediting bodies.

Head and neck surgical field fires from the use of monopolar electrocautery while open supplemental oxygen is administered are a significant risk that can be reduced, particularly with attention to readily available valuable instructional materials.

The immediate postoperative recovery period can be an even greater danger to the facial plastic surgery patient than the surgical anesthetic, particularly in the office setting. The ACS and ASA have extensive guidelines for conduct of office-based surgery.

References

1. Eichhorn JH. Prevention of intraoperative anesthesia accidents and related severe injury through safety monitoring. Anesthesiology 1989;70(4):572–577
2. Domino K. Role of the Closed Claims Project in Improving Outcome; Fleisher LA, Prough DS, eds. Problems in Anesthesia; 2001;13:491–500
3. Caplan RA, Posner KL, Ward RJ, Cheney FW. Adverse respiratory events in anesthesia: a closed claims analysis. Anesthesiology 1990;72(5):828–833
4. Tinker JH, Dull DL, Caplan RA, Ward RJ, Cheney FW. Role of monitoring devices in prevention of anesthetic mishaps: a closed claims analysis. Anesthesiology 1989;71(4):541–546
5. Leopold NA. Prolonged metoclopramide-induced dyskinetic reaction. Neurology 1984;34(2):238–239

6. American Society of Anesthesiologists Committee. Practice guidelines for preoperative fasting and the use of pharmacologic agents to reduce the risk of pulmonary aspiration: application to healthy patients undergoing elective procedures: an updated report by the American Society of Anesthesiologists Committee on Standards and Practice Parameters. Anesthesiology 2011;114(3):495–511

7. Horton JB, Reece EM, Broughton G II, Janis JE, Thornton JF, Rohrich RJ. Patient safety in the office-based setting. Plast Reconstr Surg 2006;117(4):61e–80e

8. Stoelting RK. Pharmacology and Physiology in Anesthetic Practice. 3rd ed. Philadelphia: Lippincott-Raven; 1999

9. McLure HA, Rubin AP. Review of local anaesthetic agents. Minerva Anestesiol 2005;71(3):59–74

10. Rosenblatt MA, Abel M, Fischer GW, Itzkovich CJ, Eisenkraft JB. Successful use of a 20% lipid emulsion to resuscitate a patient after a presumed bupivacaine-related cardiac arrest. Anesthesiology 2006;105(1):217–218

11. Mulroy MF. Systemic toxicity and cardiotoxicity from local anesthetics: incidence and preventive measures. Reg Anesth Pain Med 2002;27(6):556–561

12. Casati A, Putzu M. Bupivacaine, levobupivacaine and ropivacaine: are they clinically different? Best Pract Res Clin Anaesthesiol 2005;19(2):247–268

13. Ahlstrom KK, Frodel JL. Local anesthetics for facial plastic procedures. Otolaryngol Clin North Am 2002;35(1):29–53, v–vi

14. American Society of Anesthesiologists Task Force on Sedation and Analgesia by Non-Anesthesiologists. Practice guidelines for sedation and analgesia by non-anesthesiologists. Anesthesiology 2002;96(4):1004–1017

15. Jastak JT, Peskin RM. Major morbidity or mortality from office anesthetic procedures: a closed-claim analysis of 13 cases. Anesth Prog 1991;38(2):39–44

16. Landro L. Hospitals Move to Curb Anesthesia Risk. Wall Street Journal. August 9, 2006;D:D1, D3

17. Naguib M, Lien CA. Pharmacology of Muscle Relaxants and Their Antagonists. In: Miller RD, ed. Anesthesia. Vol 1. 6th ed. Philadelphia: Churchill Livingstone; 2005:481

18. Gronert GA, Pessah IN, Muldoon SM, Tautz TJ. Malignant Hyperthermia. In: Miller RD, ed. Anesthesia. Vol 1. 6th ed. Philadelphia: Churchill Livingstone; 2005:1169

19. Eichhorn JH. Malignant hyperthermia revisited. Plast Reconstr Surg 1988;82(5):883–885

20. Leape LL, Berwick DM. Five years after To Err Is Human: what have we learned? JAMA 2005;293(19):2384–2390

21. Goldman L, Caldera DL, Nussbaum SR, et al. Multifactorial index of cardiac risk in noncardiac surgical procedures. N Engl J Med 1977;297(16):845–850

22. Davenport DL, Bowe EA, Henderson WG, Khuri SF, Mentzer RM Jr. National Surgical Quality Improvement Program (NSQIP) risk factors can be used to validate American Society of Anesthesiologists Physical Status Classification (ASA PS) levels. Ann Surg 2006;243(5):636–641, discussion 641–644

23. Eagle KA, Berger PB, Calkins H, et al; American College of Cardiology/American Heart Association Task Force on Practice Guidelines (Committee to Update the 1996 Guidelines on Perioperative Cardiovascular Evaluation for Noncardiac Surgery). ACC/AHA guideline update for perioperative cardiovascular evaluation for noncardiac surgery—executive summary: a report of the American College of Cardiology/American Heart Association Task Force on Practice Guidelines (Committee to Update the 1996 Guidelines on Perioperative Cardiovascular Evaluation for Noncardiac Surgery). Circulation 2002;105(10):1257–1267

24. Lee TH, Marcantonio ER, Mangione CM, et al. Derivation and prospective validation of a simple index for prediction of cardiac risk of major noncardiac surgery. Circulation 1999;100(10):1043–1049

25. Qaseem A, Snow V, Fitterman N, et al; Clinical Efficacy Assessment Subcommittee of the American College of Physicians. Risk assessment for and strategies to reduce perioperative pulmonary complications for patients undergoing noncardiothoracic surgery: a guideline from the American College of Physicians. Ann Intern Med 2006;144(8):575–580

26. Shiga T, Wajima Z, Inoue T, Sakamoto A. Predicting difficult intubation in apparently normal patients: a meta-analysis of bedside screening test performance. Anesthesiology 2005;103(2):429–437

27. Peterson GN, Domino KB, Caplan RA, Posner KL, Lee LA, Cheney FW. Management of the difficult airway: a closed claims analysis. Anesthesiology 2005;103(1):33–39

28. Smetana GW, Lawrence VA, Cornell JE; American College of Physicians. Preoperative pulmonary risk stratification for noncardiothoracic surgery: systematic review for the American College of Physicians. Ann Intern Med 2006;144(8):581–595

29. Gross JB, Bachenberg KL, Benumof JL, et al; American Society of Anesthesiologists Task Force on Perioperative Management. Practice guidelines for the perioperative management of patients with obstructive sleep apnea: a report by the American Society of Anesthesiologists Task Force on Perioperative Management of patients with obstructive sleep apnea. Anesthesiology 2006;104(5):1081–1093, quiz 1117–1118

30. Coldiron B, Fisher AH, Adelman E, et al. Adverse event reporting: lessons learned from 4 years of Florida office data. Dermatol Surg 2005;31(9 Pt 1):1079–1092, discussion 1093

31. Bhananker SM, Posner KL, Cheney FW, Caplan RA, Lee LA, Domino KB. Injury and liability associated with monitored anesthesia care: a closed claims analysis. Anesthesiology 2006; 104(2):228–234

32. Hanke W, Cox SE, Kuznets N, Coleman WP III. Tumescent liposuction report performance measurement initiative: national survey results. Dermatol Surg 2004;30(7):967–977, discussion 978

33. Housman TS, Lawrence N, Mellen BG, et al. The safety of liposuction: results of a national survey. Dermatol Surg 2002; 28(11):971–978

34. Rao RB, Ely SF, Hoffman RS. Deaths related to liposuction. N Engl J Med 1999;340(19):1471–1475

35. Iverson RE, Lynch DJ; American Society of Plastic Surgeons Committee on Patient Safety. Practice advisory on liposuction. Plast Reconstr Surg 2004;113(5):1478–1490, discussion 1491–1495

36. a. American College of Surgeons. Patient Safety Principles for Office-Based Surgery Utilizing Moderate Sedation/Analgesia, Deep Sedation/Analgesia, or General Anesthesia (2003). http://www.facs.org/patientsafety/patientsafety.html; b. American Society of Anesthesiologists. Continuum of Depth of Sedation: Definition of General Anesthesia and Levels of Sedation/Analgesia (2009). https://www.asahq.org/For-Healthcare-Professionals/Standards-Guidelines-and-Statements.aspx; c. American Society of Anesthesiologists. Distinguishing Monitored Anesthesia Care From Moderate Sedation/Analgesia (Conscious Sedation) (2009). https://www.asahq.org/For-Healthcare-Professionals/Standards-Guidelines-and-Statements.aspx; d. American

Society of Anesthesiologists. Guidelines for Office-Based Anesthesia, (2009). https://www.asahq.org/For-Healthcare-Professionals/Standards-Guidelines-and-Statements.aspx; e. American Society of Anesthesiologists. Statement on Granting Privileges for Administration of Moderate Sedation to Practitioners Who Are Not Anesthesia Professionals, (2011). https://www.asahq.org/Standards-Guidelines-and-Statements.aspx; f. American Society of Anesthesiologists. Statement on Granting Privileges to Non-Anesthesiologist Practitioners for Personally Administering Deep Sedation or Supervising Deep Sedation by Individuals Who Are Not Anesthesia Professionals, (2006). https://www.asahq.org/For-Healthcare-Professionals/Standards-Guidelines-and-Statements.aspx; g. American Society of Anesthesiologists. Advisory on Granting Privileges for Deep Sedation to Non-Anesthesiologist Sedation Practitioners, (2010). https://www.asahq.org/For-Healthcare-Professionals/Standards-Guidelines-and-Statements.aspx; h. American Society of Anesthesiologists. Statement on Safe Use of Propofol, (2009). https://www.asahq.org/For-Healthcare-Professionals/Standards-Guidelines-and-Statements.aspx

37. Iverson RE; ASPS Task Force on Patient Safety in Office-Based Surgery Facilities. Patient safety in office-based surgery facilities: I. Procedures in the office-based surgery setting. Plast Reconstr Surg 2002;110(5):1337–1342, discussion 1343–1346

38. Winfree CJ, Kline DG. Intraoperative positioning nerve injuries. Surg Neurol 2005;63(1):5–18, discussion 18

39. Greco RJ, Gonzalez R, Johnson P, Scolieri M, Rekhopf PG, Heckler F. Potential dangers of oxygen supplementation during facial surgery. Plast Reconstr Surg 1995;95(6):978–984

40. Lypson ML, Stephens S, Colletti L. Preventing surgical fires: who needs to be educated? Jt Comm J Qual Patient Saf 2005;31(9):522–527

41. American Society of Anesthesiologists. Practice Advisory for the Prevention and Management of Operating Room Fires. Anesthesiology 2008;108:786–801

42. American Society of Anesthesiologists. Standards for Basic Anesthetic Monitoring. https://www.asahq.org/For-Healthcare-Professionals/Standards-Guidelines-and-Statements.aspx

43. Morell RC. OBA Questions, Problems Just Now Recognized, Being Defined. *Anesthesia Patient Safety Foundation Newsletter.* 15; Spring, 2000. http://www.apsf.org/newsletters/html/2000/spring/02-morell.htm

5

Complications Involving Locoregional Flap Reconstruction of Facial Defects

David A. Sherris and Paul R. Young

The use of local and regional flap reconstruction in the repair of facial defects is a mainstay of facial plastic and reconstructive surgery. The surgeon has various options available when assessing treatment of a soft-tissue defect. Each must be considered in the context of multiple factors, such as knowledge of the anatomy, vascular supply, and tissue quality available. The surgeon is required to select a course of action tailored to the individual that may include healing by secondary intent, primary closure, skin grafts, local and regional flaps, distant flaps, and free tissue transfer.

Each patient should be assessed in terms of age, race, gender, occupation, nutrition, prior irradiation, skin type, habits, and general health. Cosmetic success and survival of a local or regional flap depend on considering all these variables. The appropriate surgical approach must be based on both the distinctive characteristics of the defect and the multiple unique factors presented by each patient. The surgeon should strive to satisfy the patient's reasonable expectations and goals, understanding that these goals may differ greatly from patient to patient, based on the individual's priorities, age, gender, and health.

No precise statistics regarding complication rates are available, but adverse outcomes involving locoregional flaps can best be avoided by meticulous preoperative planning, a frank discussion with the patient about the relative risks and benefits associated with each reconstructive approach, and sound technique. Before proceeding with treatment, the surgeon must fully evaluate the dynamic spectrum of economic, psychosocial, and general health issues, coupled with the reconstructive dilemma each patient presents. The simplest approach to repair is not always the best choice for the patient, as sometimes a more complex approach will result in a better cosmetic and functional result.

Sometimes primary closure is simple and effective. Healing by secondary intent is an excellent option for small defects involving concave skin surfaces, such as the medial canthus, temple, and occasionally the nasal alar groove.[1] Yet healing by secondary intent necessitates a long period of wound care, which some patients may not find acceptable. Conversely, wounds involving convex skin surfaces tend to heal poorly by secondary intent and are therefore more complex in their management.

Locoregional flaps typically provide excellent skin color and texture match, and they may be the best option when primary closure and secondary intent closure are not the best options. Reconstruction using locoregional flaps can commonly be performed in a single stage, and the donor sites can be closed primarily with little morbidity.

Locoregional flap complications can stem from poor preoperative planning, infection, hematoma, or patient-specific factors that compromise the vascularity of the tissue or the healing of the scars. The choice of an appropriate flap to close a specific defect is complex and is not the point of this chapter. One is referred to other textbooks on reconstruction for discussion of flap choices. Yet, one must understand that surgery starts with the preoperative planning. Incisions have to be planned parallel to relaxed skin tension lines, in aesthetic unit and subunit boundaries, or in the midline of the face. An undersized flap can result in distortion of critical anatomic structures, causing ectropion, alar retraction, or retraction of other surrounding structures. Deep wounds must be reconstructed with both adequate structural support to overcome scar contracture and adequate bulk to fill the defect, but not so much bulk as to cause a contour deformity. Deep layer closure is critical to decrease the dead space where blood or scar tissue can accumulate, as well as to decrease the tension on the skin closure so that wounds heal with optimal scars. Although most complications can be avoided, others are simply the result of indiscriminate odds. This chapter will focus on the complications of locoregional flaps, ways to decrease the likelihood of a complication, and management in the event of a complication.

◆ Brief History

The term flap was derived from the Dutch word *flappe* in the 16th century, meaning something that hung broad and loose, secured by only one side. The first historical mention of flap surgery dates to a more remote time, around 600 BC, when Sushruta Samhita, believed to be part of one of the four Vedas, described what he had learned from his mentor Dhanwantri. He eloquently described using a cheek flap for nasal reconstruction. The traditional Indian technique for rhinoplasty using a flap from the adjoining forehead can be traced back to approximately 1440 AD.

Later surgical methods using flaps to repair defects progressed in distinct periods. During the First and Second World Wars, pedicled flaps were used extensively. Subsequently the procedure of axial pattern flaps (flaps with a named blood supply) was developed in the 1950s. In the 1970s, the distinction between axial and random flaps (unnamed blood supply) was first recognized. The ensuing advances include the use of cutaneous, fasciocutaneous, muscle, musculocutaneous, and osseous tissue types in flap surgeries.

◆ Vascular Anatomy

The defining characteristic of a skin flap is that its survival in the recipient bed is predicated upon a functioning intravascular circulation. Historically, the design of skin flaps was governed by a set of length-to-width ratios (5:1 for the face due to its abundant blood supply). Local flaps can easily be advanced, pivoted or interpolated, thereby allowing a greater length-to-width ratio. However, in the 1970s, Daniel showed that increasing the width of a flap did not increase the surviving length.[2,3] Rather, the amount of blood supply incorporated into a flap's width dictates the flap's surviving length. Daniel and Williams defined the blood supply to the skin as being from two types of arteries: (1) musculocutaneous arteries or (2) direct cutaneous arteries (now further subdivided[4]). The skin is supplied by two vascular plexuses. The deep vascular plexus, or subdermal plexus, is found at the junction of the dermis and subcutaneous fat. The superficial vascular plexus courses in the superficial aspect of the reticular dermis, giving off capillary loops within the dermal papillae. Musculocutaneous arteries are branches of segmental vessels arising from the aorta that supply blood to muscle and continue through the underlying muscle to the overlying dermal plexi. For the majority of their course, musculocutaneous arteries run perpendicular to the skin, supplying only small areas of the skin. Direct cutaneous arteries are branches of segmental or muscular arteries that pass through fascial septae between muscles to supply the enveloping fascia and overlying skin. Arteries run parallel to the skin, supplying a large area of the skin.[5]

Random flaps (e.g., bilobed, note, z-plasty) are the most commonly used in local flap repair of facial defects. The vascular supply to random flaps, which consist of skin and subcutaneous fat, arises mainly from multiple musculocutaneous arteries from the subdermal plexus at the flap's anatomic base. Therefore the appropriate plane of dissection is at the level of the subcutaneous fat. Axial flaps derive their blood supply from named direct cutaneous arteries. Therefore, axial flaps allow for greater length and reliability, with less concern for width or a delay procedure.[6] Surgically, the plane of dissection is deeper to incorporate fascia and must align along a distinct septocutaneous vessel. Examples of axial flaps include the paramedian forehead flap, based on the supratrochlear artery, and the nasiolabial flap, based on the angular artery.

◆ Preoperative Planning

Reconstruction of facial soft-tissue defects requires the surgeon to have knowledge of wound healing physiology, soft-tissue handling, and head and neck reconstructive surgical techniques. Poorly designed flaps can lead to an array of complications, ranging from minor cosmetic deformities to functionally debilitating abnormalities (**Fig. 5.1**). The planning of surgical incisions should adhere to the elementary principles of relaxed skin tension lines (RSTL) and lines of maximal extensibility (LME), which typically lie perpendicular to each other. Incisions heal better when placed parallel to or in the RSTLs, and wound tension is minimized if donor tissue is transferred along LMEs.[7,8] Additionally, wounds placed in aesthetic unit and subunit boundaries, along

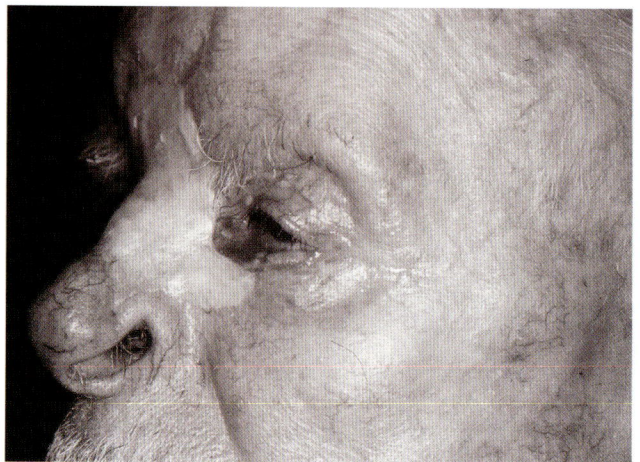

Fig. 5.1 Patient who demonstrates multiple late sequelae of poor defect repair choices, including alar retraction, ectropion, and color mismatch between the skin graft and surrounding tissue.

hairlines, and in the midline of the face heal with less perceptible scars. Wounds aligned with RSTLs are not subjected to repetitive tension and therefore reduce the risk of scar hypertrophy.[9,10]

Wound immobilization during healing will result in better cosmetic outcomes. Two techniques commonly employed to minimize wound tension during healing are undermining and using deep sutures. Undermining, however, is not always the best method to relieve excessive tension. It has been shown that beyond 4 cm, undermining has no effect on tension. Furthermore, animal studies suggest there is a correlation between excessive skin undermining and an increased incidence of flap necrosis.[11] Deep sutures help to relieve tension and make wound edge eversion easier. Wound edges that are everted at the time of closure result in better scars.

Recently, Gassner et al. have reported statistically significant results in improved scar appearance following use of botulinum toxin injections at the time of surgical repair.[12–15] Botulinum toxin decreases the tension on a wound by temporarily chemodenervating the muscles pulling on the wound. Gassner and Sherris recommend injecting the surrounding muscles at the time of wound closure to produce an improved scar. This theory has been proven in a blind, placebo-controlled trial in animals and humans with forehead defects and in an open trial with perioral wounds. Further studies using this innovative technique are underway and are promising.

Careful attention to the aforementioned principles of minimal wound tension is vital when the surgeon is designing flaps for defects involving the nasal ala, the eyelids, and the vermilion border of the mouth. These areas are extremely sensitive to unusual skin tension.[16–22] Increased tension on the nasal ala from a poorly designed flap may result in alar retraction, nasal obstruction, or both (**Fig. 5.1**). Poor flap design in the eyelid region may lead to ectropion, epiphora, or lagophthalmos, which may further result in exposure keratitis of the cornea with possible visual impairment. If the vermilion border of the lip in the perioral region is subjected to excessive tension, oral competence and speech may be compromised. These defects, aside from leading to a functional impairment, are very difficult to revise. Therefore, it is crucial to examine these anatomic structures meticulously after insetting of the flap intraoperatively. Increased tension should be relieved, even if this requires using an alternate method of closure. Consideration of placing structural grafts under the eyelid or nasal flaps to overcome the wound contracture is an effective measure to prevent contracture of these important anatomic structures.

General wound-handling principles for soft tissue should be meticulously observed during surgery of the face. Tissue should be handled with skin hooks and fine toothed forceps to minimize blunt trauma.[7,8] Tissue layers need to be properly sutured to eliminate dead space. Meticulous hemostasis should be obtained with bipolar electrocautery. Overly aggressive electrocautery, however, can increase the risk of flap necrosis. Furthermore, excessive thinning of the donor tissue reduces flap viability. Minimizing wound tension will avert damage to axial vessels and decrease the occurrence of traumatic dissection.

The design of a facial flap must always assimilate the knowledge of the underlying anatomy to avoid injury to vulnerable anatomic structures. Knowledge of the locations of the major vessels and nerves of the face, as well as the tissue layers in which they reside, is essential when considering flap elevation in these regions. Invariably, small sensory nerves will be transected at the margins of a flap, but the mild loss of cutaneous sensation is not usually clinically significant. However, the great auricular nerve, which is located anterior and superficial to the sternocleidomastoid muscle, can easily be injured unless one stays superficial to the fascia of the sternocleidomastoid muscle. If the nerve is injured, hypesthesia or paresthesia of the affected ear may occur. The infraorbital nerve, which supplies sensation to a large area of the midface, is also susceptible to injury, especially in eyelid and nasolabial flap reconstruction.

A far more serious injury can occur if the facial nerve is injured. The temporal branch of the facial nerve is very close to the surface as it crosses the zygomatic arch in the temporal region.[23–25] It is vulnerable to injury in this area, especially in elderly patients with thin skin. Transection of the temporal branch of the facial nerve can result in the loss of forehead furrows and lead to eyebrow ptosis. Injury to branches supplying the orbicularis oculi muscle may result in difficulty closing the affected eye. The zygomatic branch of the facial nerve is less vulnerable as it crosses the zygoma, because it does so in a deep plane. Transection will result in eyelid ptosis and ectropion. Injury to the buccal branch of the facial nerve along its course from the parotid gland to the orbicularis oris muscle may result in facial asymmetry, an inability to pucker the lips, or synkinesis. The marginal mandibular nerve is most vulnerable at the angle of the jaw as it courses from under the parotid gland. Facial nerve damage can result in both cosmetic deformity and significant functional impairment, particularly around the corner of the mouth. To avoid these devastating consequences of facial nerve injury, flaps in these regions should be elevated and undermined in a subcutaneous plane to avoid disruption of the superficial musculoaponeurotic system (SMAS) or platysma muscle.

◆ Complications and Their Management

Ischemia

Generally, the blood supply to the skin far exceeds the skin's nutritional demands. Blood flow to the skin is integral for thermoregulatory function and therefore fluctuates widely as demand varies. This oversupply allows for random flap viability. The face, in particular, has a rich blood supply from the subdermal plexus. Therefore, local random flaps on the face survive with fewer complications due to vascular compromise than local flaps in other regions of the body. As previously mentioned, axial flaps in the face are based on the superficial temporal, supraorbital, supratrochlear, transverse facial, and facial angular arteries, which ensure a robust vascular supply, so axial flaps can therefore be designed with a longer flap length than random flaps.[26–32]

Probably the most common complication of locoregional flap reconstruction is postoperative ischemia. Ischemia, by definition, is a compromise of the vascular supply that is inadequate to provide sufficient tissue oxygenation and results in lessened flap viability. Flap ischemia may be caused by multiple factors, including poor flap design, infection, venous congestion, excess tension, or underlying vascular disorders.[33,34] Ischemia may lead to tissue compromise due to hypoxia, complicated by dehiscence, infection, free radical production, and ultimately flap necrosis.[35–39] Smoking greatly increases the risk of flap ischemia. Thus, patients are encouraged to stop smoking two weeks before and two weeks after flap surgery.

Active bleeding at a flap's distal margin during surgery is typically a good sign of tissue perfusion.[40–42] However, perfusion cannot be correlated with adequate tissue oxygenation.[43] Tissue requirements and hemoglobin saturation change in response to trauma, the presence of free radicals, acidosis, and thromboxane A$_2$.[44–46] In the first 48 hours after surgery, there is a surge in local catecholamine release and vasoconstricting mediators in the inflammatory cascade, resulting in local vasoconstriction and edema. These factors all contribute to ischemia or direct injury to the flap. In addition, temperature, wound tension, bleeding, and atherosclerosis all affect oxygen transport within the tissue. Flaps that are shorter, with an abundant blood supply, usually do well. In the face, there are multiple large subcutaneous vessels allowing for longer flaps, such that widening a flap in proportion to the length is not necessary. The capillary perfusion pressure at the distal tip is critical, driven by the subcutaneous vessels in random facial flaps.[47–49] A delay procedure has been shown to increase flap vascularity and, as a result, flap length and viability. Baker et al. have described increased flap survival lengths through use of tissue expanders even greater than the increase in survival length seen with the delay technique.[50]

Previously irradiated skin may have a compromised blood supply, with increased fragility and propensity for injury. Skin irritation and breakdown are not uncommon following radiation. The damage in pattern of blood flow and soft-tissue architecture due to radiation radically changes the prospects for flap survival. Scarring from prior radiation and increased fibrous tissue

lead to impaired wound healing and an increased risk of scar contracture.[51] An area of irradiated skin that may have marked damage to the subdermal plexus due to obliterative endarteritis should not be used to reconstruct a soft-tissue defect.[52,53]

The most common and most avoidable causes of ischemic flap failure in healthy nonsmoking patients are technical errors in design and poor surgical techniques, including insufficient undermining, improper distribution of wound tension, torsion on the proximal pedicle and tension at the distal wound margin. In general, one should avoid tension at the site of the defect and more leeway should be used at the donor site where one is encountering healthy, well-vascularized tissue. The ability to recognize that a flap is undergoing clinically significant ischemia requires astute observation and an experienced surgeon. Ominous signs include lack of bleeding at the edges, edema, venous congestion, and a delayed capillary refill with digital compression. When a flap loses perfusion for a prolonged period, hypoxia leads to incremental loss of the underlying dermis as well as the epidermis. Epidermolysis results from early ischemia, where the epithelium desiccates and sloughs as the underlying tissue re-epithelializes (**Fig. 5.2A,B**). Local wound care is sufficient in treating epidermolysis, and the wound tends to heal without significant scarring. However, entirely necrotic tissue that is clinically demarcated should be debrided to promote re-epithelialization and minimize the potential for excessive scar formation (**Fig. 5.3A,B**). Healing by secondary intention can lead to a cosmetically acceptable outcome in areas such as the temple, forehead and concave surfaces of the face, allowing for a less aggressive approach if the reconstruction falters and debridement is necessary. Areas more susceptible to wound contraction, deformity, and functional impairment, such as the nasal ala, eyelid margin, or oral commissure, should be closed using a new flap or a skin graft soon after debridement.[54–57] Cosmetic deformities alone can be addressed in a delayed fashion if no functional impairment is inevitable.

Postoperatively, the surgeon should employ measures to reduce edema, such as ice pack application, bed rest with head elevation, no strenuous activity, and at times systemic steroids to reduce the risk of flap necrosis. Davis et al. have described the application of topical oxygen free radical scavengers (and combinations of these) in random pattern skin flaps with statistically significant success in reducing the rates of flap ischemia.[58] Oral agents have been a standard therapy although topical agents confer the benefit of a better side effect profile due to decreased systemic absorption. Medicinal leech therapy for flaps with venous congestion can result in salvage of an ischemic flap. Hyperbaric oxygen is an important option in preventing full-thickness tissue necrosis and has proven to decrease edema in healthy tissue by inducing vasoconstriction and stimulating

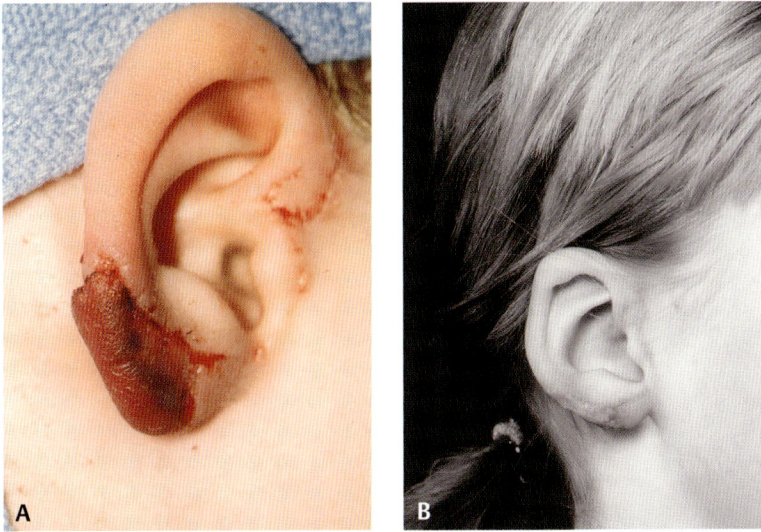

Fig. 5.2 (A) Patient one week after dog bite injury with nearly complete earlobe avulsion. Note the epidermolysis (dark purple) in the photograph. **(B)** One month later, the wound has healed without significant tissue loss.

capillary ingrowth as well as decreasing tissue hypoxia. Hyperbaric oxygen itself has associated risks, such as barotrauma, pneumothorax, increased risk of cataract formation, and seizures.

Infection

Postoperative wound infections, manifest by local erythema, edema, tenderness and drainage, occur most frequently in contaminated wounds (up to 20%). Clean wounds have a significantly lower incidence of infection (1–4%), and clean-contaminated wounds carry a 8–10% risk of postoperative infection.[59] Prophylaxis is not indicated for clean wounds but may be used in clean-contaminated wounds and should always be used in contaminated wounds (trauma, infected cyst excision). Choice of regimen is guided by knowledge of the probable contaminating flora associated with the operative site.[60] The activity of the chosen agents, therefore, should encompass the pathogens likely to contaminate the wound and the agents should be administered in a dose sufficient to achieve optimal tissue concentration prior to the initial incision.[61] Patients at high risk for wound infection should be treated prophylactically to cover *Staphylococcus aureus* (most common etiology of skin wound infections) and *Streptococcus viridans* (a common pathogen of oral flora). Most commonly, a cephalosporin or penicillin may be used. Amoxicillin with clavulanate or clindamy-

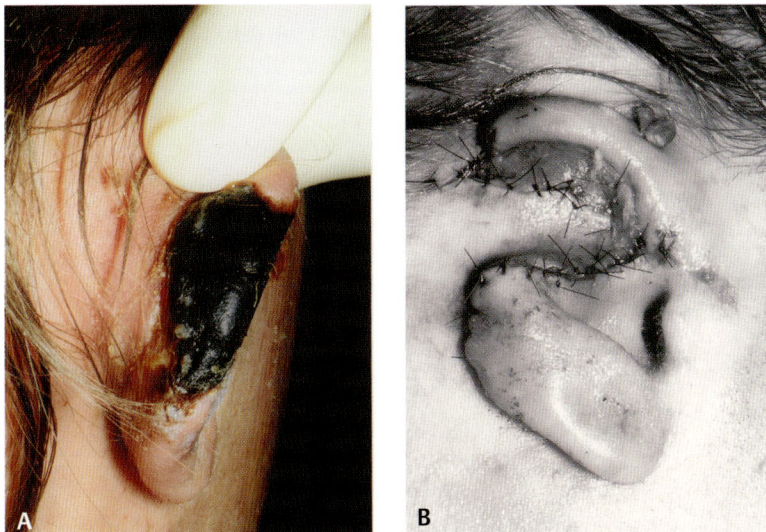

Fig. 5.3 (A) Complete tissue necrosis (black) after reattachment of a full-thickness ear wound. **(B)** The necrotic tissue was debrided and the raw surfaces were covered with a local flap until delayed, definitive reconstruction.

cin (for enhanced anaerobic coverage) is also widely used. *Pseudomonas aeruginosa* must be covered when exposed cartilage or bone near the ear canal is involved. A dated fluoroquinolone, Ciprofloxacin, is still often the drug of choice in these circumstances.[62,63]

Strict adherence to aseptic surgical technique is critical to prevent infection and to avoid compromising local host immune defenses by interfering with blood flow or causing local inflammation. A well-approximated wound, with adequate hemostasis and a minimal amount of devitalized tissue, is more resistant to infection. Excessive manipulation of wound edges, poor tissue handling, and inappropriate suture placement can impair dermal capillary blood flow, leading to ischemia and an increased risk of infection. Other factors associated with an increased risk of infection include prolonged procedures lasting more than 2 hours, complicated operative sites (ulcerated tumor, irradiated lesion, inflamed cyst, reexcision of recent biopsy site), and the presence of drains. Patient profiles, including advanced age, presence of diabetes mellitus, immunocompromise, obesity, or substance abuse, also predispose to infection (**Fig. 5.4**). Areas around the nose, mouth, and ears have a relatively high bacterial count and are similarly prone to infection. Suture materials are foreign bodies that incite a local immune response, thereby increasing infectious risk due to compromising local infection-fighting abili-

ty. The surgeon should use the smallest adequate suture and needle. It has been shown in a mouse model that monofilament sutures are less susceptible to bacterial adherence than braided sutures.

If an infection arises, patients are placed on oral antibiotics. Topical antibiotics are applied to the affected area three to four times a day. If the infection fails to respond to conservative management, flap viability is threatened by the release of proteolytic enzymes that cause local cell death and vascular thrombosis. Ischemia is exacerbated by physical stretch of the wound secondary to abscess formation as well as restricting blood flow (**Fig. 5.4**). Abscesses should be drained, expeditiously cultured, and thoroughly irrigated. Drainage is accomplished by removing some of the distal flap sutures, compressing and exploring the wound. In addition to draining the abscess, relieving the tension on the distal flap will reduce the probability of flap necrosis. The wound can then be packed with gauze and a Penrose drain or wick can be placed until drainage ceases.

Bleeding

Bleeding may be precipitated by uncontrolled hypertension, an occult drug, or congenital coagulopathy contributing to difficult hemostasis.[64,65] Bleeding during surgery should be meticulously controlled using electrocautery. It has been shown that bipolar cautery causes less tissue damage due to less thermal energy release than seen with monopolar cautery. Excessive cauterization can lead to alopecia in hair-bearing areas and increased scar formation. It will also cause the margins of the flap to be more conspicuous and less attractive cosmetically.

If a wound has persistent oozing at the time of surgery, fibrin glue can be sprayed in a thin coat, and the flap held in place over the wound for a few minutes. The fibrin glue promotes clotting and will incite flap adherence to the underlying tissue bed. Pressure dressings and drains (rubber band or Penrose) can help minimize the risks of hematoma or seroma formation, but care must be taken not to cause ischemia with their placement. A closed suction drain may be necessary in large defects. A hematoma can cause increased tension on the wound closure, potentially resulting in ischemia, dehiscence, infection and circulatory compromise. Hematomas should be expeditiously evacuated by either needle aspiration or by creating an opening at the distal wound margin and performing manual compression and lavage. Irrigation should be continued until all residual clots are removed. Packing the wound or closing with a few interrupted sutures at the distal margin should be done only after adequate hemostasis has been achieved and should not apply excess tension at the wound edges. Medications associated with increased bleeding times including aspirin, NSAIDs, and herbal remedies (vitamin E, garlic, feverfew) and should be discontinued 7–10

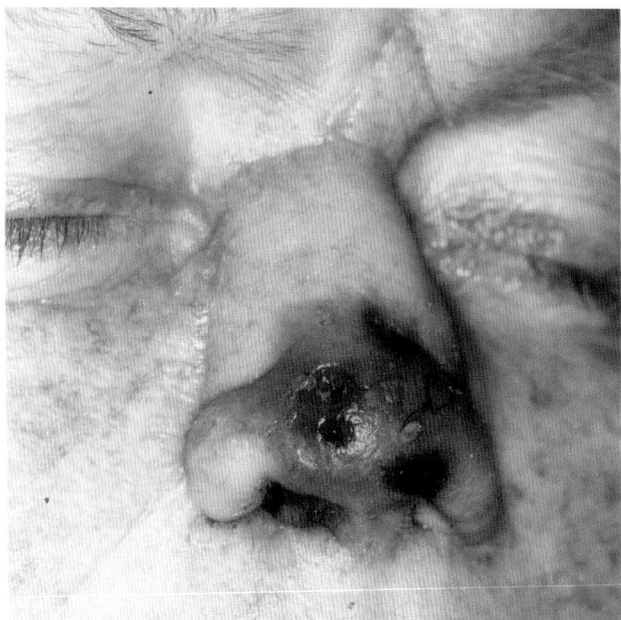

Fig. 5.4 Infected cartilage grafts with fistula formation and tissue necrosis in a diabetic patient who underwent forehead flap nasal reconstruction a month prior to the infection. The wound was treated with debridement and healed adequately after intravenous antibiotics and wound care.

days prior to surgery and for at least 7 days postoperatively. As a precautionary measure, patients should be provided preoperatively with a list of contraindicated medications and detailed wound care instructions.

Dehiscence

Dehiscence results when a wound fails to heal in apposition. In the first week after surgery, the healing wound has only 3–5% of its original tensile strength. Although re-epithelialization occurs rapidly (within 24–48 hours), subsequent collagen deposition is delayed until approximately day five. Collagen remodeling increases the tensile strength of the wound over several months. Wound dehiscence can be due to systemic factors, such as age older than 65, hypoalbuminemia, obesity, malignancy, hypertension, Cushing's disease, thyroid disease, liver disease, history of radiation therapy to the site, and congestive heart failure (CHF). Additionally, the use of tobacco, anticoagulants, systemic corticosteroids, and cytotoxic chemotherapeutics have an adverse effect on wound healing, thereby predisposing a patient to wound dehiscence. Prevention of wound dehiscence is best achieved by good surgical technique. Buried absorbable sutures should provide adequate tensile strength and last long enough to prevent dehiscence. In choosing suture material, the practitioner should take into account the tensile strength retention properties of the material used. Anti-tension taping (e.g., Steri-strips) and a bulky dressing provide wound immobilization and some protection for the area. If wound dehiscence occurs due to premature suture removal or trauma without evidence of infection, the wound can be resutured immediately after debriding devitalized tissue. In cases of delayed hematoma or infection, the wound is best treated by allowing it to heal by secondary intention. Scar revision can then be planned after adequate healing has occurred, usually no sooner than eight weeks.

Scar Contracture, Hypertrophic Scars, and Keloids

Hypertrophic scars (HTS) and keloids represent a pathologic response to tissue injury. By definition, a hypertrophic scar is a fibrous tissue outgrowth with excessive scarring that remains within the confines of the wound.[66,67] A keloid is characterized by its ability to extend outside the boundaries of the original lesion. Scar contracture results when a contractile wound-healing process occurs in a scar that has already re-epithelialized and satisfactorily healed. Each of these processes can cause cosmetic disfigurement and functional disability (**Fig. 5.5**). Management of these physiologically distinct processes differs because of their different patterns of evolution. Therefore, the surgeon must differentiate among these categories, as they require different treatments. Although the exact mechanism for

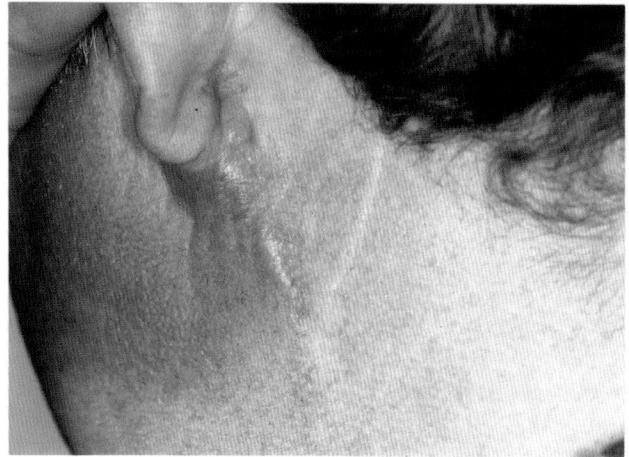

Fig. 5.5 Hypertrophic scar at the earlobe cheek junction.

the formation of HTS and keloids is poorly understood, the common belief is that trauma is the precipitating event. Furthermore, mechanical tension and strain on wound edges is one of the most important factors linked to the formation of HTS and keloids.[66,67] This has been confirmed by the fact that wounds at right angles in relaxed skin tension lines develop HTS and keloids at an increased rate. It is therefore crucial to design flaps for facial defects in a way that minimizes tension and positions incisions in RSTLs parallel or as near parallel to them as possible. The majority of these abnormalities are asymptomatic, although pruritus is the most common associated symptom and is hypothesized to be due to increased mast cells and increased histamine levels.

As mentioned previously, the best way to avoid complications is meticulous preoperative planning and sound surgical technique. In known keloid-formers, the incisions should be as short as possible, and the wounds closed with monofilament deep sutures, using either running intracuticular suturing technique or tissue glue. However, even under the best of circumstances, HTS and keloids still occur. Surgical revision generally yields a positive outcome when performed after the initial wound healing phase is completed, but it does not guarantee that there will not be a recurrence. Following revision, is it important to use pressure and range of motion exercises to prevent contractures from recurring. Management of HTS and keloids has included intralesional steroid injections, surgical removal, silicone sheeting, silicone gel, and nonsilicone occlusive dressings. The 585-nm pulsed dye laser has also shown variable results in reducing symptoms and improving appearance.[68] Other treatments that have been used are topical retinoids, cryosurgery, interferon α2b, and low-dose ionizing radiation.

Site-Specific Complications

Site-specific complications include ectropion of the lower eyelid with scleral show, causing an inability to close the eyes fully. Contributing factors include excessive vertical tension on the lower eyelid, lid laxity, injury to the orbicularis oculi muscle, nerve injury, or (most commonly) poor surgical technique. If upward massage of the eyelid fails to improve eyelid function over several weeks, surgical repair is indicated. Eclabium is a similar condition of the perioral area, causing eversion of the lip. Alar retraction is a similar condition of the alar rim of the nose (**Fig. 5.1**). Retraction of the ala is best prevented by placing a cartilage graft at the planned alar margin and placing the flap over the structural graft support. If these measures fail, revision surgery may be necessary.

The ear, a complex anatomic structure, is also susceptible to unique postoperative complications. Inflammation of the cartilage, including perichondritis, can progress to chondronecrosis and external auditory canal stenosis or external ear deformity. Infection is the most common cause and should always be aggressively treated with systemic antibiotics with *Pseudomonas* coverage. External canal stenosis lends itself to immediate reconstruction.

Other Complications

Milia are tiny epidermal inclusion cysts that can appear in the suture line after excisional surgery. They are caused by epidermal implantation into the dermis. Treatment consists of extraction and exfoliation of the skin with a hydroxyl acids or other means.

Telangiectasias also commonly appear around the suture lines in a wound with excess tension. Many will spontaneously resolve if the patient is counseled to avoid exposure to sunlight. If treatment is desired, the 532-nm potassium titanyl phosphate laser, the 532-nm diode copper vapor laser, and the 585-nm pulsed dye laser all have comparable efficacy, but the copper vapor laser is more acceptable to patients (it does not produce purpura). Intense pulsed light (IPL) also reduces telangiectasias, as does platinum-tipped electrocautery ablation of the vessels themselves.

Depressed scars and pincushioning are additional wound-specific problems that can be avoided with proper surgical technique. Depressed scars result from the spreading and inversion of the scar as the wound heals. The surgeon must make sure to undermine the recipient site, so that the flap and the recipient site can be closed with proper wound edge eversion. Additionally, the surgeon must make sure to decrease tension on the wound with deep sutures and well-designed flaps, so that the wound does not widen and flatten to a depression as healing takes place. Pincushioning is caused by persistent edema, usually at the distal portion of the flap. Edema is trapped in the dependant portion of the flap, causing the flap margins to contract and elevate the soft tissue as the wound heals.[66,69,70] The characteristic raised defect is called a trap door deformity (**Fig. 5.6**). To avoid trap door deformity, the surgeon should make sure the flap is the correct thickness and size to fill the recipient site. If the flap is too large or too thick, it should be trimmed before inset. If pincushioning occurs, it is best treated with an intralesional steroid injection and the use of silicone products, like the methods for treating keloids and hypertrophic scars. If persistent trap door deformity occurs, revision surgery may be necessary in a year or later.

◆ Conclusion

Facial defects represent a challenge that requires a high level of expertise and familiarity with the complex anatomy of the region. Locoregional flap reconstruction commonly affords the patient a good cosmetic and functional outcome. Attention to detail in the workup and preoperative planning, as well as during the procedure itself, will prevent most complications. Factors outside of the surgeon's control must be taken into account, including the aggressiveness of the underlying disease, prior irradiation, and the nutritional and immune status of the patient. When postoperative problems, such as ischemia and hematoma, are anticipated and receive the available interventions, it will help patients return to an optimal quality of life.

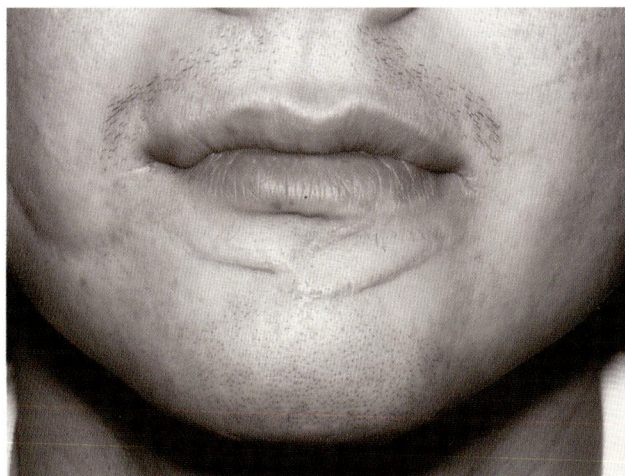

Fig. 5.6 Trap door deformity of the chin and depressed scar of the cheek in a patient with a traumatic wound repaired in the emergency room.

References

1. Zitelli J. Wound healing for the clinician. Adv Dermatol 1987;2:243–267

2. Daniel RK. The anatomic and hemodynamic characteristics of the cutaneous circulation and their influence on skin flap design. In: Grabb WC and Myers MB, eds., Skin Flaps. Boston: Little, Brown & Company; 1975:111–134

3. Daniel RK. Letter: Toward an anatomical and hemodynamic classification of skin flaps. Plast Reconstr Surg 1975;56(3): 330–332

4. Daniel RK, Williams HB. The free transfer of skin flaps by microvascular anastomoses. An experimental study and a reappraisal. Plast Reconstr Surg 1973;52(1):16–31

5. Pearl RM, Johnson D. The vascular supply to the skin: an anatomical and physiological reappraisal—Part II. Ann Plast Surg 1983;11(3):196–205

6. Milton SH. Pedicled skin-flaps: the fallacy of the length: width ratio. Br J Surg 1970;57(7):502–508

7. Borges AF. Elective Incisions and Scar Revision. Boston: Little, Brown, & Company; 1973

8. Borges AF, Alexander JE. Relaxed skin tension lines, Z-plasties on scars, and fusiform excision of lesions. Br J Plast Surg 1962;15:242–254

9. Burget GC, Menick FJ. The subunit principle in nasal reconstruction. Plast Reconstr Surg 1985;76(2):239–247

10. Menick FJ. Aesthetic refinements in use of forehead for nasal reconstruction: the paramedian forehead flap. Clin Plast Surg 1990;17(4):607–622

11. Burgess LP, Morin GV, Rand M, Vossoughi J, Hollinger JO. Wound healing. Relationship of wound closing tension to scar width in rats. Arch Otolaryngol Head Neck Surg 1990;116(7): 798–802

12. Gassner HG, Sherris DA. Chemoimmobilization: improving predictability in the treatment of facial scars. Plast Reconstr Surg 2003;112(5):1464–1466

13. Gassner HG, Sherris DA, Otley CC. Treatment of facial wounds with botulinum toxin A improves cosmetic outcome in primates. Plast Reconstr Surg 2000;105(6):1948–1953, discussion 1954–1955

14. Sherris DA, Gassner HG. Botulinum toxin to minimize facial scarring. Facial Plast Surg 2002;18(1):35–39

15. Gassner HG, Brissett AE, Otley CC, et al. Botulinum toxin to improve facial wound healing: A prospective, blinded, placebo-controlled study. Mayo Clin Proc 2006;81(8): 1023–1028

16. Grabb WC, Myers MB. Skin Flaps. Boston: Little, Brown & Company; 1975

17. Becker FF. Facial Reconstruction with Local and Regional Flaps. New York: Thieme-Stratton; 1985

18. Jackson IT. Local Flaps in Head and Neck Reconstruction. St. Louis: Mosby Year Book; 1985

19. Stauch B, Vasconez LO, Hall-Findlay EJ, eds. Grabb's Encyclopedia of Flaps. Boston: Little, Brown, & Company; 1990

20. Thomas JR, Holt GR, Eds. Facial Scars: Incision, Revision and Camouflage. St. Louis: Mosby Year Book; 1989

21. Tromovitch TA, Stegman S, Glogau RG. Flaps and Grafts in Dermatologic Surgery. St. Louis: Mosby Year Book; 1989:74

22. Dzubow LM. Facial Flaps: Biomechanics and Regional Application. Norwalk, CT: Appleton and Lange; 1990

23. Loeb R. Technique for preservation of the temporal branches of the facial nerve during face-lift operations. Br J Plast Surg 1970;23(4):390–394

24. Robbins TH. The protection of the frontal branch of the facial nerve in face-lift surgery. Br J Plast Surg 1981;34(1): 95–96

25. Bernstein L, Nelson RH. Surgical anatomy of the extraparotid distribution of the facial nerve. Arch Otolaryngol 1984;110(3):177–183

26. Herbert DC, DeGeus J. Nasolabial subcutaneous pedicle flaps. Br J Plast Surg 1964;28:63

27. Conley JJ, Price JC. The midline vertical forehead flap. Otolaryngol Head Neck Surg 1981;89(1):38–44

28. Conley JJ, Donovan DT. A new technique for total reconstruction of the lower lip in a patient with malignant melanoma. Otolaryngol Head Neck Surg 1986;94(3):393–397

29. Thomas JR, Griner N, Cook TA. The precise midline forehead flap as a musculocutaneous flap. Arch Otolaryngol Head Neck Surg 1988;114(1):79–84

30. Ohtsuka H. Nasolabial skin flaps to the cheek. In: Strauch B, Vasconez LO, Hall-Findlay EJ, eds. Grabb's Encyclopedia of Flaps. Boston: Little, Brown, & Company, 1990, pp 348–351.

31. Burget GC. The axial paramedian forehead flap. In: Strauch B, Vasconez LO, Hall-Findlay EJ, eds. Grabb's Encyclopedia of Flaps. Boston: Little, Brown, & Company; 1990:204–215

32. Cormack GC, Lamberty BGH. The Arterial Anatomy of Skin Flaps. New York: Churchill Livingstone; 1986:113–130

33. Larrabee WF Jr, Holloway GA Jr, Sutton D. Wound tension and blood flow in skin flaps. Ann Otol Rhinol Laryngol 1984;93(2 Pt 1):112–115

34. Myers MB, Combs B, Cohen G. Wound tension and wound sloughs—A negative correlation. Am J Surg 1965;109: 711–714

35. Angel MF, Narayanan K, Swartz WM, et al. The etiologic role of free radicals in hematoma-induced flap necrosis. Plast Reconstr Surg 1986;77(5):795–803

36. Angel MF, Mellow CG, Knight KR, O'Brien BM. The effect of deferoxamine on tolerance to secondary ischaemia caused by venous obstruction. Br J Plast Surg 1989;42(4):422–424

37. Knight KR, MacPhadyen K, Lepore DA, Kuwata N, Eadie PA, O'Brien BM. Enhancement of ischaemic rabbit skin flap survival with the antioxidant and free-radical scavenger N-acetylcysteine. Clin Sci (Lond) 1991;81(1):31–36

38. Knight KR, Angel MF, Lepore DA, et al. Secondary ischaemia in rabbit skin flaps: the roles played by thromboxane and free radicals. Clin Sci (Lond) 1991;80(3):235–240

39. Knight KR, Mellow CG, Abbey PA, et al. Interaction between thromboxane and free radical mechanisms in experimental ischaemic rabbit skin flaps. Res Exp Med (Berl) 1990;190(6):423–433

40. Mosely LH, Finseth F, Goody M. Nicotine and its effect on wound healing. Plast Reconstr Surg 1978;61(4):570–575

41. Reus WF, Robson MC, Zachary L, Heggers JP. Acute effects of tobacco smoking on blood flow in the cutaneous micro-circulation. Br J Plast Surg 1984;37(2):213–215

42. Webster RC, Kazda G, Hamdan US, Fuleihan NS, Smith RC. Cigarette smoking and face lift: conservative versus wide undermining. Plast Reconstr Surg 1986;77(4):596–604

43. Reinisch JF. The role of arteriovenous anastomoses in skin flaps. In: Grabb WC, Meyers MB, eds. Skin Flaps. Boston: Little, Brown & Company; 1975:81–92

44. Angel MF, Ramasastry SS, Swartz WM, Basford RE, Futrell JW. Free radicals: basic concepts concerning their chemistry, pathophysiology, and relevance to plastic surgery. Plast Reconstr Surg 1987;79(6):990–997

45. Angel MF, Haddad JJ Jr, Abramson M. A free radical scavenger reduces hematoma-induced flap necrosis in Fischer rats. Otolaryngol Head Neck Surg 1987;96(1):96–98

46. Angel MF, Ramasastry SS, Swartz WM, et al. The critical relationship between free radicals and degrees of ischemia: evidence for tissue intolerance of marginal perfusion. Plast Reconstr Surg 1988;81(2):233–239

47. McFarlane RM, Heagy FC, Radin S, Aust JC, Wermuth RE. A study of the delay phenomenon in experimental pedicle flaps. Plast Reconstr Surg 1965;35:245–262

48. Meyer MB, Cherry G. Augmentation of tissue survival by delay: An experimental study in rabbits. Plast Reconstr Surg 1969;39:397–401

49. Cherry GW, Austad E, Pasyk K, McClatchey K, Rohrich RJ. Increased survival and vascularity of random-pattern skin flaps elevated in controlled, expanded skin. Plast Reconstr Surg 1983;72(5):680–687

50. Baker SR. Fundamentals of expanded tissue. Head Neck 1991;13(4):327–333

51. Miller SH, Rudolph R. Healing in the irradiated wound. Clin Plast Surg 1990;17(3):503–508

52. Stearner SP, Sanderson MH. Mechanisms of acute injury in the gamma-irradiated chicken: effects of a protracted or a split-dose exposure on the fine structure of the microvasculature. Radiat Res 1972;49(2):328–350

53. Patterson TJS, Berry RJ, Hopewell JW, et al. The effect of x-radiation on the survival of experimental skin flaps. In: Grabb WC, Myers MB, eds. Skin Flaps. Boston: Little, Brown, & Company; 1975:39

54. Tromovitch TA, Stegman S, Glogau RG. Flaps and Grafts in Dermatologic Surgery. St. Louis: Mosby Year Book; 1989:74

55. Zitelli JA. Secondary intention healing: an alternative to surgical repair. Clin Dermatol 1984;2(3):92–106

56. Burget GC. Aesthetic restoration of the nose. Clin Plast Surg 1985;12(3):463–480

57. Becker GD, Adams LA, Levin BC. Nonsurgical repair of perinasal skin defects. Plast Reconstr Surg 1991;88(5):768–776, discussion 777–778

58. Davis RE, Wachholz JH, Jassir D, Perlyn CA, Agrama MH. Comparison of topical anti-ischemic agents in the salvage of failing random-pattern skin flaps in rats. Arch Facial Plast Surg 1999;1(1):27–32

59. Fairbanks DF. Antimicrobial Therapy in Otolaryngology—Head and Neck Surgery. Alexandria, VA: American Academy of Otolaryngology—Head and Neck Surgery; 1991

60. Sebben JE. Prophylactic antibiotics in cutaneous surgery. J Dermatol Surg Oncol 1985;11(9):901–906

61. Burke JF. The effective period of preventive antibiotic action in experimental incisions and dermal lesions. Surgery 1961;50:161–168

62. DiPiro JT, Record KE, Schanzenbach KS, Bivins BA. Antimicrobial prophylaxis in surgery: Part 1. Am J Hosp Pharm 1981;38(3):320–334

63. Simmons BP. Guideline for the prevention of surgical wound infections. Infect Control 1982;2:188–196

64. Fisher HW. Surgery on patients receiving anticoagulants. J Dermatol Surg Oncol 1977;3(2):210–212

65. Hicks PD Jr, Stromberg BV. Hemostasis in plastic surgical patients. Clin Plast Surg 1985;12(1):17–23

66. Sherris DA, Larrabee WF Jr, Murakami CS. Management of scar contractures, hypertrophic scars, and keloids. Otolaryngol Clin North Am 1995;28(5):1057–1068

67. Brissett AE, Sherris DA. Scar contractures, hypertrophic scars, and keloids. Facial Plast Surg 2001;17(4):263–272

68. Paquet P, Hermanns JF, Piérard GE. Effect of the 585 nm flash-lamp-pumped pulsed dye laser for the treatment of keloids. Dermatol Surg 2001;27(2):171–174

69. Webster RC, Benjamin BJ, Smith RC. Treatment of "trap door deformity." Laryngoscope 1978;88(4):707–712

70. Holt GR. Treatment of the trapdoor scars. In: Thomas JR, Holt GR, eds. Facial Scars: Incisions, Revision and Camouflage. St. Louis: Mosby Year Book; 1989:271

6

Challenges in Skin Resurfacing

Gary D. Monheit and Randolph B. Capone

Contemporary skin resurfacing procedures—chemoexfoliation, laser resurfacing, and dermabrasion—have been in continual evolution since their inception over 65 years ago and in general represent safe and efficacious techniques for the rejuvenation of aging skin. Like all surgical procedures, resurfacing has associated complications (**Table 6.1**). Most complications, however, are avoidable if the physician thoroughly understands this family of treatments, including the pharmacokinetics of different wounding agents on various skin types, the histology of depth wounding, normal wound healing, and laser physics. Each modality has a particular mechanism to injure skin and the physician must know how an agent or technique can be used to produce the favorable results desired.

By convention, resurfacing procedures are divided by depth of injury into superficial, medium, and deep. The depth of wounding determines the level of destruction and thus the degree of rejuvenation, as well as length of time for wound healing and risk of complications. While superficial wounding will heal within 24 to 48 hours with little risk of problems, medium and deep resurfacing may take considerably longer, and can produce many of the complications to be discussed. In general, resurfacing below the mid-reticular dermis causes destructive necrosis and scarring and should not be performed. Much has been published regarding resurfacing and is available in the literature for physicians to develop a better understanding of its principles and procedures.[1,2] When resurfacing devices or peel solutions are overused, inappropriately used, or mismatched with a skin type, unintended injuries and complications may occur.[3] Such injuries are the focus of this chapter.

◆ Timing of Adverse Events

Resurfacing complications can be divided by the timing of their occurrence. Intraoperative problems inadvertently occur during the procedure, and for dermabrasion, an example would be overly aggressive use of the mechanical abrader, creating a wound too deep to heal without a scar. There are documented cases of the wire-brush dermabrader piercing through skin or ripping a lip or eyelid due to lack of surgical control or sudden movement of the patient. One must also be careful not to overuse a freezing agent, which can cause a freeze-burn injury that will create textural scarring or pigmentary alteration.

Intraoperative laser complications include laser-induced fires and laser energy deposition outside the operative field. Proper laser safety precautions should always be mandated, such as keeping wet towel drapes around the operative field and keeping O_2 sources and combustible products out of range. The surgeon must give the procedure his full attention so that there are not unwanted laser impacts. Laser-impermeable scleral shields should be used for all facial CO_2 or erbium resurfacing cases, especially when performed around the periorbital area. Chemical peel solutions—whether TCA or phenol—are caustic and can cause significant problems if they are inadvertently dripped into the eye or sensitive cutaneous surfaces. The surgeon should per-

Table 6.1

Complications Seen with All Types of Resurfacing
Dyspigmentation
Scarring
Infection
Prolonged erythema or pruritus
Contact dermatitis
Textural changes
Milia
Acne
Cold sensitivity
Worsened doctor-patient relationship

sonally check the acid and strength before applying and never pass the application over the patient's central face or eyes. Accidents of this sort have resulted in disastrous corneal damage and cutaneous scars. Over all, however, scarring after all resurfacing procedures—chemical peeling, laser resurfacing, and dermabrasion—has a reported incidence of less than 1%.

Once a resurfacing procedure is completed, the recovery and regrowth of new skin should occur in a controlled environment in which noxious external factors—trauma, allergy, and infection—should be minimized to prevent serious complications. The final common pathway for a resurfacing complication is scarring. This dreaded result can be avoided by careful observation and follow-up during the recovery period, as well as early intervention to reguide the skin to normal healing.[4]

◆ Patient Expectations Associated with Resurfacing

The most common risk of skin resurfacing is patient dissatisfaction with the procedure. While it is not a complication in the strictest of terms, many authors view this undesirable outcome as such. This can be avoided by carefully analyzing the patient's perceived problem and deciding how to realistically treat it with a particular type of procedure.[5] It is best to give a patient a mirror and allow them to show you the specific problem that bothers them. Their concern may be fine wrinkles, abnormal color, or inappropriate texture (all effectively treated with erbium laser or medium-depth chemical peeling), or volume defects that require fillers rather than resurfacing. The physician must address the procedure most applicable to achieve the results desired. Repetitive light chemical peels or microdermabrasion can correct pigmentary change but not significant rhytids, which may require a deeper resurfacing procedure. One must then look at patient-specific risks for particular complications, such as hypo- or hyperpigmentation, or the potential for scarring in previously irradiated skin or in the penumbra of a course of isotretinoin.[6]

It is also important for the physician to distinguish a true complication from an expected side effect of resurfacing and educate the patient appropriately. For example, most ablative resurfacing procedures have expected side effects of transient erythema, flushing, increased skin temperature, pruritus, edema, milia formation, and acne. These are consequences of the new skin formation and should be addressed (as with patient expectations) before the procedure so their appearance will not alarm the patient. Patient reassurance is usually all that is necessary since these problems will resolve spontaneously. Overtreatment of these side effects alone can lead to overtreatment complications.

◆ Chemoexfoliation: The Workhorse of Resurfacing Procedures

The most common resurfacing procedure performed under the direction of a physician is chemical peeling. Generally, light chemical peels have fewer complications than any of the others. These peels are "lunch time" procedures designed to exfoliate the upper epidermis with minimal dermal inflammation. Healing is usually uncomplicated, occurring in 1 to 3 days. Untoward problems can occur with overcoating low-dose trichloracetic acid (TCA), leaving glycolic acid in place for prolonged periods without proper neutralization, or over-aggressive degreasing of the skin prior to the peel.[7] These can result in edema, prolonged erythema, excessive pain, prolonged exfoliation, and delayed healing. Hyperpigmentation and scarring can occur. Practitioners should be especially concerned with sensitive-skinned patients, such as those with atopy, or patients using regular exfoliating programs or retinoids or other skin-care programs that may thin the stratum corneum. Most of these problems are reversible with skin protection, bland emollients and appropriate treatment, such as topical corticosteroids and bleaching agents. In well-trained hands, unmet expectation is the prime risk associated with light chemical peels.

If medium or deep resurfacing is chosen as the procedure to solve a patient's skin problem, the physician must discuss the patient's expected down time, temporary side effects such as erythema, pruritus, and skin sensitivity, as well as care instructions for for 7–14 days of healing. Doing so will likely yield a favorable result with a happy patient. Not doing so can produce complications—reversible or irreversible—and an unhappy patient. Medium and deep resurfacing create full-thickness destruction of the epidermis along with partial necrosis and inflammation of varying levels of dermis. With medium depth chemical peeling, aggressive overcoating with 35% of TCA or combination TCA peels can drive a medium peel into a much deeper destructive procedure and potentially cause scarring (**Fig. 6.1**).[7] The most common complication, though, is hyperpigmentation, which can last up to 3 months, depending on skin type and postoperative care. Medium and deep chemical peels along with deep resurfacing procedures, such as CO_2 resurfacing or dermabrasion, must be considered more serious surgical procedures and deserve the appropriate preoperative consultation and informed consent with a thorough understanding of the postoperative care and sequelae.

◆ Dyspigmentation

Alterations in pigmentation after resurfacing procedures can be either desirable or constitute a complication. Desirable pigmentary changes include lightening

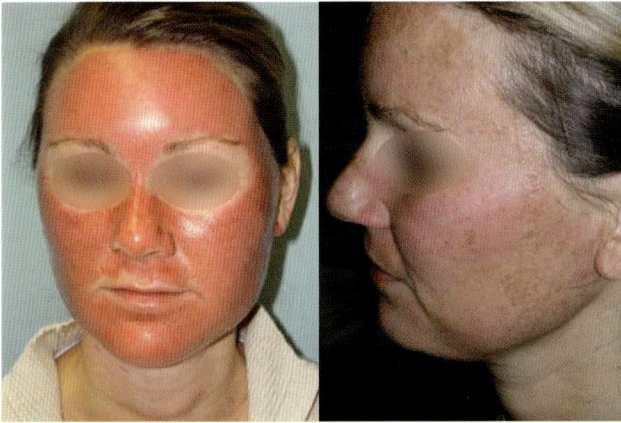

Fig. 6.1 Excess skin wounding from overcoating with Jessner's solution.

Table 6.2

Common Photosensitizing Medications

Antibiotics

- fluoroquinolones (ciprofloxacin, levofloxacin, gatifloxacin)

- tetracyclines (tetracycline, doxycycline, minocycline)

- sulfonamides (sulfamethoxazole, trimethoprim, cotrimoxazole)

Antihistamines

- diphenhydramine

Antimalarials

- quinine

- chloroquine

- hydroxychloroquine

Chemotherapeutic agents

- 5-fluorouracil

- vinblastine

- dacarbazine

Cardiac agents

- amiodarone

- nifedipine

- quinidine

- diltiazem

Diuretics

- furosemide

- hydrochlorothiazide

Diabetic agents

- sulfonylureas (chlorpropamide, glyburide)

Analgesics

- nonsteroidal anti-inflammatory drugs (naproxen, piroxicam)

Skin medications

- 5-aminolevulinic acid (Levulan, DUSA Pharmaceuticals, Wilmington MA)

Acne medications

- isotretinoin (Accutane, Hoffman-LaRoche, Palo Alto CA)

Antipsoriatic agents

- acitretin (Soriatane, GlaxoSmithKline)

Psychiatric drugs

- phenothiazines (chlorpromazine)

- tricyclic antidepressants (desipramine, imipramine)

uneven dyschromias or correcting conditions such as melasma or age-related hyperpigmentation. Unintended pigmentation changes, such as streaks or irregular lines of demarcation, can occur from uneven degreasing, inhomogeneous chemical application, or inappropriate choice of wounding agent. TCA 50%, for example, has fallen out of favor as a resurfacing treatment because of its increased complication profile, including dyspigmentation and scarring. Post-peel pigmentary inhomogeneity typically occurs around the eyes, mouth, or jawline margin adjacent to the untreated neck. Such irregularities are not specific to chemical resurfacing, but also occur as a result of uneven laser resurfacing or dermabrasion. With all modalities of resurfacing, care must be taken to ensure an even and homogeneous treatment.

Dyspigmentation can occur after any depth chemical peel, but deeper peel procedures harbor risk of greater problems. In general, patients with light complexions (Fitzpatrick skin types I–II) have lower risks for this complication, while Fitzpatrick IV–VI skin must be approached with caution due to the elevated risk of hyperpigmentation. Patients taking photosensitizing drugs or hormone replacement therapy (estrogen) are also at greater risk for pigmentary complications from resurfacing procedures (**Table 6.2**), and therefore it is unwise to proceed until these medications have been stopped completely and the risk profile has decreased sufficiently (12 months after Accutane, for example).

Reactive dyschromia (postinflammatory hyperpigmentation, PIH) occurs by postoperative weeks 3 or 4, but may appear earlier. PIH usually responds to topical therapy (**Table 6.3**) and is therefore viewed as a less troublesome complication than hypopigmentation. PIH is more common after superficial and medium-depth peels, whereas hypopigmentation typically is a risk after deep peels (e.g., Baker-Gordon) and laser resurfacing. PIH is often initiated by minimal sun exposure during the erythematic phase of healing, and broad spectrum sunscreen protection and/or sun avoidance is imperative after resurfacing procedures for 3–6 months. Fortunately, PIH usually responds well to lightening agents, tretinoin, and corticosteroids as outlined above.[8] Treatment for hyperpigmentation should begin in susceptible skin types directly after re-epithelialization is complete and continue for 4 to 6 weeks. It is also helpful to pretreat susceptible skin types IV to VI with hydroquinone 6 to 8 weeks prior to peeling as a preventive measure. Skin lightening agents are then resumed after re-epithelialization.

It should be emphasized that factors promoting hyperpigmentation after resurfacing procedures include birth control pills and exogenous estrogens, photosensitizing drugs, steroids, and excessive sun or tanning bed exposure prior to and after peeling (**Fig. 6.2**). If post-peel hyperpigmentation does not respond to topical treatments alone, repeated light chemical peels can be a helpful adjunct. Selective lasers such as Q-switch YAG 532 and intense pulse-light sources can also be helpful in treating resistant post-peel or resurfacing pigmentation or resurfacing pigmentary problems.[9]

Hypopigmentation can be a normal event in resurfacing to a degree. The removal of photodamaged, dyschromic epidermis evens a "muddy complexion" and brightens skin. Thus, in fair-complected skin, a medium depth chemical peel will restore a lighter color, pre-sun damaged complexion. In both superficial- and medium-depth chemoexfoliation, the removal of the epidermis

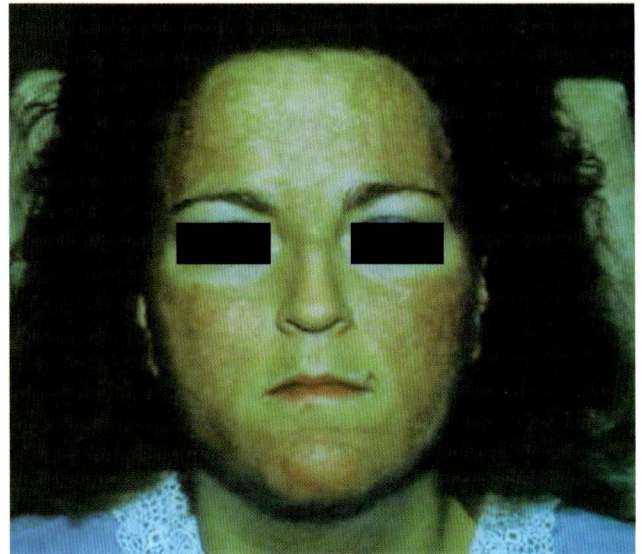

Fig. 6.2 Diffuse facial hyperpigmentation after full face laser resurfacing.

and its melanin will temporarily lighten the skin but color will return as migrating melanocytes from pilosebaceous complexes re-pigment the new skin. This is especially apparent in types IV through VI skin.[10] Therefore, reactive hyperpigmentation is a greater risk in darker skin types than is prolonged hypopigmentation.

Protracted (even permanent) hypopigmentation can be the result of deep peeling or aggressive resurfacing in darker skin types. This is especially true with CO_2 laser and occluded phenol peels which may destroy the reserve of melanocytes in pilosebaceous apparatus needed to resurface the epidermis. A "melanotoxic" effect of the deeply penetrating phenol on melanocytes has been purported, but this perhaps is a direct result of deep-depth injury, since it is also seen after ablative laser resurfacing, overly aggressive dermabrasion or laser hair removal, and deep chemical peeling without phenol. In addition to hypopigmentation, the skin can assume an atrophic or 'plastic' appearance with deep peeling due to destruction of the papillary dermis.[11] Although this was an acceptable side effect of deep phenol peeling in past decades, it is no longer tolerated by patients today and resurfacing at this depth should be avoided.

◆ Scarring

The most feared complication associated with all resurfacing procedures is scarring. Factors that lead to this unfortunate result are myriad and at times additive. Contributing factors are classified as intrinsic, preoperative, or postoperative as outlined in **Table 6.4**. The re-

Table 6.3

Treatment of Postinflammatory Hyperpigmentation (PIH)
1. hydroquinone 4 to 8%—inhibits melanogenesis
2. retinoic acid—enhances pigment exfoliation
3. mild corticosteroids—reduce inflammation
4. non-inflammatory, light chemical peeling:
a. salicylic acid—20%
b. glycolic acid—30 to 40%

Table 6.4

Factors Associated with Scarring after Deep Resurfacing

I. Intrinsic causes

  A. Hereditary skin type

    1. Discoid lupus erythematosus

    2. Scleroderma

    3. Atopic

    4. Ehler-Danlos syndrome

    5. Keloid tendency

  B. Compromised skin healing

    1. Irradiated skin (absence of pilosebaceous apparatus)

    2. Poikilodermatous atrophy

    3. Undermined skin before surgery

    4. Isotretinoin therapy within last six months

    5. Poor health and nutritional status

    6. Active infection or open wounds, excoriations, and inflammatory acne

    7. Inflammation from active skin disease or retinoid dermatitis

II. Operative causes

  A. Overtreatment creating a wound beyond the mid reticular dermis

    1. Repeated overcoating with 25–40% of TCA

    2. Use of 50% or above TCA

    3. Overly aggressive use of phenol

  B. Aggressive treatment of scar-prone areas on the face—forehead, malar prominence, eyelids, jaw line

  C. Aggressive treatment of nonfacial skin, especially neck, chest, shoulders

III. Postoperative causes

  A. Infection

    1. Bacterial—*Staphylococcus*, *Pseudomonas*, *E. coli*

    2. Fungal—*Candida*

    3. Viral—Herpes simplex

  B. Trauma: Irritants, allergens, physical factors that wound skin, and picking or scratching

  C. Idiopathic prolonged wound healing

  D. Idiopathic prolonged erythema

sultant scars themselves can be divided into 3 variants based on extent of wound injury: textural, atrophic/hypopigmented, and contractile. Textural scarring occurs with the ablation of superficial skin structure and is characterized by a "grainy" skin texture (**Fig. 6.3A**). Enlarged pores are also common in textural scarring after resurfacing due to inflammation of the high papillary dermis with widening of the pore exit to the skin surface. Dermal atrophy and hypopigmentation with irregular contours can be seen with wounds extending through the upper/mid-dermis, while contractile (or pulling) scars are seen after full-thickness dermal injuries with deep dermal scarring. Contractile scars create the worst deformities and include such problems as lower eyelid ectropion, lip deformities, and nasal alar distortions (**Fig. 6.3B**).

Early identification and intervention can help prevent scarring complications, and knowledge of the normal timetable of each healing phase is imperative to detect an impaired healing process. Early evidence for the development of scarring can be erythema or pruritus, though these are typical in the fibroplasia phase of wound healing. When they persist for a prolonged time or appear in a particularly aggressive fashion, it should be a red flag to the physician. Prolonged erythema should be treated with mild topical steroids and/or systemic steroids to reduce the inflammation triggering the problem. Pruritus can be a part of this problem and the symptoms should be treated with antihistamines, as scratching the delicate new skin can lead to skin breakdown and scarring. Mild topical steroids and bland emollients will protect the newly formed skin and control symptoms.

Skin breakdown is also an abnormality that needs the physician's attention. The wound should be cultured immediately to rule out the presence of a post-procedure infection. Non-epithelialized areas may be covered with a biologic dressing [e.g., Flexzan (Bertek Pharmaceuticals) or Vigilon (Bard Medical)], and changed daily. Antibiotic, antifungal, or antiviral agents should be used where appropriate.

Other causative factors leading patients down the scarring pathway can include trauma (chemical or mechanical irritations) or contact allergy. These external factors should be eliminated with fastidious post-procedural patient education. Patients should be instructed to use only bland emollients (Vaseline, Aquaphor) and non-caustic cleansers. Early use of irritating makeup or glycolic acid-containing skin products, for example, can induce this erythematous phase and thus all topicals, including sunscreens, bleaches, and retinoids, should be discontinued until the skin is fully healed and no longer inflamed.

If the affected areas of erythema begin to thicken, intralesional injections of corticosteroids (Kenalog, triamcinolone acetonide) may be injected throughout the area and repeated weekly if needed. Care must be taken,

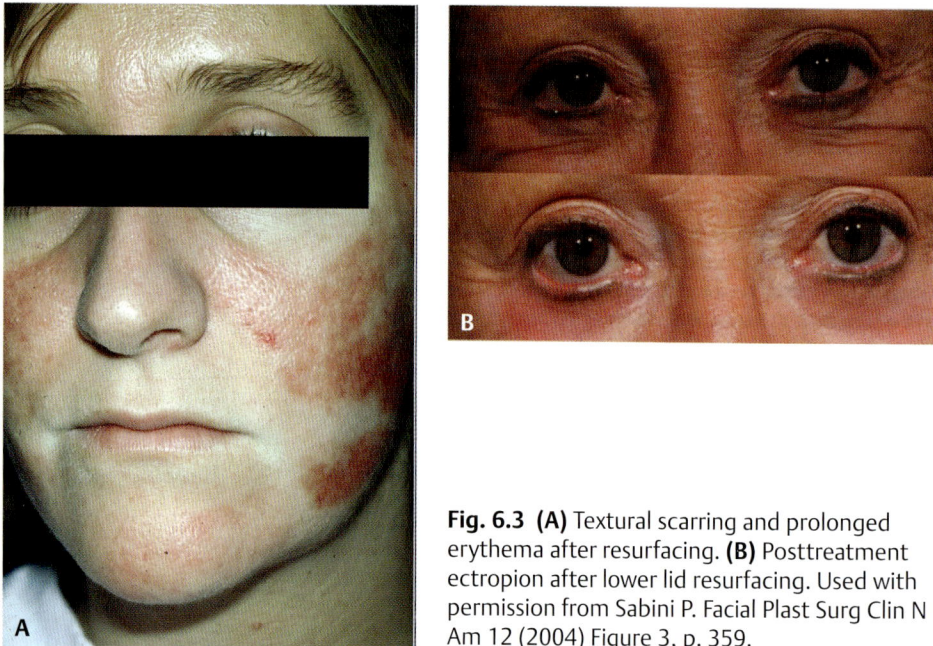

Fig. 6.3 (A) Textural scarring and prolonged erythema after resurfacing. **(B)** Posttreatment ectropion after lower lid resurfacing. Used with permission from Sabini P. Facial Plast Surg Clin N Am 12 (2004) Figure 3, p. 359.

however, not to induce steroid atrophy or telangiectasia formation; thus it may be more judicious to use a short course of systemic steroids. This can be delivered as 40 mg of intramuscular triamcinolone acetonide or 60 mg of oral prednisone tapered gradually over 2 to 3 weeks.

If left unchecked, scar formation can follow different pathways, dependent on the dermal level of injury, the region of the face or body cavity and the injury and the nature of the skin; i.e., eyelid versus neck versus jaw line. Resurfacing by laser or deep peel of the lower eyelid skin induces significant collagen contraction which can produce scleral show or even ectropion in susceptible patients. If the patient has a poor Snap Test, the resurfacing procedure should be very conservative. These patients should be seen regularly because ectropion can occur 1 to 2 weeks after re-epithelialization—when the physician feels all is well. Intervention with intralesional steroid therapy, silicone sheeting, and even mechanical debridement of early adhesions can be productive in preventing and correcting early ectropion.

◆ Infection (Table 6.5)

During wound healing, compromised skin is undoubtedly susceptible to infection. Factors contributing to bacterial or yeast infection are inadequate debridement of necrotic tissue and occlusive ointments such as petrolatum and moisturizers. The mineral and vegetable fats used for occlusive healing can serve as a culture medium, promoting the growth of pathogens, including *Streptococcus*, *Staphylococcus*, and *Pseudomonas* species (**Fig. 6.4A–D**). Regular, gentle debridement of exudate, necrotic tissue, and ointment using a 0.25% acetic acid solution [1 tablespoon (15 cc) of white vinegar in 1 pint (473 cc) of sterile water] is necessary to encourage the normal phases of wound healing—granulation, epithelialization, and fibroplasia. Systemic antibiotics are usually not necessary in open healing with good debridement, because bacterial infection is rare if good hygiene, postoperative soaks, and careful observation are enforced.[12] It is important for the physician to see the patient regularly during the postoperative period to catch the signs of early bacterial infection. Any suspicious exudate should be cultured, and the patient should be placed on the appropriate antibiotic. If an infection is neglected and left untreated, it will lead to delayed wound healing and scarring.

Table 6.5

Infections after Resurfacing
Bacterial pyoderma
Herpes simplex virus
Epstein-Barr virus keratitis
Candidiasis
Toxic shock syndrome

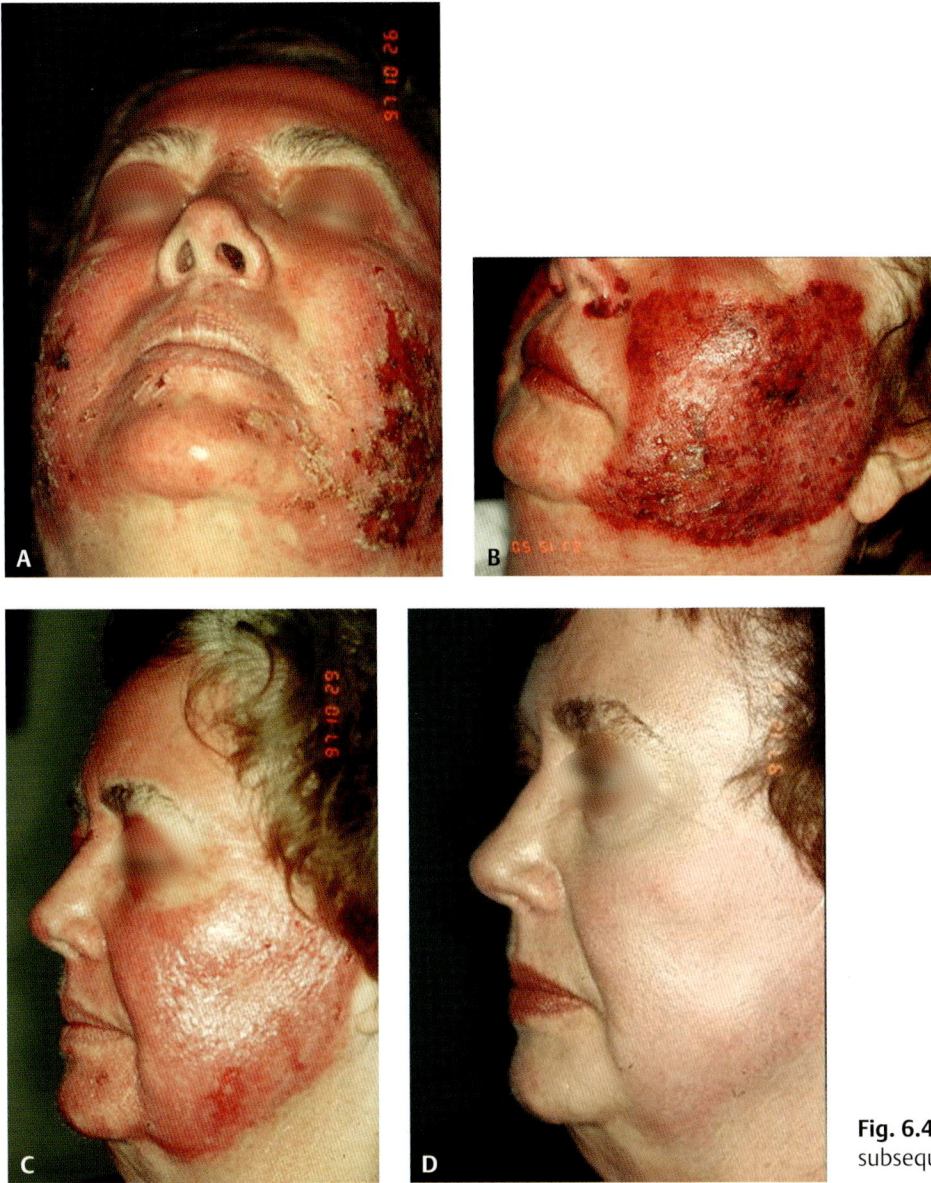

Fig. 6.4 (A–D) Staphylococcal infection and subsequent healing after deep chemical peel.

It has been noted that some patients develop *Candida* infections after occlusive healing without debridement while on systemic antibiotics. They have been reported more frequently after dermabrasion and CO_2 laser resurfacing, because the nonviable epidermis after a peel has been thought to be somewhat protective. Yeast overgrowth should be treated aggressively with soaks and debridement, plus oral ketoconazole and fluconazole.[13] Daily dressing changes and debridement performed by the physician or a trained staff member are advisable during the first three to five days after a resurfacing procedure.

Herpes simplex outbreaks can be triggered by the resurfacing procedure itself. A careful history of prior herpes simplex virus I or II outbreaks will reveal those patients who require prophylactic therapy. Because many patients do not know if they have had HSV and are carriers, all patients having medium-depth and deeper resurfacing procedures should receive prophylactic therapy, such as Valcyclovir, 500 mg twice a day for 10 days, starting 4 days prior to the procedure. If HSV infection occurs during the postoperative phase, the vesicular infection can spread over the entire peeled area and has the potential for devastating sequelae and scarring (**Fig. 6.5A–C**). Vesicles are rare on denuded skin, but the sudden onset of pain in the midst of uneventful wound healing is the classic sign of HSV infection and mandates skin swab culture and prompt initiation of antiviral therapy (Valcyclovir, 500 mg TID or QID)[14] and prolonged skin care.

Epstein-Barr virus keratitis can manifest with vision changes, fever, and arthralgias; it is a rare complication seen after chemoexfoliation with a solution containing croton oil. EBV reactivation and replication can be induced by croton oil in up to 10% of otherwise healthy EBV seropositive patients.[15] The condition can be treated with steroid-containing eye drops, parenteral antiviral agents, and ophthalmologic consultation.

Toxic shock syndrome has also been described after facial resurfacing.[16] Toxic shock is a severe toxin-mediated condition that affects multiple organ systems, with predominant signs being sudden fever, rash, desquamation, and hypotension. It occurs in both males and females and is not related to the menstrual period. The resurfaced area does not usually appear infected as with other types of infections seen after a peel. Early recognition and prompt therapy are the hallmarks of successful intervention. Patients need symptomatic therapy, with aggressive administration of fluids and IV antistaphylococcal antibiotics.

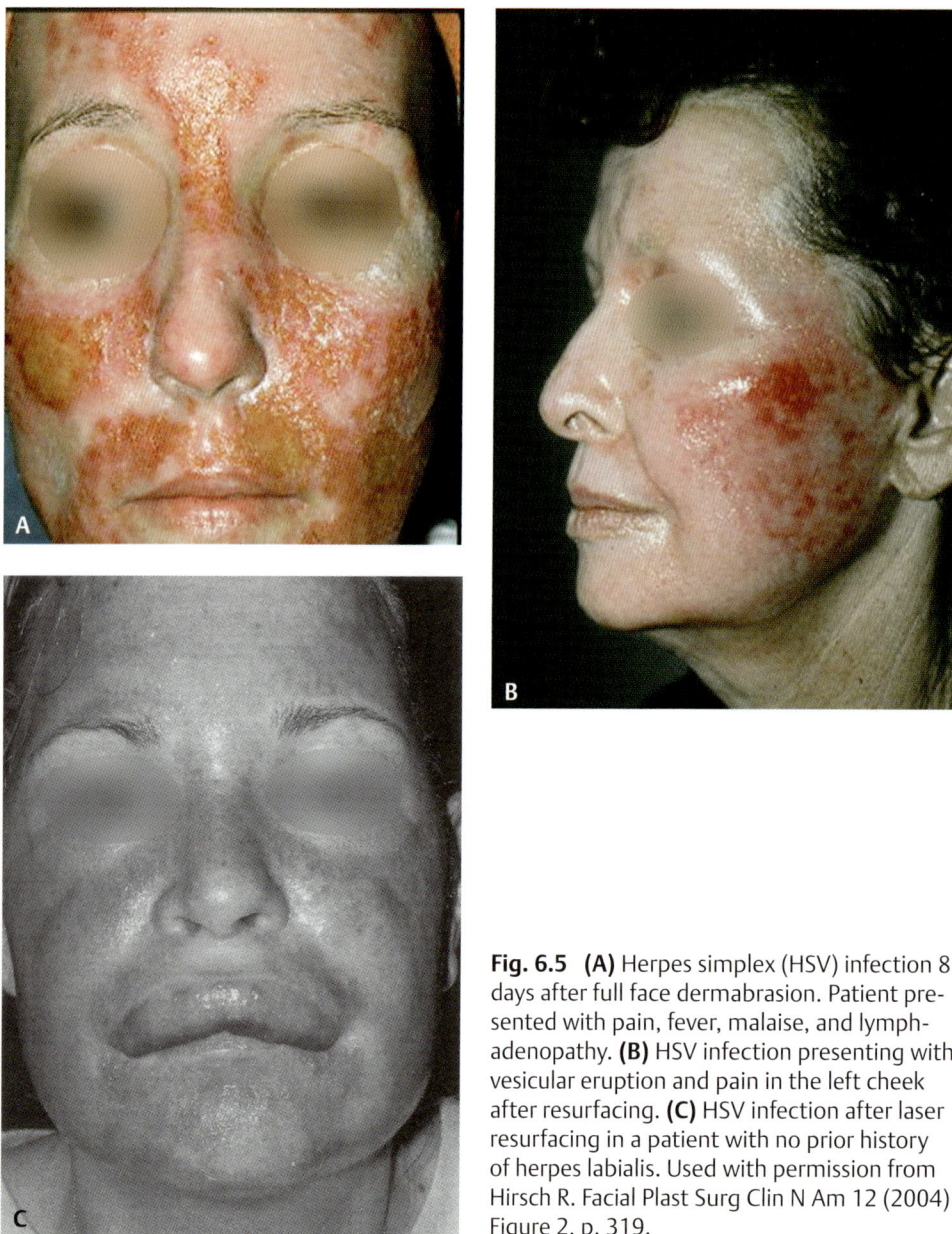

Fig. 6.5 (A) Herpes simplex (HSV) infection 8 days after full face dermabrasion. Patient presented with pain, fever, malaise, and lymphadenopathy. **(B)** HSV infection presenting with vesicular eruption and pain in the left cheek after resurfacing. **(C)** HSV infection after laser resurfacing in a patient with no prior history of herpes labialis. Used with permission from Hirsch R. Facial Plast Surg Clin N Am 12 (2004) Figure 2, p. 319.

◆ Delayed Wound Healing

It is important to recognize delayed wound healing after a resurfacing procedure has been performed. Patients may present with painful open erosions with friable granulation tissue well beyond the time epithelialization should be completed. The symptoms of delayed healing can occur during the second or third weeks after a resurfacing procedure and continue for weeks. Rarely they can surface four to six weeks after full healing. Prolonged granulation phase is a stimulus for scarring and should be treated aggressively to complete epithelialization and healing. Empiric antimicrobial therapy to cover the possibility of an underlying bacterial, yeast, or herpetic infection should be instituted until culture results are available. The treatment of choice is close follow-up with daily dressing changes, using a commercial biosynthetic membrane such as Vigilon (C.R. Bard, Inc., Covington, GA).[17] The protection and coverage of the granulating wound allow the tissues to progress to normal healing.

◆ Persistent Erythema

All patients undergoing a resurfacing procedure will have some degree of erythema for a variable period of time. The degree and extent of redness are dependent on the depth of injury and procedure type. Laser resurfacing generally has a more prolonged period of erythema than does chemical peeling. Although superficial peels are erythematous for two to three days, medium depth peels are normally erythematous for two to three weeks, deep peels for four to six weeks, and CO_2 resurfacing for up to 12 weeks. Erythema that lasts beyond the normal duration is defined as persistent erythema and should signal the physician that there is a potential problem. Persistent erythema is often accompanied by prolonged pruritus, burning or stinging sensations, and irregularities in skin texture. It may represent sensitivity to topical agents such as an allergy to antibiotic ointment or irritation from lanolin, makeup, moisturizer, SPF, or early usage of a retinoid. It may also be an indication of intrinsically sensitive skin, such as atopic dermatitis, seborrheic dermatitis, or rosacea. The surgeon should attempt to identify and correct any underlying factors that may be contributing to the problem. This is most important because persistent erythema may indicate the impending development of scar formation.[18] It should be recognized that neglect of these symptoms and signs is now considered failure to meet the standard of good medical care.

Therapy directed at persistent erythema should emphasize protection of the skin from noxious and irritating agents, as well as the use of corticosteroids and anti-inflammatory agents—topical and/or systemic—to halt any emerging cicatricial process. If the erythematous area begins to feel firm and indurated, it is a sign that scar formation is beginning. If scarring is treated early, it can be prevented and corrected. In many cases, the early fibroplasia stage exhibited by induration and erythema can be reversed, preventing the final results of scar formation and deformity. If, however, prevention fails and a scar forms, the various treatment options—intralesional corticosteroids, topical corticosteroids under occlusion, silicone sheeting, and pulse dye laser treatment—must be considered.

◆ Conclusion

Although cosmetic resurfacing procedures, like all surgical procedures, have associated complications and the potential for adverse sequelae, these can be minimized with a strong knowledge base, careful technique, close patient observation, and appropriate intervention when necessary. Proper physician training for this family of procedures should encompass optimal patient selection, conservative and safe performance of the appropriate resurfacing method, and knowledge of untoward sequelae and their treatment. A skilled physician with such knowledge and experience will make skin resurfacings—whether with chemicals, lasers, or dermabrasion—the safe, efficacious, and successful treatments they are meant to be.

PEARLS OF WISDOM

Always maintain an eyewash station and have it readily available before starting any chemical peel.

Mineral oil, not water, should be used as a flushing medium if phenol inadvertently splashes in a patient's eye.

For all resurfacing modalites, always take additional care to blend the transition from the face to the neck to prevent unsightly demarcation.

Dermabrasion is not an appropriate resurfacing technique for eyelid rejuvenation.

The use of newer resurfacing modalities, such as fractionally ablative CO_2 resurfacing, can be enticing, but the risk-benefit profile of emerging technologies often lags.

References

1. Matarasso SL, Glogau RG. Chemical face peels. Dermatol Clin 1991;9(1):131–150
2. Coleman WP, Lawrence N, eds. Skin Resurfacing. Philadelphia: Williams and Wilkins; 1998:42–66
3. Brody HJ. Complications of chemical peeling. J Dermatol Surg Oncol 1989;15(9):1010–1019
4. Demas PN, Bridenstine JB. Diagnosis and treatment of postoperative complications after skin resurfacing. J Oral Maxillofac Surg 1999;57(7):837–841
5. Duffy DM. Cosmetic surgery and informed consent. Dermatol Surg 1993;5:369–370
6. Rubenstein R, Roenigk HH Jr, Stegman SJ, Hanke CW. Atypical keloids after dermabrasion of patients taking isotretinoin. J Am Acad Dermatol 1986;15(2 Pt 1):280–285
7. Monheit GD. The Jessner's–TCA peel. Facial Plast Surg Clin North Am 1994;2:21–22
8. Brody HJ. Complications of chemical resurfacing. Dermatol Clin 2001;19(3):427–438, vii–viii
9. Monheit GD, Zeituni MC. Skin resurfacing for photoaging; Laser resurfacing vs. chemical peeling. Cosmetic Dermatol 1997;10:11–22
10. Ho C, Nguyen Q, Lowe NJ, Griffin ME, Lask G. Laser resurfacing in pigmented skin. Dermatol Surg 1995;21(12): 1035–1037
11. Hetter GP. An examination of the phenol-croton oil peel: part IV. Face peel results with different concentrations of phenol and croton oil. Plast Reconstr Surg 2000;105: 1061–1083
12. Coleman K, Coleman W. Complications in Skin Resurfacing. Philadelphia: Wilkins and Wilkins; 1998:244–268
13. Giandoni MB, Grabski WJ. Cutaneous candidiasis as a cause of delayed surgical wound healing. J Am Acad Dermatol 1994;30(6):981–984
14. Monheit GD. Facial resurfacing may trigger the herpes simplex virus. Cosmetic Dermatol 1995;8:9–16
15. Brody HJ. Chemical Peeling and Resurfacing. St. Louis: Mosby; 1997:161–193
16. LoVerme WE, Drapkin MS, Courtiss EH, Wilson RM. Toxic shock syndrome after chemical face peel. Plast Reconstr Surg 1987;80(1):115–118
17. Alt TH. Avoiding complications in dermabrasion and chemical peeling. In Skin Allergy News; 1990:2
18. Maloney BP, Millman B, Monheit G, McCollough EG. The etiology of prolonged erythema after chemical peel. Dermatol Surg 1998;24(3):337–341

7

Complications of Upper Eyelid Blepharoplasty

Tom D. Wang and Andrew A. Winkler

Upper eyelid blepharoplasty can have a dramatic restorative affect on the eyes and the face as a whole. However, care must be taken during this delicate operation to prevent its many possible complications. As experience with upper eyelid blepharoplasty has grown over the last century, so has the list of complications. This chapter discusses avoidance and management of complications that may be encountered before, during, and after this surgery.

◆ Preoperative Complications

The treatment of complications begins with careful preoperative assessment of the patient. Certain preexisting conditions are more likely to result in complications or disappointing outcomes. The initial encounter with the patient provides an opportunity to identify and avoid the sources of potential future complications. These conditions do not necessarily prohibit upper eyelid surgery but may need to be addressed before surgery.

Psychiatric History

Determining the patient's desires, motivations, and expectations of blepharoplasty is an essential component of the initial consultation. Properly motivated patients have a healthy self-esteem and seek restorative changes. The surgeon must determine exactly what bothers the patients about their eyes and whether these conditions can be corrected with surgery. If inappropriate desires, motivations, or expectations exist preoperatively, the procedure is likely to fail to satisfy the patient.

A brief psychiatric assessment should be part of every cosmetic preoperative evaluation. Cosmetic surgery patients may have concomitant psychiatric disorders, but this rarely precludes surgery. Body dysmorphic disorder (BDD) is a preoccupation with an imagined or slight defect in appearance that leads to excessive concern and significant impairment in social, occupational, or other areas of functioning.[1] In one prospective study, the prevalence of BDD in patients seeking cosmetic eyelid rejuvenation was 13%.[2] The authors found that cosmetic surgery patients are no more dissatisfied, critical, or preoccupied with their overall appearance than a nationwide sample of Americans. This contrasts with the common portrayal of cosmetic surgery patients as excessively vain. Most patients seek blepharoplasty to restore their eyes to a previous state and are likely to cope with the postoperative change in appearance. However, patients desiring to dramatically change the shape of the eye must be approached with caution, and a preoperative psychiatric consultation may be indicated.[3]

Past Medical History

When obtaining a past medical history, the surgeon should pay close attention to past bleeding problems and the use of anticoagulant or herbal medications. Those with bleeding disorders or who use anticoagulant medications have an increased risk of bleeding complications following blepharoplasty. Many commonly used herbal medications, such as echinacea, ephedra, garlic, ginkgo, ginseng, kava, St. John's wort, and valerian, pose a perioperative bleeding risk.[4] In particular, garlic,[5] ginkgo,[6] and ginseng[7] have been shown to decrease coagulation parameters. The authors request their blepharoplasty patients stop taking all herbal medications 10 days before surgery.

During the initial consultation, the surgeon must also inquire about disorders that may lead to poor healing. Diabetes, malnutrition, and immunosuppression constitute relative contraindications for elective surgery. A discussion regarding wound healing preoperatively will help avoid litigation should poor healing lead to a complication postoperatively. A careful medical history allows the surgeon to filter out candidates whose preoperative health may produce complications and poor outcomes.

Physical Examination

A meticulous physical examination can identify many potential causes of blepharoplasty complications. While patients commonly present with a desire to remove redundant eyelid skin, close examination often reveals that skin redundancy is caused at least in part by descent of the eyebrows. To make this assessment, it is helpful to understand the anatomic position of the eyebrows in youth. The youthful brow in women lies just above the supraorbital rim and is a gentle arc.[8,9] In men, the brow is flatter and lies at the level of the supraorbital rim.[10] The surgeon evaluates the contribution of the brow to eyelid skin redundancy by manually elevating the eyebrows to these positions in the office. This often leads to a dramatic decrease in the amount of skin laxity. If the brow position is corrected to the level of the orbital rim, much, if not all, of the skin redundancy is often reduced. After the contribution of the eyebrows to eyelid skin redundancy has been determined, the surgical steps to correct the problem can more accurately be suggested. Excision of the upper eyelid skin without addressing preexisting eyebrow ptosis results in further brow descent and prevents the desired opening of the eyes.

Dry Eye Syndrome

Symptoms of soreness, burning, foreign body sensation, or mucoid discharge should raise red flags during an assessment of blepharoplasty patients (**Fig. 7.1**). Blepharoplasty surgery in those with tear deficiency can aggravate subclinical symptoms into full-blown dry eye syndrome.[11] An understanding of the tear film allows the physician to differentiate the causes of dry eye syndrome. The tear film is a trilaminar fluid barrier that bathes the exposed cornea. It contains antibacterial agents, oxygenates the corneal epithelium, maintains a smooth refractive surface, and provides lubrication for

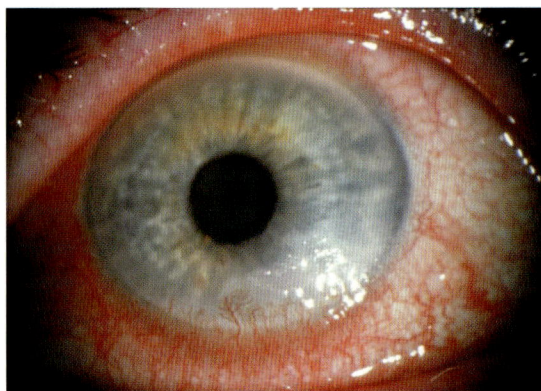

Fig. 7.1 Clinical appearance of a dry eye.

eyelid movement.[12] The outermost layer of the tear film is a hydrophobic oil layer produced by the meibomian glands and accessory sebaceous glands (the palpebral glands of Zeiss and Moll) that reduces evaporation of the tear film. When this layer is disrupted, evaporative losses may increase 10 to 20 times.[13] The middle layer is aqueous and has the largest volume. It is produced by basal secretion from numerous accessory glands (lacrimal exocrine glands of Kraus and Wolfring) plus a stimulated secretion from the lacrimal gland. Basal aqueous secretion decreases with age, leading to a loss in tear volume.[11] The deep layer of the tear film is a mucous barrier produced by goblet cells of the conjunctiva. The secretion of mucin by the goblet cells of the conjunctiva increases in response to inflammation.

Keratoconjunctivitis sicca is the term used to describe eye irritation caused by decreased tear production or increased tear film evaporation. There are many pathophysiologic causes of dry eye, but the most common one is a reduction of the aqueous portion of the tear film. Many systemic disorders are associated with keratoconjunctivitis sicca, including systemic lupus erythematosus, scleroderma, Wegener's granulomatosis, hyperthyroid states, and rheumatoid arthritis. It is important to identify preoperatively those patients who are likely to develop dry eye symptoms. In one study of blepharoplasty, those more likely to develop postoperative keratoconjunctivitis sicca included men, postmenopausal females, and patients with hypertension.[14]

The tear deficiency is diagnosed through inquiring about dry eye symptoms and confirming abnormal tear film production. One may be clued into the presence of a dry eye by observing the corneal surface in preoperative photographs: it should appear glass-like. If the light reflex appears rough, as if there is debris on the cornea, further workup should be sought. On exam, an abnormal tear film is recognized by rapid tear evaporation and increased mucus on the eyelid margins.

Schirmer testing is perhaps the most useful and easily performed test to establish the diagnosis of keratoconjunctivitis sicca in the preoperative setting.[14] The eye is first topically anesthetized to prevent eliciting reflex secretion and the patient is placed in a moderately illuminated room facing away from direct light. Filter paper 35 mm long × 5 mm wide is partially folded at one end and the folded end is placed on the lateral one-third of the lower lid conjunctiva. The patient is then asked to fixate on an object above the direct line of gaze for 5 minutes. Hyposecretion is defined by less than 10 mm of wetting. Normal wetting is between 10 and 30 mm.[15] Unfortunately, the results of the Schirmer test in a given patient may vary greatly and it is necessary to perform several tests for each patient. Those who consistently fall below 10 mm of wetting should be suspected of having dry eye syndrome and warrant a complete ophthalmologic workup.

Hypothyroidism

Hypothyroidism causes soft-tissue changes throughout the body, including the periorbital soft tissues. In one study, 2.6% of patients seeking a consultation for blepharoplasty were found to have undiagnosed hypothyroidism.[16] These patients will attribute the skin changes of their eyelids to aging and excessive fatigue. When examined, they will have characteristic skin laxity and periorbital edema leading to a puffy appearance. Swelling of the periorbital tissues is due to local deposition of mucopolysaccharides. These patients should undergo further evaluation, because the orbital changes generally resolve with adequate treatment of the hypothyroidism.[17] Although iodine deficiency is the most common cause of hypothyroidism worldwide, Hashimoto's thyroiditis, which is caused by anti-thyroid peroxidase (anti-TPO) antibodies, is the most common cause in the United States. If patients suspected of having hypothyroidism have an elevated TSH level on initial screening, a total serum T_4 should then be evaluated. Once the diagnosis is made, the patient's primary care physician may institute treatment.

Lacrimal Gland Prolapse

Occasionally, prolapse of the lacrimal gland is encountered on initial examination. This must not be mistaken for fat prolapse and should be evaluated to exclude a malignant, inflammatory, or thyroid hormone-related pathology of the lacrimal gland. Patients with undiagnosed lacrimal gland lymphoma, adenocarcinoma, and metastatic cancer have all presented requesting cosmetic eyelid surgery. The lacrimal gland lies in the superotemporal quadrant of the orbit and is separated into the orbital and palpebral lobes. These lobes are divided by the lateral horn of the levator aponeurosis, through which run the lacrimal ductules. Lacrimal gland prolapse can be diagnosed by everting the upper eyelid and asking the patient to look down. This will accentuate prolapse of the palpebral portion of the lacrimal gland. Comparison between sides and during globe ballottement should also be performed. Repositioning of the lacrimal gland, if necessary, may be performed to elicit a satisfying cosmetic result in upper blepharoplasty. Suturing techniques as well as removal of the orbital fat that surrounds the lacrimal gland have been described.[18,19]

Surgical Planning

Poor postoperative results can often be attributed to poor preoperative surgical planning. It is important for both the patient and the surgeon to reach a congruent understanding of the goals for surgery and to share reasonable expectations of the outcome. One of the most common errors in preoperative planning is not taking into account the patient's ethnicity. The surgeon must respect the patient's desires for maintaining ethnic traits in the appearance of the upper eyelid

Patients are often unaware of asymmetries in their eyelids, and taking standard preoperative blepharoplasty photographs is an important practice. These photographs are reviewed with the patient to demonstrate the small degrees of asymmetry between the upper eyelids. The most important landmark in upper eyelid blepharoplasty is the upper lid crease. When inherent asymmetry exists, attempts to create symmetry between the upper eyelid creases may change the shape and overall appearance of the eyes. It is imperative to identify asymmetries and discuss them with the patient preoperatively to avoid a situation where the patient believes the preexisting condition was caused by the surgery.[20]

Preexisting Upper Eyelid Ptosis

Patients seeking blepharoplasty are often unaware of preexisting upper eyelid ptosis. Blepharoptosis is classified by the extent of superior limbus coverage by the lid margin. It is defined as mild (2 mm or less), moderate (2–4 mm), or severe (4 mm or more).[21] Beard classified acquired ptosis by etiology into neurogenic, myogenic, traumatic, and mechanical categories.[22] The levator aponeurosis, which normally inserts on the anterior tarsal surface, can become disinserted or dehiscent. Eyelid trauma, ocular surgery, recurrent lid edema of any etiology (i.e., allergic, inflammatory), and idiopathic atrophy of the levator aponeurosis may all lead to upper eyelid ptosis. In the elderly population, acquired ptosis is most often due to senile atrophy of the levator aponeurosis, which is often accompanied by varying amounts of dermatochalasis. Excess skin exaggerates the degree of ptosis and leads the patient to seek surgical correction.

In evaluating a patient with eyelid ptosis, the surgeon should inquire about a history of eyelid trauma, recurrent lid edema or inflammation, previous eyelid surgery, or congenital ptosis. The surgeon must also document the onset, duration, and progression of the ptosis. Reviewing old photos of the patient can be useful to illustrate the progress of ptosis. The position of the eyelid relative to the superior limbus in primary gaze should be noted. The superior eyelid margin is normally positioned 1 mm below the superior limbus. If the eyelid falls below this level, the upper eyelid is ptotic.[23] The degree of levator aponeurosis function can be documented with a millimeter ruler in front of the eye. Using one or two fingers of pressure over the brow to prevent use of the frontalis muscle, the patient is asked to look down and then upward. The amount of excursion of the eyelid margin is due to levator function. Movement of 4 mm or less is classified as poor function, 6 mm is fair, and 8 mm is considered good levator function.[24] In some cases, preexisting ptosis may actually be exaggerated by tightening of the eyelid skin.[25] If upper eyelid ptosis is asymmetric, the surgeon should consider Herring's phenomenon. Herring's law states that there is equal and symmetric innervation to the frontalis muscle. If asymmetric ptosis is corrected, the stimulus to raise the eyebrows via contraction of the frontalis muscle decreases bilaterally, which then unmasks ptosis on the less affected side.

Myasthenia gravis is an autoimmune phenomenon mainly affecting young women that causes upper eyelid ptosis. Ptosis that gets worse as the day progresses is the hallmark of this condition. While the Tensilon test is the standard method for diagnosis, a simple method of testing for myasthenia in the office is to place a few drops of phenylephrine in the eye. Immediate improvement of the ptosis suggests the presence of underlying myasthenia. This finding should prompt a referral to a neurologist for further treatment and work-up.

A high upper eyelid crease suggests the most common cause of upper eyelid ptosis, levator aponeurosis dehiscence. Levator aponeurosis dehiscence can have several causes, including senile aging and intraoperative stretching. It is important, therefore, for the surgeon to be careful to avoid manipulation of an atrophic levator aponeurosis.[26] In patients with levator aponeurosis dehiscence, the eyelid crease must be marked inferior to the existing crease and the ptosis repaired by advancement of the levator aponeurosis in a superior direction. The eyelid crease may then be reformed at the desired level, taking small bites of the orbicularis muscle when closing the skin.[27]

Orbital Tumors

Asymmetric swelling of the upper eyelids should prompt further attention. Palpation of the upper eyelids may quickly identify a lacrimal gland mass. As the previous discussion indicated, potential tumors in this location include glandular tumors, lymphomas, and metastatic tumors from other sites. In addition, unilateral eyelid edema can be the presenting symptom of retroorbital tumors that impair lymphatic flow from the eyelid.

Preexisting Visual Complaints

A visual acuity examination is warranted in blepharoplasty patients with new visual obstructive complaints. In those who wear prescription eyeglasses, the surgeon should obtain recent documentation of visual acuity from the patients' ophthalmologist. In a national survey, surgeons were asked what percentage of their blepharoplasty patients received an eye examination. Overall, only 50% of the patients undergoing eyelid surgery had an eye examination.[28] It is important to document vi-

sual acuity preoperatively, because patients are often unaware of poor vision in one eye. If they first notice decreased vision postoperatively, they may attribute this inappropriately to the surgical procedure. For this reason, before the operation the surgeon should test the patient's vision, then discuss and document any visual acuity issues with the patient.

◆ Intraoperative Complications

Corneal Abrasion

Corneal abrasion commonly occurs following blepharoplasty, though its true incidence is unknown. Corneal eye shields offer excellent protection against unforeseen events and accidents. If they are used, eye shields must be generously lubricated on the concave surface with a petrolatum-based agent to minimize the risk of abrasion. During surgery, cotton-tipped applicators should be used instead of gauze sponges to avoid inadvertent injury to the cornea. Only the surgeon or the assistant should instrument around the surgical field, and extraneous movements should be minimized.

Throughout the procedure and at its end, balanced saline solution should be used frequently to wash out bits of suture and other debris.[29] The first complaint of patients who have sustained a corneal abrasion is eye pain. If an abrasion is suspected, it is prudent to obtain an ophthalmologic consultation for a fluorescein dye and a slit lamp exam. Patients with poor Bell's phenomenon are at risk for postoperative corneal abrasion in the setting of a transient lagophthalmos. For such patients, the use of eye drops and ointment, especially at night, helps to avoid injury.

Chlorhexidine concentrations of 2% and 4% have been shown to be toxic to corneal epithelium. In a rabbit study, MacRae et al. found that a single drop caused sloughing of the entire corneal epithelium in three hours.[30] In contrast, povidine iodine solution (without detergent) caused no de-epithelialization or increase in corneal thickness compared to the saline control. Affected corneas returned to normal within one week. Should accidental spillage into the eye occur, immediately irrigate the eye with balanced salt solution and consider an ophthalmologic consultation.

Corneal Thermal Injury

Thermal injury to the cornea during cosmetic blepharoplasty from electrocautery has been reported.[31] The resultant contraction of stromal collagen can cause significant astigmatism. Patients under general anesthesia may sustain greater damage to the corneal epithelium because of a lack of Bell's phenomenon and other protective reflexes. Treatment of corneal thermal injury begins with antimicrobial prophylaxis with broad-spectrum antibiotic drops and pain management using cycloplegic agents and analgesics. After re-epithelialization, topical steroids are used to limit inflammation and scarring. If significant astigmatism persists, some patients may benefit from corrective astigmatic keratotomy.

Transient Ophthalmoplegia/Mydriasis

Transient mydriasis and ophthalmoplegia is common following blepharoplasty.[32] This condition is caused by the effects of local anesthetic on the short ciliary nerves and the oculomotor nerve. As such, it is a benign, self-limiting condition that must not be confused with the mydriasis caused by retrobulbar hematoma (see below). Recognition of the cause of these findings prevents unnecessary treatment.

In the patient with a shallow anterior chamber any condition that causes pupillary dilation may precipitate acute glaucoma.[33] The stress of surgery plus the sympathetic action of vasoconstrictive agents in local anesthetics can lead to closure of the anterior chamber drainage angle. In susceptible patients, this precipitates acute glaucoma. Patients with elevated intraocular pressure should undergo a slit lamp examination before surgery. Acute angle closure glaucoma is successfully treated with instillation of pilocarpine drops.

◆ Immediate Postoperative Complications

Bleeding

Of all immediate postoperative complications, bleeding is potentially the most devastating. There are numerous causes of postoperative bleeding, including needle injection trauma, rough handling of orbital fat, and patient-related factors, such as coagulopathies or Valsalva maneuvers while coming out of anesthesia.[34] Every patient will have some degree of periorbital ecchymosis following upper lid blepharoplasty, so this should not necessarily raise concern (**Fig. 7.2**). On the other hand, retrobulbar bleeding is a feared complication that can lead to one of the most devastating complications of blepharoplasty: blindness. Retrobulbar bleeding can lead to a compartment syndrome within the bony orbital boundaries. Though the exact mechanism is unknown, two theories exist to explain this phenomenon. One theory focuses on occlusion of the central retinal artery, which can occur through the following sequence of events.[35–37] As retroorbital hemorrhage proceeds, blood dissects into the orbital fat, muscles, and other structures. Pressure then builds in the rigid confines of the bony orbit. As intraorbital pressure reaches that of the systolic blood pressure, bleeding from the contributing artery halts. However, blood flow also ceases in the central retinal artery. The body responds to increased intraocular pressure by increasing the systolic

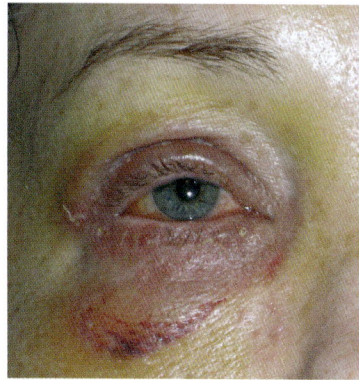

Fig. 7.2 Periorbital ecchymosis and edema are common after upper eyelid blepharoplasty, as is demonstrated in this patient two days after surgery.

blood pressure, which promotes continued bleeding into the orbital space and increased pressure. Some authors dispute this hypothesis, citing visual evoked response data that is more consistent with optic nerve injury rather than retinal ischemia.[38,39] In the opposing theory, pressure becomes great enough to occlude the vasa nervorum of the optic nerve and cause permanent visual impairment.

Retrobulbar hemorrhage generally occurs during the first few hours after surgery, but it has been reported days after surgery.[40] The characteristic findings include stone-hard proptosis, chemosis, mydriasis, increased intraocular pressure, and severe eye pain.[35] Acute retrobulbar hemorrhage is common in ophthalmologic surgery and occurs in perhaps 0.03–0.05% of all blepharoplasties.[41] The rate of blindness following blepharoplasty surgery is probably underreported but is estimated to be 0.04%.[28] When loss of vision accompanies retrobulbar hemorrhage, it is almost always transient.[37] In 2004, members of the American Society of Ophthalmic Plastic and Reconstructive Surgery were surveyed to ascertain the incidence of postoperative retrobulbar hemorrhage and blindness.[41] Among 269,433 cosmetic eyelid cases, there were 149 orbital hemorrhages (0.055%). Only 12 of these (0.0045%) were associated with permanent visual loss. Though visual loss is more likely to be a complication of lower eyelid blepharoplasty, there have also been reports of blindness after upper blepharoplasty alone.[39]

Treatment of retrobulbar hemorrhage is generally conservative and includes ice packs and monitoring of the retinal circulation by an ophthalmologist.[39] In these cases, changes in visual acuity should determine the course of action, not intraocular pressure alone. Uncomplicated cases may be managed by medications, which include intravenous osmotic agents, acetazolamide, and β-blocker eye drops. However, retrobulbar hematoma associated with visual changes requires aggressive and immediate treatment. Frequent monitoring of vision establishes the necessity for a surgical procedure. If there are any signs that vision has deteriorated, the orbit should be surgically decompressed via lateral canthotomy and cantholysis, and the wound explored.[40,42]

Blepharoptosis

Eyelid ptosis is a relatively common complication of upper eyelid blepharoplasty, though it is rarely permanent. There are several potential etiologies of this complication, including local anesthesia, postoperative edema, direct injury, and levator-septal adhesion. Deep penetration of local anesthesia can cause blockade of the sympathetic innervation of the levator superioris muscle. This blockade produces a ptosis lasting an hour or two after surgery, depending on the agent used. Postoperative swelling, which causes a temporary ptosis, occurs in nearly every patient undergoing upper eyelid blepharoplasty.[43] The patients can be quite concerned about this swelling, but they can be reassured that it will resolve over the next several days. Cool compresses can help to hasten the resolution of edema.

The levator aponeurosis can be injured directly during surgery, resulting in blepharoptosis. This generally occurs from inadvertent sharp dissection during skin-muscle excision or during excision of orbital fat.[44,45] At the lower half of the skin-muscle excision, the levator is merging with the septum and orbicularis muscle and is more vulnerable to injury. To prevent injury at this location, the surgeon should perform the septal excision superiorly, where the preaponeurotic fat pad is thick and protects against direct levator injury.[44] As well, pulling on the upper lid orbital fat pulls the aponeurosis into the wound, where it is vulnerable to surgical damage. Gentle ballottement of the globe with careful and conservative fat excision will help to prevent injury to the levator complex.

Ptosis may also occur if the orbital septum is inadvertently sutured to the levator apparatus during closure.[45] This will occur only if the orbital septum is attached to the levator superior to the original insertion of the septum. In effect, this causes a reduction of the mechanical advantage of the levator, resulting in ptosis.

Chemosis

Chemosis is common in the immediate postoperative period following upper lid blepharoplasty. It is seldom of concern to the patient, but in rare cases it can persist for several weeks. The cause of chemosis following cosmetic upper eyelid blepharoplasty is unknown. Eyelid lymph vessels consist of a superficial system that drains the skin of the lids and the orbicularis oculi muscle, along with a deep system that drains the tarsal and conjunctival region. Chemosis is probably caused by interruption or compression of lymphatic outflow secondary to local edema and postoperative changes. Chemosis generally resolves by five months, and its resolution does not appear to be hastened by any specific treatment.[46,47]

◆ Late Postoperative Complications

Infection

Like any procedure that penetrates the skin barrier, upper lid blepharoplasty carries with it a risk of infection, albeit quite low. There have, however, been reports of very serious infections stemming from cosmetic upper blepharoplasty, and the surgeon should be cognizant of them. Necrotizing fasciitis, a life-threatening soft-tissue infection caused by group A α-hemolytic *Streptococcus*, has been reported following blepharoplasty.[48–50] Necrotizing fasciitis typically occurs in the setting of trauma, immunosuppression, malnutrition, and other conditions that cause poor wound healing.[51] The characteristic findings are those of a tense dusky-gray eyelid with violaceous bullae and necrosis across fascial planes. Proper and rapid identification of necrotizing fasciitis is crucial, as immediate intravenous antibiotics and debridement of necrotic tissue are essential to achieving a positive outcome. Ancillary treatment modalities include hyperbaric oxygen therapy and intravenous gamma globulin therapy.

Orbital abscess has also been reported following upper eyelid blepharoplasty.[52] An orbital abscess will typically present on the fifth to seventh postoperative day, and *Staphylococcus aureus* is the most common bacterium isolated. Typical findings include lid inflammation, diplopia, and proptosis. Computed tomography or ultrasound can be useful in making the diagnosis. As in other areas of the body, treatment includes surgical drainage of the abscess cavity and administration of intravenous antibiotics.

Visual Complaints/Astigmatism

The risk of astigmatism after eyelid surgery or from eyelid tumors such as hemangiomas has been well documented.[53–55] Studies have indicated that astigmatism and blurred vision may occur following upper eyelid blepharoplasty as well.[56] Removal of skin repositions the eyelid and alters its relationship to the cornea. This in turn leads to changes in corneal curvature, which may affect the patient's refraction. In one study, the average refractive error at one month and three months after surgery was 0.62 diopters (D) and 0.45 D, respectively.[56] This study also revealed that one month after blepharoplasty 16% of patients showed astigmatic changes greater than 1.00 D. Surgeons should therefore inform patients that changes in their refractive status may occur. However, visual changes of less than 0.50 D are perceived only by those whose activities require a higher standard of visual acuity. These patients should know that they may require a change in their lens prescription to account for refractive change after blepharoplasty.

Lagophthalmos

A small degree of scleral show, especially during sleep, is an expected outcome in the acute postoperative setting following blepharoplasty. Scleral show is often accentuated by concurrent brow lift, but it will gradually improve over the first few postoperative weeks. Lagophthalmos occurs when scleral show persists longer than two to three weeks. Upper eyelid lagophthalmos is caused by excessive skin removal or by fibrosis of the orbital septum. Patients who develop lagophthalmos complain of eye pain and fluctuating vision, which results from corneal exposure and keratopathy. Corneal infections can develop, and the patient may even experience permanent vision loss.[57,58]

Full-thickness upper eyelid skin grafting may be used to replace insufficient skin, and often it is the only cure for a shortened upper eyelid anterior lamella. Skin grafting is the only surgical procedure that directly addresses earlier excessive removal of skin.[58]

Eyelid Skin Abnormalities

Epicanthal folds can occur if the line of skin excision in the nasal portion of the upper lid is carried too far into the thicker skin of the nasal sidewall near the canthal angle. The resulting contracture of the scar creates a tight band across the canthus that can be quite conspicuous postoperatively. In mild cases, massage and time may resolve the epicanthal fold formation. A V-to-Y relaxation incision can be performed to restore the contour of the upper lid crease and medial canthal region. Lateral epicanthal folds can also occur if the incision is carried past the level of the lateral canthus. Separating the upper and lower blepharoplasty incisions by at least 5 mm will help to prevent this complication.[59]

Hypesthesia occurs in most patients following blepharoplasty, but it is seldom a complaint in the postoperative period. Recovery of eyelid sensation occurs over two to six months, although in rare cases this change is permanent.[60]

Milia

Milia are epidermal inclusion cysts that result from the entrapment of glandular ducts or epithelial debris in the operative wound (**Fig. 7.3**). The formation of milia along the fresh scar is frequently seen in the upper eyelid, and less frequently in the lower lid. The rate of milia formation is approximately 2% with wound closure using either a permanent subcuticular or fast-absorbing gut skin suture.[61] Milia often resolve spontaneously, so they do not require immediate treatment. However, if

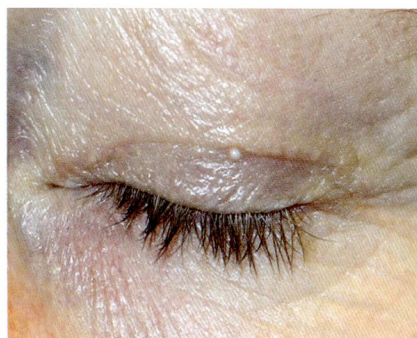

Fig. 7.3 Milia result from entrapment of epithelial tissue in the wound closure.

persistent, they may be easily treated by unroofing the thin epithelium with a #11 blade scalpel tip or a fine needle.[29]

Other incisional complications include dyspigmented scars, hypertrophic scars, or visible suture tracks (**Figs. 7.4, 7.5**). These can be difficult to predict and to manage once present. Strict adherence to meticulous suture technique (wound edge apposition, not constriction) and timely suture removal (five to six days) can help limit these issues. Silicone sheeting can be used without problems on the upper eyelids, but the use of topical steroids and hydroquinone is not advisable.

◆ Conclusion

If the surgeon performs a careful analysis of the prospective upper blepharoplasty patient and responsibly discusses postoperative expectations, it can prevent many complications. In addtion, careful technique with a mastery of eyelid surgical anatomy will help to prevent complications during the procedure. In the postoperative setting, prevention or treatment of infections and anticipation of the vagaries of healing maximize patient satisfaction with upper eyelid blepharoplasty. A properly performed blepharoplasty is a satisfying procedure that results in a very high percentage of grateful patients.

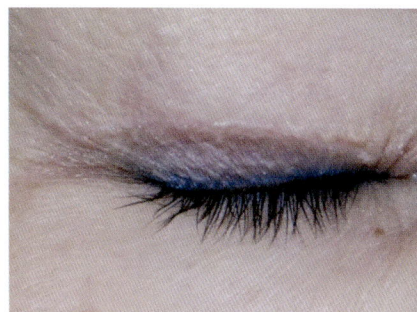

Fig. 7.4 Hypertrophic upper blepharoplasty scar.

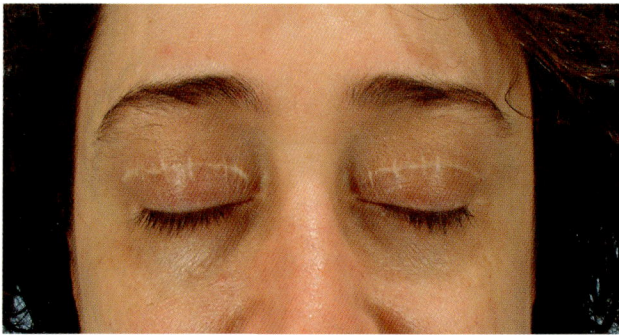

Fig. 7.5 Hypopigmented upper blepharoplasty scars with visible suture tracks, one year after surgery.

PEARLS OF WISDOM

Complications in upper eyelid blepharoplasty can occur in all phases of patient care: preoperatively, intraoperatively and postoperatively.

Patients undergoing blepharoplasty should halt all herbal medications 10 days before the procedure because they increase the risk of bleeding complications.

Brow ptosis commonly occurs concomitantly with upper eyelid aging and must be addressed separately.

Dry eye symptoms should be evaluated during the initial consultation and explained to the patient.

Preexisting eyelid ptosis and asymmetries should be identified and pointed out to the patient.

Visual acuity should be documented preoperatively.

Corneal abrasions occur commonly, so attempts should be made to prevent this complication intraoperatively.

Retrobulbar hemorrhage is a rare complication of blepharoplasty that warrants an immediate consultation with an ophthalmologist.

Visual loss in the setting of retrobulbar hematoma necessitates lateral canthotomy, cantholysis, and surgical exploration.

Chemosis and upper eyelid ptosis can commonly occur following upper eyelid blepharoplasty and usually resolve without intervention.

A small degree of astigmatism is almost universally present following blepharoplasty and generally resolves without intervention.

Lagophthalmos occurs when scleral show persists for more than two weeks, and it is caused by excessive skin removal.

References

1. American Psychiatric Association. Diagnostic and Statistical Manual of Mental Disorders. Washington DC: American Psychiatric Association; 1994
2. Sarwer DB, Wadden TA, Pertschuk MJ, Whitaker LA. Body image dissatisfaction and body dysmorphic disorder in 100 cosmetic surgery patients. Plast Reconstr Surg 1998;101(6):1644–1649
3. Goin MK, Goin JM. Psychological effects of aesthetic facial surgery. Adv Psychosom Med 1986;15:84–108
4. Ang-Lee MK, Moss J, Yuan CS. Herbal medicines and perioperative care. JAMA 2001;286(2):208–216
5. Srivastava KC. Evidence for the mechanism by which garlic inhibits platelet aggregation. Prostaglandins Leukot Med 1986;22(3):313–321
6. Chung KF, Dent G, McCusker M, Guinot P, Page CP, Barnes PJ. Effect of a ginkgolide mixture (BN 52063) in antagonising skin and platelet responses to platelet activating factor in man. Lancet 1987;1(8527):248–251
7. Kimura Y, Okuda H, Arichi S. Effects of various ginseng saponins on 5-hydroxytryptamine release and aggregation in human platelets. J Pharm Pharmacol 1988;40(12):838–843
8. Westmore MG. Facial Cosmetics in Conjunction with Surgery. Aesthetic Plastic Surgical Society Meeting. Vancouver, British Columbia; 1975
9. Whitaker LA, Morales L Jr, Farkas LG. Aesthetic surgery of the supraorbital ridge and forehead structures. Plast Reconstr Surg 1986;78(1):23–32
10. Goldstein SM, Katowitz JA. The male eyebrow: a topographic anatomic analysis. Ophthal Plast Reconstr Surg 2005;21(4):285–291
11. Rees TD, Jelks GW. Blepharoplasty and the dry eye syndrome: guidelines for surgery? Plast Reconstr Surg 1981;68(2):249–252
12. Graham WP III, Messner KH, Miller SH. Keratoconjunctivitis sicca symptoms appearing after blepharoplasty. The "dry eye" syndrome. Plast Reconstr Surg 1976;57(1):57–61
13. Mishima S, Maurice DM. The oily layer of the tear film and evaporation from the corneal surface. Exp Eye Res 1961;1:39–45
14. Rees TD, LaTrenta GS. The role of the Schirmer's test and orbital morphology in predicting dry-eye syndrome after blepharoplasty. Plast Reconstr Surg 1988;82(4):619–625
15. Pflugfelder SC, Solomon A, Stern ME. The diagnosis and management of dry eye: a twenty-five-year review. Cornea 2000;19(5):644–649
16. Klatsky SA, Manson PN. Thyroid disorders masquerading as aging changes. Ann Plast Surg 1992;28(5):420–426
17. Wortsman J, Wavak P. Palpebral redundancy from hypothyroidism. Plast Reconstr Surg 1980;65(1):1–3
18. Smith B, Lisman RD. Dacryoadenopexy as a recognized factor in upper lid blepharoplasty. Plast Reconstr Surg 1983;71(5):629–632
19. Petrelli RL. The treatment of lacrimal gland prolapse in blepharoplasty. Ophthal Plast Reconstr Surg 1988;4(3):139–142
20. Wiggs EO. Blepharoplasty complications. Trans Sect Ophthalmol Am Acad Ophthalmol Otolaryngol 1976;81(4 Pt 1):OP603–OP606

21. Lee V, Konrad H, Bunce C, Nelson C, Collin JR. Aetiology and surgical treatment of childhood blepharoptosis. Br J Ophthalmol 2002;86(11):1282–1286

22. Beard C. Ptosis. St. Louis: Mosby; 1981

23. Wilkins RB, Patipa M. The recognition of acquired ptosis in patients considered for upper-eyelid blepharoplasty. Plast Reconstr Surg 1982;70(4):431–434

24. Hornblass A. Ptosis and pseudoptosis and blepharoplasty. Clin Plast Surg 1981;8(4):811–830

25. Millay DJ, Larrabee WF Jr. Ptosis and blepharoplasty surgery. Arch Otolaryngol Head Neck Surg 1989;115(2):198–201

26. Lisman RD, Hyde K, Smith B. Complications of blepharoplasty. Clin Plast Surg 1988;15(2):309–335

27. Glavas IP. The diagnosis and management of blepharoplasty complications. Otolaryngol Clin North Am 2005;38(5):1009–1021

28. DeMere M, Wood T, Austin W. Eye complications with blepharoplasty or other eyelid surgery. A national survey. Plast Reconstr Surg 1974;53(6):634–637

29. Adams BJ, Feuerstein SS. Complications of blepharoplasty. Ear Nose Throat J 1986;65(1):6–18

30. MacRae SM, Brown B, Edelhauser HF. The corneal toxicity of presurgical skin antiseptics. Am J Ophthalmol 1984;97(2):221–232

31. Chou B, Boxer Wachler BS. Astigmatism after corneal thermal injury. J Cataract Refract Surg 2001;27(5):784–786

32. Perlman JP, Conn H. Transient internal ophthalmoplegia during blepharoplasty. A report of three cases. Ophthal Plast Reconstr Surg 1991;7(2):141–143

33. Gayton JL, Ledford JK. Angle closure glaucoma following a combined blepharoplasty and ectropion repair. Ophthal Plast Reconstr Surg 1992;8(3):176–177

34. Mahaffey PJ, Wallace AF. Blindness following cosmetic blepharoplasty—a review. Br J Plast Surg 1986;39(2):213–221

35. Hartley JH Jr, Lester JC, Schatten WE. Acute retrobulbar hemorrhage during elective blepharoplasty. Its pathophysiology and management. Plast Reconstr Surg 1973;52(1):8–15

36. Kelly PW, May DR. Central retinal artery occlusion following cosmetic blepharoplasty. Br J Ophthalmol 1980;64(12):918–922

37. Moser MH, DiPirro E, McCoy FJ. Sudden blindness following blepharoplasty. Report of seven cases. Plast Reconstr Surg 1973;51(4):364–370

38. Goldberg RA, Marmor MF, Shorr N, Christenbury JD. Blindness following blepharoplasty: two case reports, and a discussion of management. Ophthalmic Surg 1990;21(2):85–89

39. Heinze JB, Hueston JT. Blindness after blepharoplasty: mechanism and early reversal. Plast Reconstr Surg 1978;61(3):347–354

40. Cruz AA, Andó A, Monteiro CA, Elias J Jr. Delayed retrobulbar hematoma after blepharoplasty. Ophthal Plast Reconstr Surg 2001;17(2):126–130

41. Hass AN, Penne RB, Stefanyszyn MA, Flanagan JC. Incidence of postblepharoplasty orbital hemorrhage and associated visual loss. Ophthal Plast Reconstr Surg 2004;20(6):426–432

42. Callahan MA. Prevention of blindness after blepharoplasty. Ophthalmology 1983;90(9):1047–1051

43. Castañares S. Complications in blepharoplasty. Clin Plast Surg 1978;5(1):139–165

44. Baylis HI, Sutcliffe T, Fett DR. Levator injury during blepharoplasty. Arch Ophthalmol 1984;102(4):570–571

45. Smith B. Postsurgical complications of cosmetic blepharoplasty. Trans Am Acad Ophthalmol Otolaryngol 1969;73(6):1162–1164

46. Levine MR, Davies R, Ross J. Chemosis following blepharoplasty: an unusual complication. Ophthalmic Surg 1994;25(9):593–596

47. Enzer YR, Shorr N. Medical and surgical management of chemosis after blepharoplasty. Ophthal Plast Reconstr Surg 1994;10(1):57–63

48. Goldberg RA, Li TG. Postoperative infection with group A beta-hemolytic *Streptococcus* after blepharoplasty. Am J Ophthalmol 2002;134(6):908–910

49. Ray AM, Bressler K, Davis RE, Gallo JF, Patete ML. Cervicofacial necrotizing fasciitis. A devastating complication of blepharoplasty. Arch Otolaryngol Head Neck Surg 1997;123(6):633–636

50. Suñer IJ, Meldrum ML, Johnson TE, Tse DT. Necrotizing fasciitis after cosmetic blepharoplasty. Am J Ophthalmol 1999;128(3):367–368

51. Bisno AL, Stevens DL. Streptococcal infections of skin and soft tissues. N Engl J Med 1996;334(4):240–245

52. Rees TD, Craig SM, Fisher Y. Orbital abscess following blepharoplasty. Plast Reconstr Surg 1984;73(1):126–127

53. Robb RM. Refractive errors associated with hemangiomas of the eyelids and orbit in infancy. Am J Ophthalmol 1977;83(1):52–58

54. Stigmar G, Crawford JS, Ward CM, Thomson HG. Ophthalmic sequelae of infantile hemangiomas of the eyelids and orbit. Am J Ophthalmol 1978;85(6):806–813

55. Schwartz SR, Kodsi SR, Blei F, Ceisler E, Steele M, Furlan L. Treatment of capillary hemangiomas causing refractive and occlusional amblyopia. J AAPOS 2007;11(6):577–583

56. Brown MS, Siegel IM, Lisman RD. Prospective analysis of changes in corneal topography after upper eyelid surgery. Ophthal Plast Reconstr Surg 1999;15(6):378–383

57. Rees TD. The "dry eye" complication after a blepharoplasty. Plast Reconstr Surg 1975;56(4):375–380

58. Shorr N, Goldberg RA, McCann JD, Hoenig JA, Li TG. Upper eyelid skin grafting: an effective treatment for lagophthalmos following blepharoplasty. Plast Reconstr Surg 2003;112(5):1444–1448

59. McCord CD. (1982). Complications of Upper Eyelid Blepharoplasty. In Putterman AM, Cosmetic Oculoplastic Surgery. New York: Grune & Stratton, Inc.; 1982:249–274

60. Black EH, Gladstone GJ, Nesi FA. Eyelid sensation after supratarsal lid crease incision. Ophthal Plast Reconstr Surg 2002;18(1):45–49

61. Joshi AS, Janjanin S, Tanna N, Geist C, Lindsey WH. Does suture material and technique really matter? Lessons learned from 800 consecutive blepharoplasties. Laryngoscope 2007;117(6):981–984

8

Complications of Lower Eyelid Blepharoplasty

Robert A. Goldberg

Complications are an inevitable part of surgery, and eyelid surgery is no exception. Despite the best efforts during preparation, events may not unfold as planned, and unanticipated complications unavoidably occur. A thorough knowledge of potential complications in order of likelihood and importance is paramount for achieving the best possible outcome, not simply to minimize the occurrence of these events but also to provide the best evaluation and management of such events should they arise.

A meticulous preoperative evaluation is important, including an appropriate ocular examination and an assessment of the patient's expectations. The practitioner should assess and document any factors that may affect surgical outcome, such as previous surgery, orbicularis and facial nerve function, lagophthalmos, tear film instability, prominent eye configuration, and preexisting chemosis or edema. If possible, the use of anticoagulation should be discontinued to decrease the risk of intraoperative and postoperative bleeding.

◆ Diplopia

Diplopia after blepharoplasty may be a consequence of edema, and it often resolves with time.[1] Diplopia may also occur from extraocular muscle injury from anesthesia, intramuscular hemorrhage and edema, and cicatricial changes within the muscle or adjacent connective tissues.[1-3] Management of postblepharoplasty diplopia should be conservative, with the use of corticosteroids as appropriate. In rare cases the diplopia may be permanent and require muscle surgery to reduce the symptoms of double vision.

◆ Hematoma

Postoperative hemorrhage can occur with blepharoplasty, with sequelae ranging from annoyance to loss of vision. The bleeding is most often from the vessels associated with the orbicularis.[4] Only in rares cases are the deep orbital vessels the source of postoperative bleeding.

◆ Superficial Hematoma

Following cutaneous lower blepharoplasty, bleeding can lift the flap from the underlying septum and orbital fat. This presents as a superficial hemorrhage or organized hematoma. It can be differentiated from orbital hemorrhage by the absence of proptosis, decreased extraocular motility, bloody chemosis, and deep orbital pain. Hemorrhage below the skin flap results in increased postoperative inflammation. If there is substantial inflammation in the plane of the orbicularis and orbital septum, the risk of postoperative fibrosis and of eyelid retraction is increased.

Treatment of superficial hematoma is primarily conservative. The use of orticosteroids should be considered to break the cycle of inflammation and decrease the risk of lower eyelid retraction. After five to seven days, eyelid massage with lower eyelid stretch elevation can be employed, and for early chemosis with lower eyelid retraction in the first week, temporary tarsorrhaphy with eyelid suspension sutures to the eyebrow should be considered.

A substantial localized hematoma that is organizing should be drained, consistent with surgical principles of any facial flap surgery (**Fig. 8.1**).

◆ Deep Orbital Hemorrhage and Vision Loss

The deep orbital hemorrhage is the most worrisome postoperative complication of blepharoplasty: arterial pressure can build up in the closed compartment of

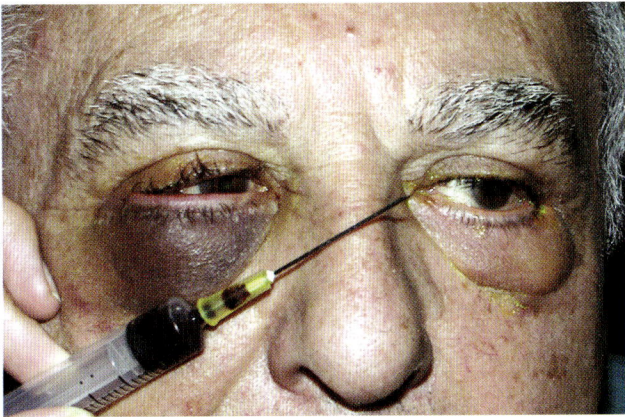

Fig. 8.1 A superficial hematoma usually resolves spontaneously, but an organized hematoma should be drained. Used with permission from Regents of the University of California, Copyright 2009.

the orbit.[5] If the orbital pressure rises above the capillary filling pressure of the posterior ciliary arteries (or less likely, the central retinal artery), there is potential for ischemia of the optic nerve and retina, which can lead to loss of vision. Treatment of orbital hemorrhage is emergent. Permanent ischemic damage can occur in 90 minutes or perhaps even less. The symptoms of orbital hemorrhage include severe deep orbital pressure, pain, and nausea; firm orbit with proptosis; limitation of extraocular movement; hemorrhagic chemosis; and decreased or lost vision with unresponsive pupils (afferent pupillary defect). When orbital hemorrhage is causing ischemic optic or retinal changes, urgent treatment to decrease the orbital pressure and restore capillary perfusion is required. Opening the wound and releasing any clots is the first-line treatment and is almost always effective; it may be necessary to spread gently within the orbital tissues to release any loculated hemorrhage. Lateral cantholysis with complete release of the lateral canthal tendon is the next step in the ladder of treatment. In rare cases, bony orbital decompression could be considered. Pericentesis (removing fluid from the anterior chamber) should be considered only as a last resort. Pain and anxiety should be treated. Hypertension should be treated, although an abrupt severe reduction in blood pressure could theoretically compromise arterial filling pressure. Medical treatment of the orbital pressure, including steroids, osmotics such as mannitol, and diuretics such as acetazolamide, can be started, but their use should not delay the implementation of surgical reduction of orbital pressure. Because of the importance of early treatment, both the patient and the staff should understand the significance and urgency of the symptoms of orbital hemorrhage.

◆ Dry Eye and Chemosis

Dry eye symptoms are common after blepharoplasty, and chemosis occurs in a significant percentage of patients with dry eye after blepharoplasty.[6–8] Risk factors include previous history of dry eye or ocular surface disorders, previous LASIK refractive surgery, and mechanical factors predisposing the patient to poor blink function (prominent eye, lower eyelid laxity, orbicularis weakness, neurologic or myogenic conditions affecting blinking or eye movements, or Graves' orbitopathy). In this setting, the term dry eye is a misnomer, because these patients usually have adequate tear production. In fact, their eyes are often wet or tearing because of reflex tear production in response to irritation. The mechanism of surface irritation and dry eye symptoms following blepharoplasty relates to dysfunction of the tear-spreading or "windshield wiper" function of the eyelid. Loss of the squeegee effect of the normal blink leads to disruption of the smooth tear film, abnormal evaporation of tears, symptoms of blurred vision (related to loss of the smooth tear film surface), and foreign body sensation or burning pain. The resulting inflammation, potentially combined with generalized postoperative swelling, leads to conjunctival swelling or chemosis. When the conjunctiva becomes chemotic, it creates an additional mechanical impediment to the ability of the eyelid to create a smooth tear film. A vicious cycle of increasing chemosis can occur, leading to mechanical disruption and drying out of the ocular surface (**Fig. 8.2**).

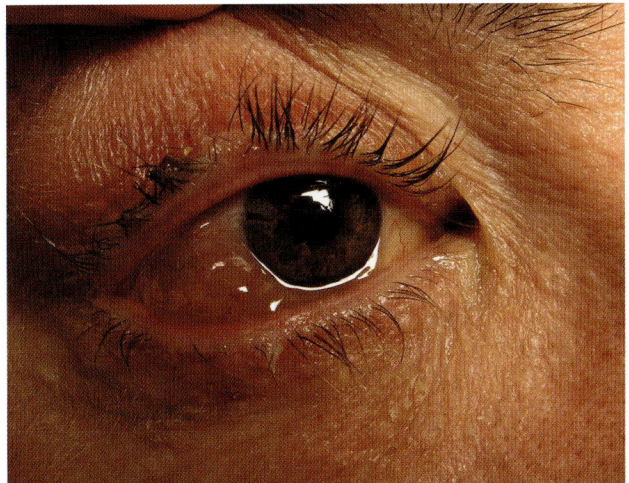

Fig. 8.2 Conjunctival chemosis relates to general edema and also to abnormal eyelid tone with failure of mechanical protection. Used with permission from Regents of the University of California, Copyright 2009.

Treatment of dry eye after blepharoplasty is accomplished in stepladder fashion. Prevention is important: appropriate lubrication of the ocular surface during and immediately after surgery is critical. Corneal shields protect the cornea from inadvertent injury, and their use is reasonable. However, because the shields can also irritate the cornea, some surgeons prefer to avoid their use. Protective shields should be used with copious lubrication. Neither soap nor betacaine should collect under the shield, and care should be taken to avoid inadvertently leaving the shield in after surgery. If dry eye develops, the first step in treatment is lubrication of the ocular surface with artificial teardrops and nocturnal ointment. Steroid eyedrops and ointments may provide some therapeutic anti-inflammatory effect, and oral steroids should be considered. (Be alert to the possibility of an allergic reaction to topical eye drops or ointments, which can exacerbate the inflammation and confound the diagnosis.) Humidifiers or plastic wrap dressings can be used at bedtime to maintain a moist ocular surface. More severe cases might require closing the eyelids, for example with a carefully applied patch or suture tarsorrhaphy.

◆ Wound Granulomata

The differential diagnosis of wound granulomata includes foreign body (including sutures), ointment granuloma related to the oily vehicle retained inside the tissues, and atypical infection (including mycobacteria).[8,9] Postoperative granulomata can be initially managed conservatively, for example with steroids or 5-FU injections, but persistent or atypical granulomata should be cultured for mycobacteria (**Fig. 8.3**).

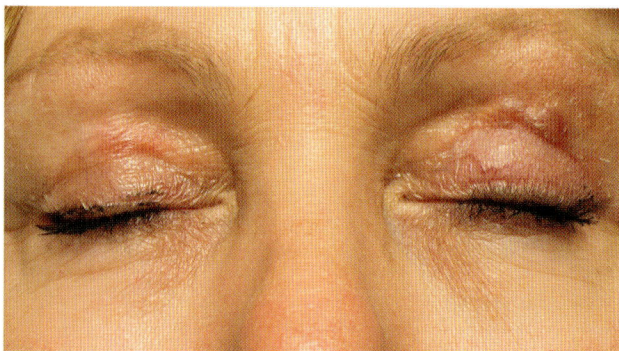

Fig. 8.3 Eyelid granulomas appearing two weeks after blepharoplasty surgery; I&D with culture revealed atypical mycobacteria. (*Used with permission from Regents of the University of California, Copyright 2009.*)

◆ Lower Eyelid Retraction

Lower eyelid retraction following blepharoplasty is a difficult problem. I am not aware of good data to assess the incidence of this complication accurately, but certainly it is the most frequent postsurgical referral in an urban ophthalmic plastic surgery practice: I see three to five new patients every week for consultation regarding management of eyelid malposition, contour problems, or ocular surface problems after blepharoplasty or midface surgery. These patients may be angry, frustrated, or despondent; in my experience, eyelid complications are a particularly difficult type of aesthetic surgery complication, because they not only change the appearance of the critically important periorbital aesthetic unit of the face but also create ophthalmic symptoms that can range from annoying to vision threatening.

In approaches to the patient with lower eyelid retraction after blepharoplasty, accurate diagnosis is the prelude to appropriate treatment. Every case must be individualized. The unique anatomy and physiology of every case will dictate a treatment plan that may draw from a wide spectrum of medical and surgical treatment options. There are many variations, but I suggest that the etiology of lower eyelid retraction following blepharoplasty can be divided into seven main categories, each of which should be assessed when the patient is evaluated:

1. Orbicularis paralysis
2. Anterior lamellar tightness
3. Middle lamellar tightness
4. Volume collapse
5. Relationship of the globe to its bony support
6. Horizontal laxity
7. Psychological stability and realistic expectations

In this section, I will review each of these mechanisms with particular attention to diagnosis and management. In managing the individual patient, the practitioner should assess the contribution of each of the various factors and then design an individualized treatment plan that treats each factor in proportion to its participation in the problem.

Orbicularis Paralysis

The physiology of the orbicularis oculi is one of Nature's wonders. Acting on the supple, independently functioning eyelid lamella, the delicate concentric rings of the orbicularis provide the blink reflex that spreads the corneal tear film to allow clear vision, drive the tear pump that drains tears out of the eye into the nasal lacrimal outflow system, and provide static tonic support for the lower eyelid. Although there is typically a fair amount of reserve strength, subtle weaknesses the orbicularis oculi can substantially affect eyelid position and function, especially in the face of postsurgical tightness or unfavorable globe to bony orbit relationship. I often note subtle or occasionally substantial orbicularis weakness in patients after blepharoplasty eyelid retraction. I believe that the orbicularis can be easily denervated by eyelid or midface procedures that cut across the lateral innervation. This is particularly true in patients who receive multiple operations: I presume that each surgical insult causes temporary weakness, with return of function in the months following surgery, but there would also be some degree of permanent loss of function that can accumulate with multiple operations.

Orbicularis paralysis is diagnosed by careful study of eyelid closure. Advanced paralysis is easily identified (but, in my experience, often overlooked). When the patient forcefully closes the eyelids, the examiner notes failure of the orbicularis muscle to bunch up, and the eyelid is easily distracted away from the globe by the examiner's finger (**Fig. 8.4**). More subtle orbicularis weakness can be identified by careful observation and palpation of the eyelid margin during forced closure. Sometimes the eyelid will evert on forced closure (**Fig. 8.5**). This type of "fish mouthing" is more common if there is some degree of coexisting horizontal laxity.

There is no great treatment for orbicularis paralysis. Fortunately, in a postsurgical setting the muscle function tends to regenerate, but this process can take many months. Therefore, in cases of orbicularis paralysis, time is on the patient's side, and often a conservative approach will reward the surgeon and patient with spontaneous improvement as the muscle function returns. For

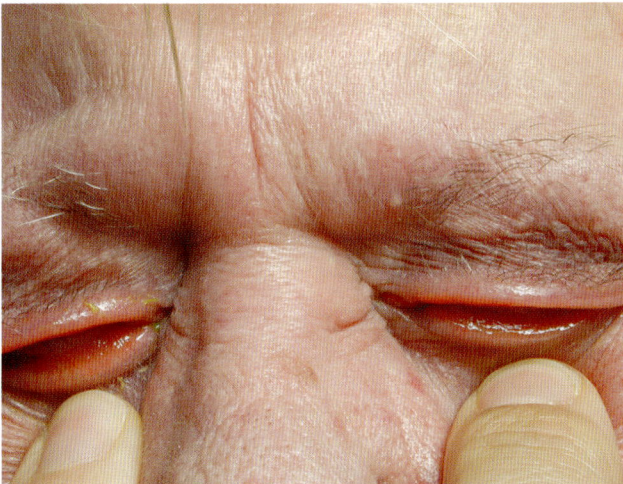

Fig. 8.5 Orbicularis weakness: The upper eyelid margin spontaneously everts during forced closure, suggesting weakness of the pretarsal orbicularis combined with static horizontal laxity. Used with permission from Regents of the University of California, Copyright 2009.

persistent orbicularis weakness, static horizontal slings and upper eyelid gold weights can sometimes be useful, but frankly no treatment is great or long lasting. Perhaps most importantly, if significant orbicularis paralysis is recognized, any further surgical interventions must be meticulously constructed to avoid further weakening of the muscle or interruption of the nerve supply.

Volume Collapse

In traditional blepharoplasty, skin, muscle, and fat are removed in various combinations. In the case of puffy or full eyelids, this can improve the patient's appearance. However, volume in the eyelid is important aesthetically and functionally, and volume collapse can not only create the aesthetic problem of a hollow, surgical appearing eyelid but also lead to functional problems.

If we remember the answer to the brain teaser that involves letting air out of the tires of the truck so that it could fit beneath the overpass, we will understand the role that a full inflated lower eyelid has in supporting the lower eyelid margin. Deflation of the eyelid, just like deflation of the truck tire, leads to lowering of the eyelid margin.

Volume of the eyelid affects function in another way. The eyelid is composed of multiple delicate lamellae that need to slide against each other and function independently for proper eyelid mechanics. When fat is removed, this buffer function can be lost, so that the eyelid lamellae no longer function independently. In the upper eyelid, this can lead to tethered ptosis or lagoph-

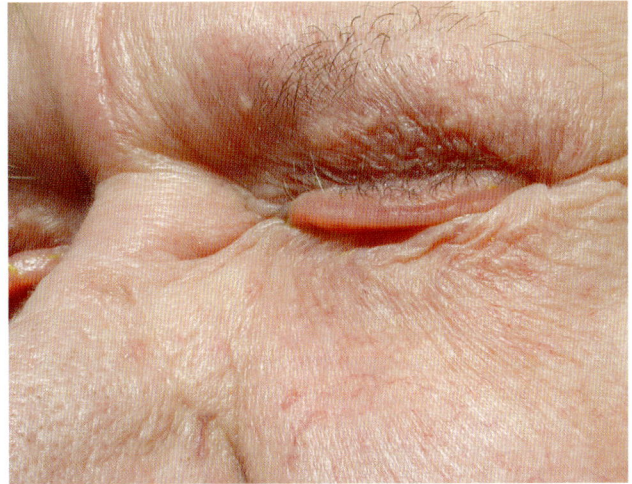

Fig. 8.4 Orbicularis weakness: The eyelid is easily distracted from the globe during attempted closure. Used with permission from Regents of the University of California, Copyright 2009.

thalmos. In the lower eyelid, it can lead to retraction and lagophthalmos, related to loss of excursion of the eyelid relative to the orbital rim and lower eyelid retractors.

Volume collapse is recognized clinically by noting a hollow or long eyelid (**Fig. 8.6**). By digitally elevating the lower eyelid, the examiner can sometimes sense the collapse of the various eyelid lamellae, so that the eyelid is rigid (cardboard eyelid). In the extreme situation, volume collapse is indistinguishable from shortening of the anterior and posterior lamellae, with the full-thickness eyelid plastered down to the orbital rim.

Treatment of volume collapse is difficult because we do not have technology to recreate the delicate lamellar layers of the eyelid. However, tissue grafts, carefully and delicately inserted, can sometimes allow improvement. Injected fat is difficult to use effectively in my experience; I have had better success using small pearls of free fat, placed in the plane of the lower eyelid retractors with minimal incisions (**Fig. 8.7A–D**). An alternative to surgery is the use of injectable synthetic fillers, such as hyaluronic acid gel. Although these are temporary, they can produce improvement of the eyelid hollowing that can last six months or more, the procedure is repeatable, and patients are often receptive to the idea of minimally invasive procedures that can be repeated over time (**Fig. 8.6**).

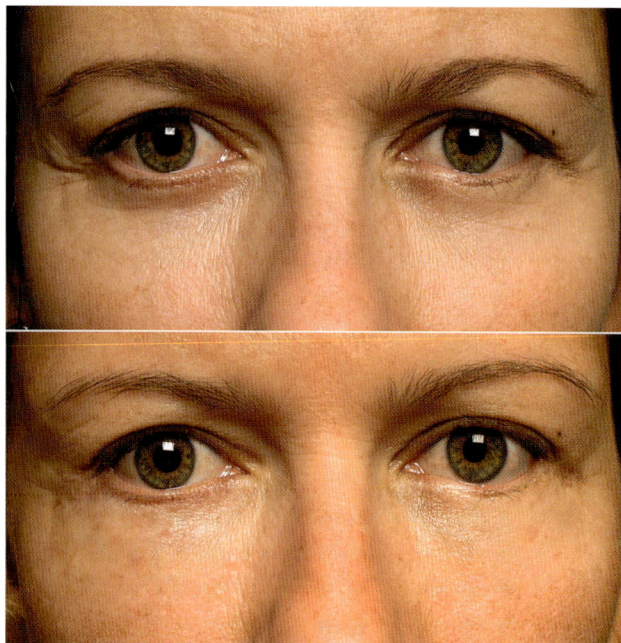

Fig. 8.6 *Top*: Volume collapse of the lower eyelid, recognized as a long eyelid with orbital hollowing. *Bottom*: Following hyaluronic acid gel filling of the retractor plane, improvement in eyelid support and volume is demonstrated. Used with permission from Regents of the University of California, Copyright 2009.

Horizontal Laxity

In the older patient population, horizontal eyelid laxity can play a role in lower eyelid retraction (**Fig. 8.8**). The diagnosis is straightforward: the snap test (distracting the eyelid from the globe and noting the rapidity with which it snaps back into position) and the distraction test (grasping the eyelashes and pulling the eyelid away from the globe) identifying abnormally lax eyelids. The normal eyelid should snap back, without blink, in a few seconds, and should not distract from the globe more than 5 to 7 mm.

If horizontal eyelid laxity is the primary cause of lower eyelid retraction, then horizontal eyelid shortening by tightening the lateral canthus should be curative. Unfortunately, after the patient has had blepharoplasty, it is rare in my experience that horizontal laxity is the primary culprit. Instead, vertical inadequacy, volume collapse, and orbicularis paralysis are usually contributing factors. For that reason, horizontal shortening alone typically provides only partial or minimal improvement and can even make things worse if the surgery further damages the function of the orbicularis. Tightening the "clothesline" when there are lots of clothes hanging on it will predictably fail: the lateral canthal tendon will not heal under excessive surgical tension, and the vertical forces will win the war (**Fig. 8.9**).

To help provide additional elevating power to the horizontal shortening, some surgeons place the canthal angle superiorly on the lateral orbital rim. There is some virtue to the physics of this, because the artificially elevated canthal tendon will drag the lower eyelid upward, reducing scleral show inferiorly. However, the resulting canthal dystopia is not only functionally suboptimal for the upper and lower eyelid function but distressingly disfiguring to the sophisticated patient, especially if it is asymmetric (**Fig. 8.10**).

If canthoplasty is to be performed, it should be conservative (over-tightening simply creates a wound under tension that will not heal properly) and should spare tissue (removing the tarsus leads in the long run to phimosis; **Fig. 8.11**). The approach should be designed to minimize extensive cutting across the orbicularis and its nerve supply: often there is already some orbicularis paralysis that reduces the available reserve function, and even subtle additional loss of orbicularis function can be significant. I most often use an upper eyelid crease incision, which allows access to the common tendon at the lateral rim; the retinaculum can be released as needed, and the cut end of the tendon can be re-attached to the arcus marginalis using sutures placed directly into the tendon, through the gray line with a double-armed suture (**Fig. 8.12**).

Anterior Lamellar Shortening

The lower eyelid anterior lamella consists of the skin and the orbicularis. Vertical inadequacy of the anterior lamella can be diagnosed with the forced upward

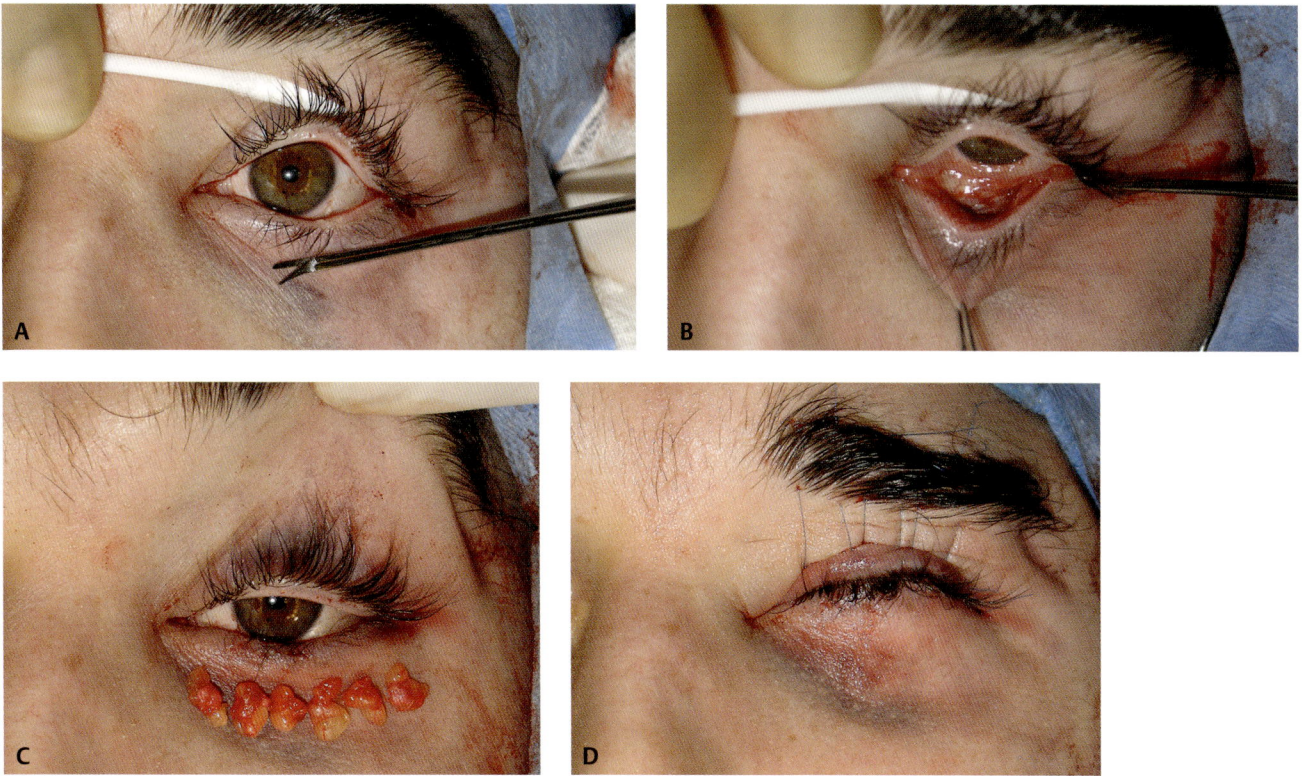

Fig. 8.7 (A–D) After en-glove lysis of the contracted middle lamellar scar, a dermis strip or pearl fat grafts are placed across the plane of the lower retractors, and the eyelid sutured to the eyebrow on stretch for seven to ten days. Used with permission from Regents of the University of California, Copyright 2009.

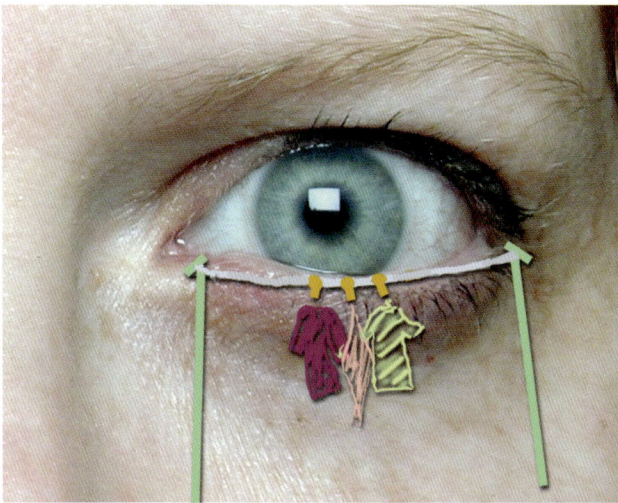

Fig. 8.8 The normal eyelid is like a clothesline with few clothes. Used with permission from Regents of the University of California, Copyright 2009.

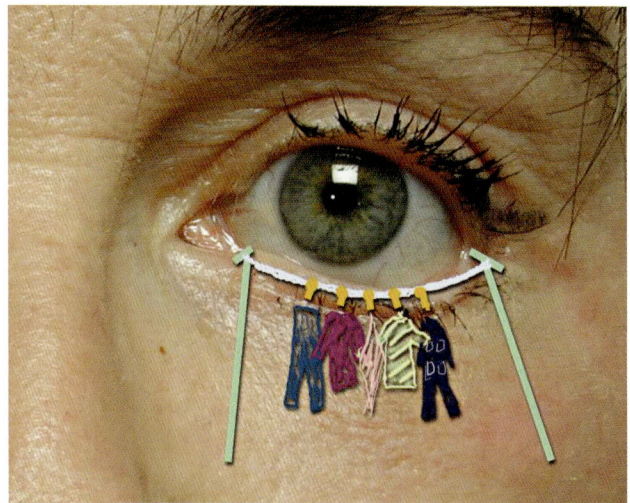

Fig. 8.9 The tight postoperative eyelid has active vertical force, like a clothesline with many clothes. Used with permission from Regents of the University of California, Copyright 2009.

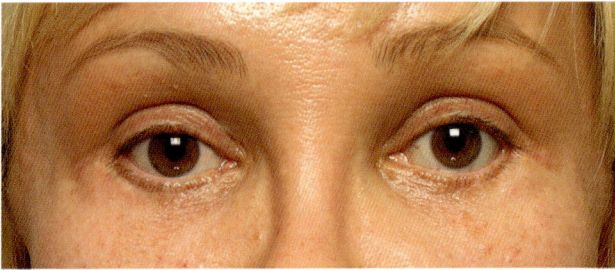

Fig. 8.10 Canthal dystopia with unnatural superior displacement to the right more than the left side, following canthoplasty with vertical placement. Used with permission from Regents of the University of California, Copyright 2009.

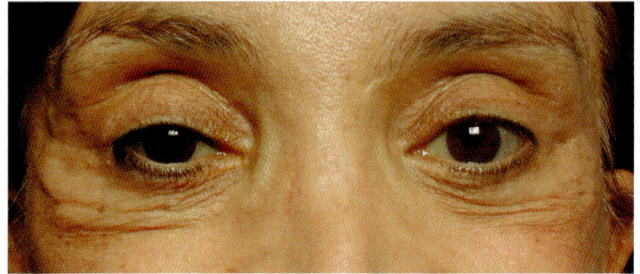

Fig. 8.11 Horizontal phimosis right side, following multiple canthoplasties with tarsal removal. Phimosis relates to inadequate lateral tarsus, so that no amount of lateral tightening will open the canthal angle. This patient also demonstrates segmental orbicularis paralysis. Used with permission from Regents of the University of California, Copyright 2009.

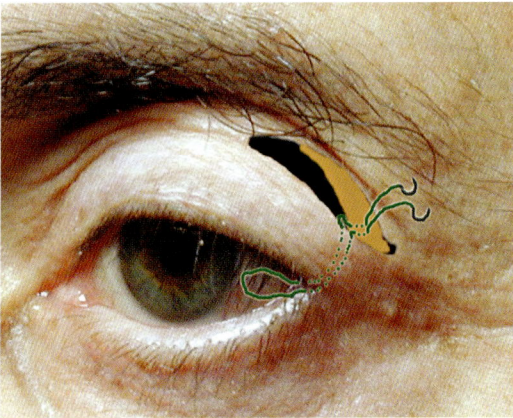

Fig. 8.12 Configuration of lateral canthal reattachment performed through a small upper eyelid crease incision, using a suture externalized through a stab incision in the gray line of the eyelid margin. Used with permission from Regents of the University of California, Copyright 2009.

phimosis is destined to fail if the tissues are tight and the wound is being closed under tension.

Treatment of anterior lamellar vertical inadequacy traditionally involves skin grafting. Skin grafting is not ideal in the aesthetic patient after blepharoplasty: although the skin graft, with luck, can heal fairly well, it is rarely invisible. Importantly, when there is some orbicularis paralysis, the skin graft can further decrease the function of the orbicularis, both because the muscle must be exposed and manipulated to place the graft, and also because the graft itself will always be stiffer than the original supple skin that it replaces, decreasing the effective functioning of the orbicularis.

Supplying anterior lamella by elevating the midface is the preferred technique for addressing anterior lamellar inadequacy in a patient after blepharoplasty. Numerous approaches have been described; I prefer the subperiosteal approach, using incisions that minimize additional trauma to the orbicularis (such as the temporal endoscopic approach) (**Fig. 8.14**). Unfortunately, severe sun damage with tissue laxity, atonicity related to the zygomatic nerve damage, or a bony disadvantage related to relatively small maxilla are factors that will decrease the success and longevity of midface lifting. The anticipation that repeat procedures might be necessary should be additional stimulus to the surgeon to identify minimally invasive approaches.

Middle Lamellar Shortening

Vertical inadequacy of the middle lamella, like anterior lamellar shortening, is diagnosed by the forced upward traction test: if the eyelid does not come up when anterior lamella is supplied, then a middle lamellar tether is present. Middle lamellar tethering occurs when the orbital septum is shortened, and it is strongly influenced by volume collapse, with loss of the orbital fat

traction test. The examiner digitally elevates the eyelid; normally, it should not take much force to lift the lower eyelid to the superior corneal limbus. If resistance is encountered, then the next step is to determine whether the vertical inadequacy is in the anterior lamella or in the middle lamella. By supplying cheek tissue, either by manually elevating the cheek or by asking the patient to smile and allowing the patient's orbicularis to do the work, the examiner can repeat the test can determine if the result normalizes (suggesting an anterior lamellar problem) or if the eyelid is still tethered (suggesting a middle lamellar tightness).

Rounding of the lateral canthal angle is often evidence of anterior lamellar inadequacy, with an inferolateral vector (**Fig. 8.13**). Tightening the canthus against an active cicatrix in an effort to improve the rounding and

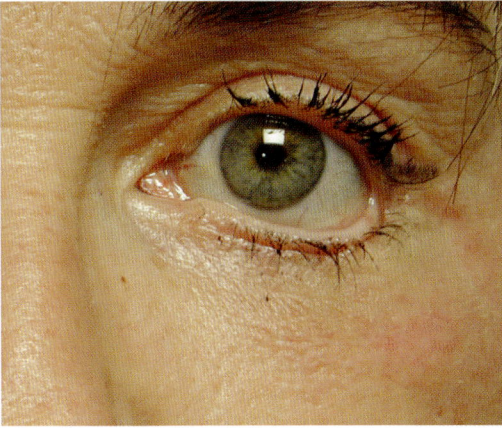

Fig. 8.13 Anterior lamella shortening with rounding of the lateral canthal angle related to inferolateral vector shortening. Used with permission from Regents of the University of California, Copyright 2009.

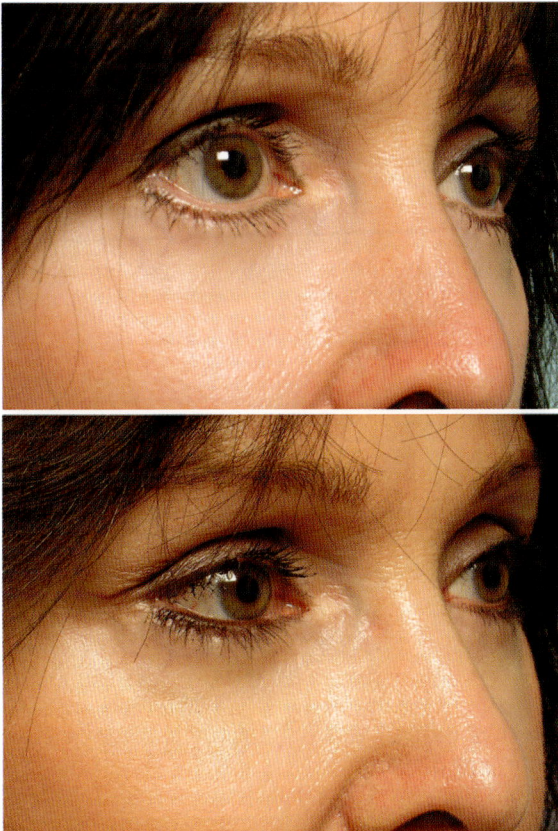

Fig. 8.14 Patient shown before and seven months after endoscopic subperiosteal midface lift, hidden temporal incision in the hair, designed to support the midface and provide anterior lamella to the lower eyelid. Used with permission from Regents of the University of California, Copyright 2009.

buffer between the septum, retractors, and orbital rim. Therefore, cutting through the septum and removing orbital fat, as performed in the standard transcutaneous blepharoplasty, is a common mechanism for production of middle lamellar tether.

It is very rare for the actual posterior lamella or conjunctiva to play a role in vertical inadequacy. The conjunctiva is quite redundant as it sweeps across the inferior fornix and onto the bulbar surface. Therefore, procedures that lengthen the posterior lamella, such as mucosal or hard palate grafts, will not by themselves address middle lamellar tether. Instead, the middle lamellar scar tissue has to be released (preferably with as little collateral damage as possible) and then both the anatomy and the biology of the situation optimally arranged to reduce the risk of further scar formation. Spacer grafts, such as hard palate mucosa or ear cartilage, may vertically stent the eyelid and decrease the early tendency for the scar to recur, but I have seen many cases in which these grafts enmeshed in recurrent scar tissue, with no improvement in retraction. Adding a volume buffer such as cheek fat or free fat may improve the situation by reinflating the eyelid and providing a buffer between the tissue planes. Unfortunately, despite nonspecific anti-inflammatories such as steroids, or anti-metabolites such as 5-FU or mitomycin C, we have no uniformly predictable tools to affect the biology of wound healing. In difficult cases that receive multiple operations, the biologic tendency for scar tissue to recur is what defeats us.

Relationship of the Globe to Its Bony Support

The mechanics of the lower eyelid are dependent on the relationship of the globe to its bony support. When the inferior-lateral orbital rim is relatively posterior to the cornea, for example related to development (congenital prominent eye), proptosis (for example Graves orbitopathy) or aging, then the lower eyelid is at a mechanical disadvantage to cover the cornea. These patients often demonstrate inferior scleral show even before any blepharoplasty is performed. The youthful eyelid that has not been operated on has enough reserve vertical elasticity and orbicularis support to protect the cornea and provide a tear pump even when the globe is relatively prominent. However, when disadvantaged by a relatively prominent globe, the eyelid has less reserve. As a result, subtle loss of orbicularis function or stiffening of the vertical elasticity will more easily create symptomatic eyelid retraction and tear film problems.

There is no easy treatment for lower eyelid retraction in the patient with prominent eyes. Recognizing this configuration preoperatively and designing conservative surgery are the take-home lesson. One option for treating lower eyelid retraction in the prominent globe patient is to address the relative proptosis via orbital surgery. Orbital decompression, using minimally invasive techniques, can be appropriately considered in selected cases. Removing fat from behind the globe reduces proptosis and provides a potential source of fat grafting to address any coexistent volume collapse of the eyelid, but with increased risk compared with removal of anterior fat (traditional blepharoplasty), including increased risk of double vision (**Fig. 8.15**).

Psychological Factors

Psychological factors play an important role in aesthetic surgical practice, as any experienced practitioner knows well. An unhappy patient after blepharoplasty with functional and aesthetic eyelid problems is particularly vulnerable. For reasons that psychologists and psychiatrists could presumably elucidate better than I, the eyes seemed to be a particularly sensitive areas not only regarding physical discomfort (if you have ever scratched your cornea, you understand this) but also regarding emotional discomfort. In my experience, these patients are often depressed, anxious, angry, and frightened. Obviously, support from the physician and staff is a critical first step in rebuilding the confidence, trust, and optimism that will allow the patient to heal over time. There should be a low threshold for obtaining consultation from professional therapists. The better the the management of the emotional state of the patient, the more likely it will be that the patient will accept the incremental improvements that we can achieve through stage treatment as positive forward steps.

Lower eyelid retraction following blepharoplasty is a difficult problem. Because of the complex physiology of the lower eyelids and the substantial variations of normal anatomy, an individualized approach to diagnosis and treatment is required. Analyzing the contributions of orbicularis paralysis, anterior and middle lamellar tightness, volume collapse, relationship of the globe to its bony support, and horizontal laxity will lead to a customized diagnosis and individualized treatment plan. Surgeries should be carefully designed to minimize the risk of additional collateral damage to the remaining normal tissues. These patients not only have delicate and fragile eyelid anatomy and physiology, but also have a delicate emotional state: a supportive environment and appropriate use of professional counseling are important.

Patient expectations have to be managed: it is not realistic to expect to cure these patients. Fortunately, by employing a thoughtful, problem-oriented, customized, stepwise approach, the surgeon can usually achieve functional and aesthetic improvement in eyelid retraction after blepharoplasty.

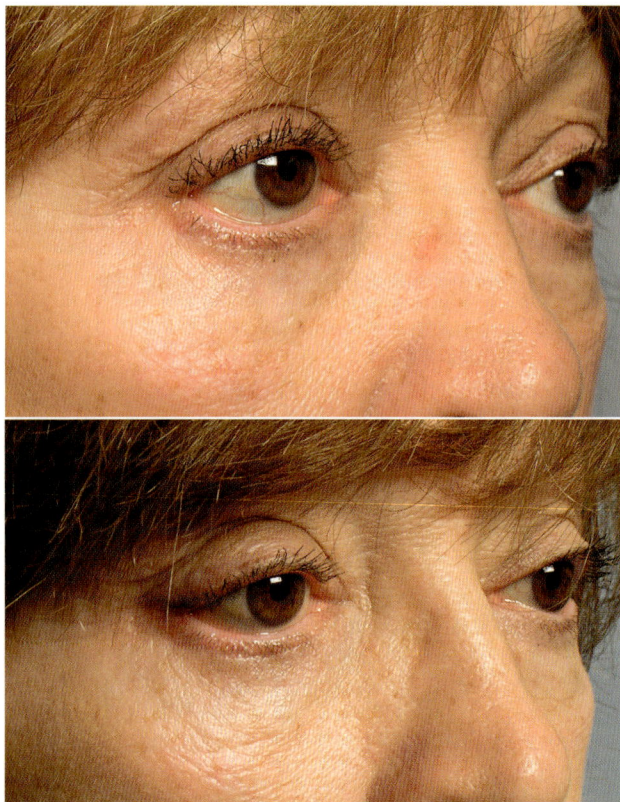

Fig. 8.15 Patient with relatively prominent globe, seen before and after intraconal fat harvest (which reduced the proptosis by 2 mm) and en-glove lower eyelid lysis with placement of the harvested intraconal fat as a free graft. Used with permission from Regents of the University of California, Copyright 2009.

◆ Conclusion

Annoying complications of blepharoplasty are common; fortunately, ocular surface irritation, early paralysis, swelling and chemosis, wound granulomas, and early asymmetries usually respond to conservative management.

The nightmare complication of blepharoplasty is blindness, produced by orbital hemorrhage. The symptoms and signs of increased orbital pressure (and their urgency) should be familiar both to the patients and their families and to the physician's staff. When increased orbital pressure that threatens vision is diagnosed, rapid treatment might save the patient's vision.

Lower eyelid retraction is the most common serious complication of lower blepharoplasty. It causes include vertical shortening of tissues, volume collapse, and orbicularis weakness. Conservative surgery decreases the risk. Treatment is complex and should be customized to the individual patient's anatomic and physiologic features.

PEARLS OF WISDOM

The doctor, the patient, and the staff should know the symptoms and significance of orbital hemorrhage (pain, firm swelling, decreased vision, nausea).

Chemosis relates to dysfunctional blink and windshield wiper mechanism of the lower eyelid; lubrication and topical anti-inflammatory medications can help break the cycle until eyelid function returns.

Lower eyelid retraction has multiple potential causes, and treatment must be individualized.

Prominent eye configuration is a strong risk factor for complications and should be identified preoperatively.

Eyelid anatomy and physiology are delicate and easily disrupted; blepharoplasty surgery should be conservatively designed and meticulously performed to avoid over-resection and to minimize collateral tissue damage

References

1. Harley RD, Nelson LB, Flanagan JC, Calhoun JH. Ocular motility disturbances following cosmetic blepharoplasty. Arch Ophthalmol 1986;104(4):542–544
2. Ghabrial R, Lisman RD, Kane MA, Milite J, Richards R. Diplopia following transconjunctival blepharoplasty. Plast Reconstr Surg 1998;102(4):1219–1225
3. Syniuta LA, Goldberg RA, Thacker NM, Rosenbaum AL. Acquired strabismus following cosmetic blepharoplasty. Plast Reconstr Surg 2003;111(6):2053–2059
4. Sutcliffe T, Baylis HI, Fett D. Bleeding in cosmetic blepharoplasty: an anatomical approach. Ophthal Plast Reconstr Surg 1985;1(2):107–113
5. Goldberg RA, Marmor MF, Shorr N, Christenbury JD. Blindness following blepharoplasty: two case reports, and a discussion of management. Ophthalmic Surg 1990;21(2):85–89
6. Hamawy AH, Farkas JP, Fagien S, Rohrich RJ. Preventing and managing dry eyes after periorbital surgery: a retrospective review. Plast Reconstr Surg 2009;123(1):353–359
7. Weinfeld AB, Burke R, Codner MA. The comprehensive management of chemosis following cosmetic lower blepharoplasty. Plast Reconstr Surg 2008;122(2):579–586
8. Enzer YR, Shorr N. Medical and surgical management of chemosis after blepharoplasty. Ophthal Plast Reconstr Surg 1994;10(1):57–63
9. Douglas RS, Cook T, Shorr N. Lumps and bumps: late postsurgical inflammatory and infectious lesions. Plast Reconstr Surg 2003;112(7):1923–1928

9

Prevention and Management of Adverse Outcomes in Brow Rejuvenation

Randolph B. Capone

Surgical rejuvenation of the aging brow is straightforward in principle, with primary goals being upward repositioning of the lateral brow/upper eyelid complex and reduction in brow depressor muscle activity. When the procedure is undertaken on a suitable patient, the combination of anatomically appropriate dissection and bitemporal fixation should be free from complications, easy to undergo, appear natural, improve the aesthetics of the upper face, and be pleasing to the patient (**Fig. 9.1A–D**).

The operation itself is one of the safer cosmetic surgical procedures, typically devoid of the devastating complications that can be seen with other facial surgeries. Even so, there is no dispute over the importance of a well-performed browlift and its significant contribution to the overall appearance of the rejuvenated patient.[1] In this chapter, both the potential pitfalls of contemporary endoscopic browlifting and straightforward mitigation strategies are reviewed.

◆ A Brief History

Modern browlifting, like many facial surgery procedures, can trace its roots to a time of human conflict when combat-related deformities were abundant, with the first description of an aesthetic foreheadplasty in 1919 by Rene Passot.[2] Early emphasis was placed upon horizontal skin excisions to improve forehead furrows and lateral brow hooding, but repositioning techniques quickly emerged. These subsequent techniques described wide skin undermining, modifications to the brow depressor muscles, and eventual subgaleal dissection. By the latter half of the 20th century, descriptions of multiplanar brow dissection became commonplace, and the coronal browlift became the procedure of choice. In 1992 Isse and Vasconez introduced a minimally invasive technique of brow rejuvenation: the endoscopic foreheadplasty.[3–5] Although no single procedure has proven definitively to be the best for forehead rejuvenation,

the endoscopic browlift or a combination of the endoscopic and open trichophytic browlift has been widely embraced, challenging their predecessors in pursuit of the procedure of choice for brow rejuvenation.[6–11] Endoscopic brow rejuvenation is the focus of this chapter.

◆ Patient Selection and General Considerations

Rejuvenation of the aging brow is not complex in nature; however, there are pitfalls to avoid in the quest for the ideal result. Prevention of a bad outcome starts with appropriate patient selection and a thorough preoperative evaluation. Poor patient selection, that is, performing the wrong operation on an inappropriate patient, is often at fault. The surgeon should always strive to avoid this situation by selecting the correct operation for an appropriate patient.

The prospective browlift patient should be healthy enough to undergo the proposed operation and the accompanying level of anesthesia, and it is incumbent upon the operating surgeon to discover any medical or psychiatric history that could lead to a contrary result. A history of poor wound healing, chronic steroid use, brittle diabetes mellitus, inability to lie supine, dry eyes, or frontal bone fibrous dysplasia may alter the surgical plan. A history of prior forehead surgery or injury (craniofacial trauma, frontal sinus fracture, forehead or temple skin cancer reconstruction, paramedian forehead flap, osteoplastic flap, CN VII injury, scalp avulsion or extensive laceration, or hair transplantation) may also require a change in the rejuvenation strategy. Communication with the patient's primary care physician or consultation with a medical specialist is important if there is any doubt regarding the patient's prior medical history. As with all surgical procedures, it is prudent to communicate any concerns regarding anesthesia (airway compromise, vocal fold motion impairment, sleep apnea, prior difficult intubation, prior cervical spine

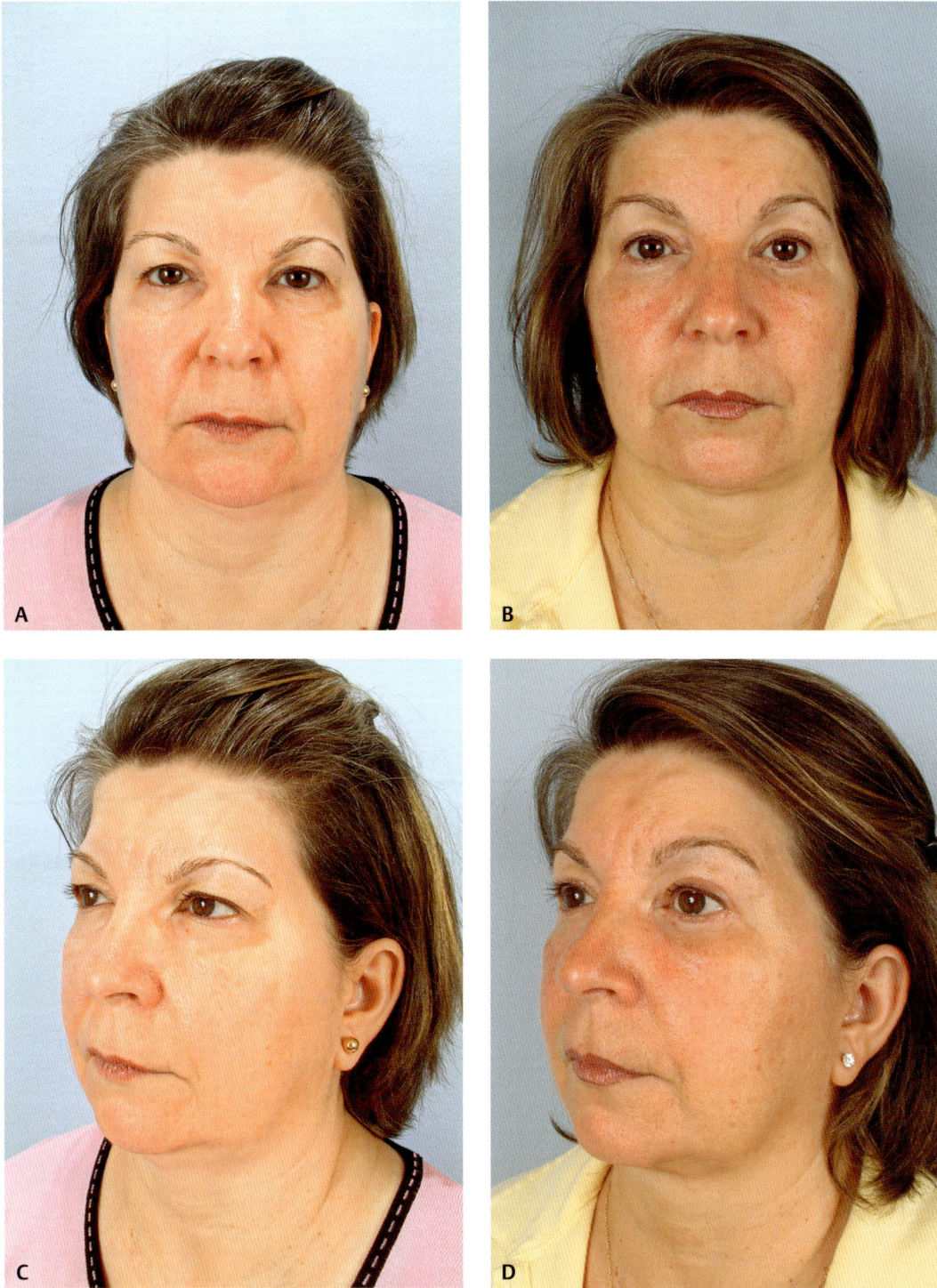

Fig. 9.1 Patient before **(A, C)** and after **(B, D)** endoscopic browlift with upper blepharoplasty.

surgery, latex allergy, family history of malignant hyperthermia or pseudocholinesterase deficiency, etc.) to the anesthesiologist. In other words, always attempt to forecast obstacles from induction to recovery. It is ultimately better to refuse to perform the browlift or to alter strategy than to proceed in an unsafe or uncertain fashion.

While talking with prospective browlift patients, obtain a sense of their motivations for and expectations of surgical rejuvenation. Do they seem appropriate and realistic? Often, the patients most enamored with their surgical experience have the most realistic expectations at the outset. Many individuals may initially be surprised by your suggestion of a browlift, thinking that their upper eyelids are the sole problem. Patients are often unaware of the link between upper eyelid aging and brow ptosis. If they have eyelid ptosis (e.g., levator dehiscence) or excess skin (blepharoptosis), the eyelids may indeed be at issue, but it is the surgeon's responsibility to educate the patient sufficiently about the effects of brow ptosis and its contribution to an aged eyelid appearance. The patient needs to know what a browlift is, why it is being proposed, how it is achieved, and what it might look like once it is performed. It is incumbent upon the surgeon to explain how a browlift augments facial rejuvenation as a whole when it is performed in concert with other procedures, especially blepharoplasty and rhytidectomy.

The surgeon must also openly discuss the effect that a browlift may have on the patient's hairline. If the patient has a high hairline, forehead shortening may need to be utilized.[12] Too often the forehead shortening modification is overlooked, contributing to inappropriate hairline elevation. If the patient has alopecia or pattern baldness, a standard endoscopic approach may not be indicated, and incision orientation and/or browlift technique may need to be altered (e.g., midforehead or transblepharoplasty). Spending time discussing these myriad topics during the consultation will go far to educate patients and crystallize their postoperative expectations, which will ultimately lead to enhanced patient satisfaction.

The Brow Exam

The old idiom "forewarned is forearmed" is particularly appropriate with regard to cosmetic surgery, and a thorough physical examination is the surgeon's early warning system. With the relaxed patient directly in front of the examiner, the position and shape of the eyebrows as well as the location of the hairline and status of hair pattern (using the Norwood classification for males) should be noted.[13] Eyebrow position should be documented relative to the underlying bony brows. Note whether the patient exhibits exophthalmos, lateral canthal dystopia with inferior eyelid rounding, or a negative vector that might predispose him or her to exposure keratitis. Skin thickness, skin condition, alopecia, and any relevant scars

should be noted. Pay particular attention to the presence of eyebrow asymmetry, blepharoptosis, and superolateral orbital hooding. Is there evidence of eyelid ptosis accompanied by compensatory brow elevation? (**Fig. 9.2**) Is ptosis absent, but brow asymmetry present? (**Fig. 9.3**)

Surgeons must recognize that browlifting does not correct eyelid ptosis (**Fig. 9.4**), and those surgeons uncomfortable with ptosis repair should consider having an oculoplastic surgeon perform this concomitantly with the browlift.

After the inspection of the patient at rest, the practitioner should perform a dynamic exam. The mobility of the soft tissue envelope and the strength of the frontalis, corrugator supercilii, procerus, and orbicularis oculi muscles should be assessed. Is there evidence of frontotemporal branch weakness, or is there skin tethering suggestive of prior trauma? Is there any evidence of forehead lipomata or cystic masses? The bony brow and the frontal skull should be palpated to ensure there are no irregularities (e.g., osteomata) that may hamper brow rejuvenation.

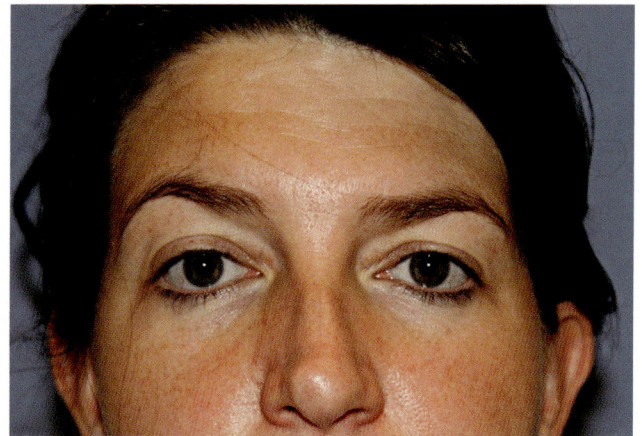

Fig. 9.2 Illustration of right-sided ptosis with compensatory frontalis muscle hyperfunction.

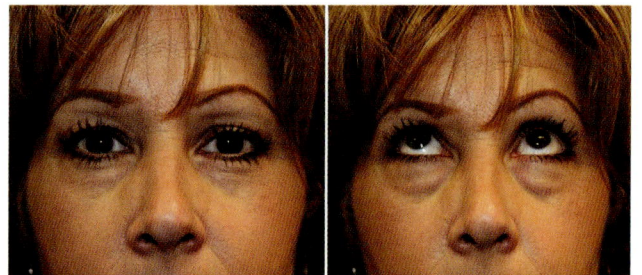

Fig. 9.3 Patient with right frontotemporal nerve palsy and brow asymmetry, elicited more dramatically on upward gaze.

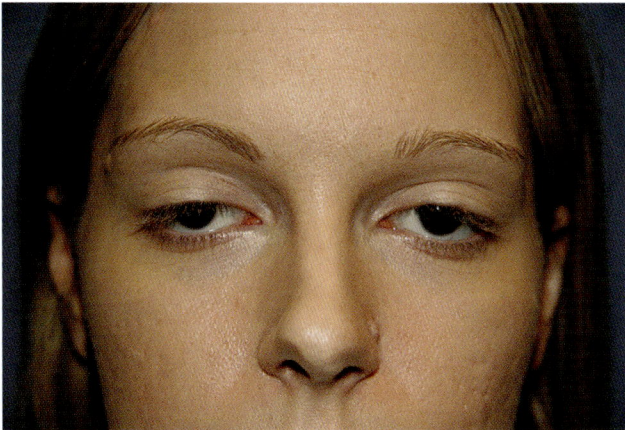

Fig. 9.4 Patient with bilateral eyelid ptosis.

Photographic documentation should be performed next. Studying the patient's preoperative photographs often provides the surgeon with additional information, as they are a good supplement to the physical examination. The images should be reviewed with the patient, and any preexisting asymmetries, ptosis, scars, alopecia, hairline position, etc. should be clearly illustrated, openly discussed, and thoroughly documented. Lastly, providing there is consent to do so, before and after photographs of *other* browlift patients should be reviewed with the patient. This review will help candidates for surgery to bring their expectations of benefit into better focus.

◆ Browlift Pitfalls

As Withey et al. pointed out in their review of 100 endoscopic browlifts, no in-depth studies of the complication rates of this operation have been published.[14] Even so, adverse outcomes do occur and are generally attributable to one or more of the following: (1) inappropriate surgical technique, (2) inappropriate surgical judgment, (3) inappropriate recovery, or (4) inappropriate patient expectations. Regarding expectations, patients must firmly understand that the goal of a browlift is not perfection but rather improvement that has a natural appearance. Therefore, preoperative discussion and counseling are absolute necessities. This allows prospective browlift patients to develop appropriate expectations and leads to increased satisfaction with the outcome. As indicated previously in this text, Dr. Eugene Kern advises that preoperative preparation should be taken a step further, by preparing the patient for a second operation (i.e., revision) before performance of the first.[15] Problems in recovery are avoided with prudent

patient selection and careful postoperative care, while solid surgical experience and careful preparation will help the surgeon avoid perturbations in judgment (for example, doing an endobrowlift without the forehead lowering modification in a patient already self-conscious about a high hairline).

Errors or inadequacies in browlift technique, which are myriad and are similarly minimized with impeccable training and increased experience with the operations, are the focus of the rest of this chapter (**Table 9.1**).

Facial Nerve Injury

In surgical brow repositioning, injury to the frontotemporal branches of the facial nerve is a serious concern; although it has not been definitively defined in the literature, its incidence is estimated at 3–5% (both transient and permanent cases). The surgeon can protect the frontotemporal branches and preserve the motion of the frontalis muscle by understanding the anatomy in this area.[16] After the main trunk of the facial nerve exits the stylomastoid foramen, the frontotemporal branch fibers depart the pes anserinus, coursing superiorly through the parotid gland and over the zygomatic arch, ultimately sending motor fibers to synapse with the frontalis and orbicularis oculi muscles (**Fig. 9.5**).

Table 9.1

Adverse Endoscopic Browlift Outcomes
Facial nerve injury (neuropraxia, axonotmesis, neurotmesis, brow ptosis)
Sensory nerve injury (paresthesias, formication, pruritus, chronic pain)
Inappropriate or inadequate fixation (quizzical look, stare, asymmetry)
Hardware failure (abrupted duration, foreign body reaction, exposure)
Infection
Forehead elongation
Alopecia
Telogen effluvium
Hairline distortion
Hematoma
Intracranial hemorrhage
Periocular venous congestion
Equipment failure

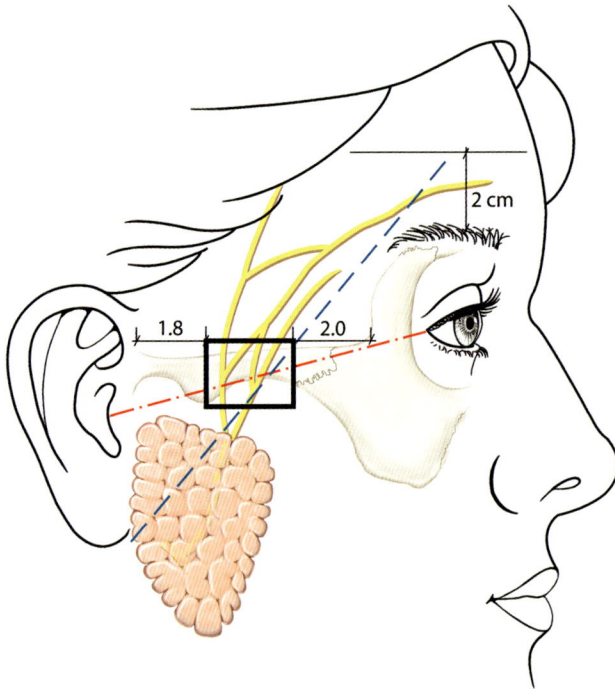

Fig. 9.5 Branches of the frontal division of the facial nerve (VII) relative to surface anatomy. The intersection of Pitanguy's line (blue) and the tragal canthal line (red) roughly approximates where the branches cross the middle third of the zygomatic arch (box). (*Illustration by Robert Brown*.)

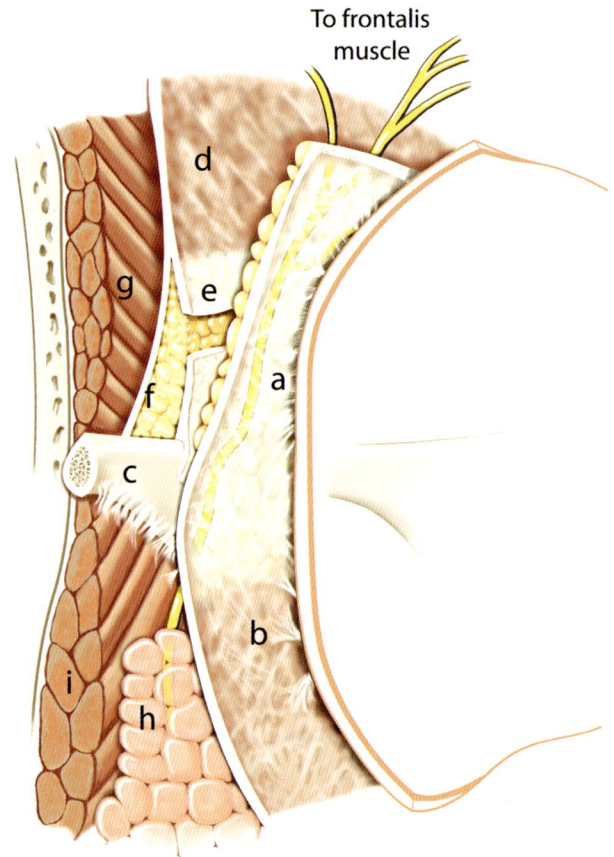

Fig. 9.6 Frontotemporal branches of the facial nerve travel from deep to superficial in their course from the pes anserinus to the frontalis muscle: (a) superficial temporal fascia, (b) SMAS, (c) zygomatic arch, (d) deep temporal fascia, (e) intermediate temporal fascia (superficial reflection of the deep temporal fascia), (f) deep reflection of the deep temporal fascia with the overlying intermediate fat pad, (g) temporalis muscle, (h) parotid gland, and (i) masseter muscle. (*Illustration by Robert Brown*.)

Anywhere from 2 to 5 rami cross superficial to the zygomatic arch at approximately the junction of the medial and middle thirds of the zygomatic arch, or approximately 2 cm lateral to the lateral orbital rim.[17–19] Neuropraxia, axonotmesis, or neurotmesis of these branches can occur from aggressive soft-tissue dissection, flap traction at the lateral brow, or dissection that strays too superficially (**Fig. 9.6**).

Injury will cause unilateral frontalis hypofunction, brow ptosis, accompanying brow asymmetry, and asymmetric relaxation of the forehead. Although complications are usually temporary (resolving in a matter of two to three months), permanent injury can also occur. Because the surgeon has little ability to manage this complication once it occurs, prevention is the key. Careful, controlled dissection in the subgaleal (subperiosteal) plane across the forehead and directly on the deep temporal fascia laterally is safe. Lysis of the conjoined tendon (where the deep temporal fascia fuses with the galea) should also be done with care, and minimal traction should be placed upon the flap during release of the arcus marginalis and lateral periorbital area. Release of these formidable periosteal reflections at the superolateral brow area can be achieved with partially open

Metzenbaum scissors in a controlled pushing fashion, rather than with excessively forceful blunt dissection. If motor nerve injury is diagnosed postoperatively, injection of botulinum toxin into the unaffected frontalis muscle can enhance symmetry while watchful waiting is undertaken. Reassuring the patient at frequent intervals while nerve function returns is mandatory.

Sensory Nerve Injury

Less worrisome to the surgeon (but not less bothersome from the patients' perspective) is injury to the supratrochlear and supraorbital nerves that convey sensation from the frontal scalp and forehead skin. Such injury can cause prolonged numbness, disturbing paresthesias (e.g., pins and needles, formication), bothersome scalp pruritus, and even chronic pain.[14] Careful understanding of the anatomic relationships of the sensory nerves, the corrugator supercilii muscle, and the frontalis muscle is essential to avoid complications. Typically, the supraorbital and supratrochlear nerves emanate from the skull via a foramen located within the supraorbital notch; however, in 10% of cases one or both nerves can emanate from a true foramen located outside of the notch (**Fig. 9.7**).[18]

Marking the supraorbital notch with a marking pen before injection of local anesthetic can be useful. Using the endoscope, the surgeon should watch for the presence of a true foramen and attempt to visualize the neurovascular bundles as they emanate from the corrugator supercilii muscles on the undersurface of the flap. Injury in a proximal location will result in altered sensorium across a wide distribution of the forehead and frontal scalp. Transient sensory loss in the vicinity of the endobrowlift incisions is expected, although the orientation of the midline and paramedian incisions should always be parallel to the nerve fibers to minimize the chance of transection. Patients should be informed of this.

If a hairline-lowering or hairline-preserving endobrowlift is performed, care must be taken to ensure that the skin excision is superficial to the frontalis muscle.[12] Almost always, however, excision of skin at the top of the forehead that accompanies this variation will result in numbness, paresthesia, and pruritus posterior to the incision, since the frontalis muscle attenuates superiorly, leaving the nerves vulnerable. Let patients know to expect this, but also inform them that it will typically become less bothersome and resolve over the course of a few months.

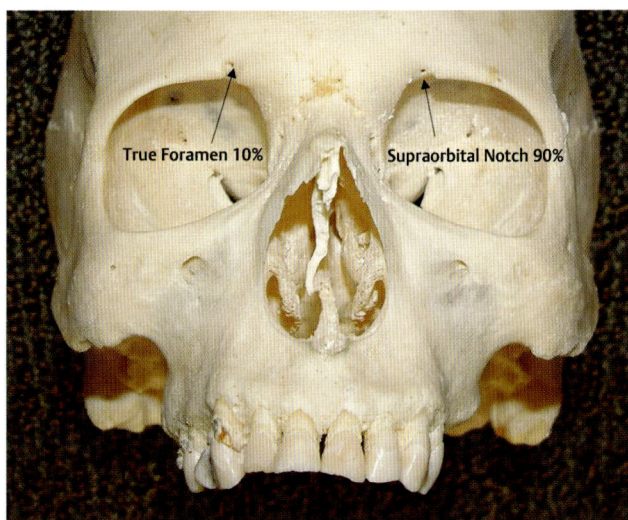

Fig. 9.7 Frontal view of human skull with a true supraorbital foramen on the right.

Venous Congestion

Another general landmark that has been described for identification of the frontotemporal branch of the facial nerve is the sentinel vein and associated bridging veins.[18,20] These veins can be observed endoscopically and course from the deep temporal fascia into the elevated flap at the temple and are associated with the position of the frontal branch. Disruption of these bridging vessels has been posited to cause another potential browlift complication: periocular venous congestion. Some authors report that this complication is significant enough to recommend preservation of these veins during endoscopic dissection.[21] No studies, however, illustrate long-term implications from periocular venous congestion after browlifting.

Hematoma and Infection

The scalp is richly vascularized, and traditional browlift methods (e.g., bicoronal incision) incurred a risk of hematoma from the lack of incisional hemostasis and persistent incisional bleeding. This typically necessitated hemostatic sutures to close the galea and scalp. Since the endoscopic browlift approach is less invasive, utilizing small incisions parallel to neurovascular structures, its chance of forming a hematoma is substantially less. Skin incision closure and gently compressive dressings placed at the conclusion of the case are typically all that are required to prevent hematoma complication. If a hematoma is recognized, it should be evacuated by opening of the closest incision or by serial aspiration.

Infection is also a rare complication of endoscopic browlift procedures. As previously mentioned, the vascular supply to the scalp is abundant and protective. Even with manipulation of hair proximate to the incision and frank insertion of hair into the wound in the presence of indwelling alloplastic or metal implants, infection is an endobrowlift complication that some surgeons never see. However, most prudent surgeons still routinely administer perioperative antibiotics against gram-positive organisms for prophylaxis.

Alopecia and Hairline Distortion

Even with meticulous hair preparation and gentle tissue handling, alopecia is often observed with browlifting, because incisional trauma can result in hair follicle injury. Mechanical avulsion, electrocautery, friction from the endoscope sheath, and manipulative stress can create ischemia that results in hair follicle death and resulting telogen effluvium along the incisional site. In the subgaleal brow lift, alopecia should not be a concern with proper tension applied at the appropriate sites. Patients should be warned, however, not to be overly anxious about seeing an inordinate amount of hair in the tub drain after the first few hair washings. Avoid overly compressive dressings.In addition, making the port incisions along (instead of across) the hair shafts preserves hair follicles. The blade should be kept orthogonal to the skin without beveling. If the forehead-shortening modification is used, however, incisions should be beveled across the hair follicles to encourage hair regrowth through the scar for camouflage (**Fig. 9.8**). Strict avoidance of electrocautery along the base of the hair follicles is another way to limit resultant alopecia.

Hairline distortion after browlifting is a significant concern, even when the procedure is performed by skilled surgeons. Without careful planning, both the cor-

onal browlift and the endoscopic browlift will increase the length of the forehead in all patients. Although this can be an acceptable or even a desirable outcome in select patients with a low hairline and short forehead, if patients have a high hairline and tall forehead, they will generally view further elongation of the forehead as unacceptable. In these patients, use of the forehead shortening modification is advisable so the hairline can be lowered to make the outcome more aesthetically pleasing. If this technique is used, it is incumbent upon the surgeon to discuss preoperatively the rationale for the longer incision and numbness that will occur. Trichophytic incisions are beveled across the hair shafts to encourage hair regrowth through the scar for camouflage, and precise closure of the incision without tension is paramount. The use of trichophytic incisions makes the incision nearly undetectable, which allows patients to wear a desired hairstyle rather than camouflaging a high forehead with bangs. The possibility of aberrant wound healing after hairline preservation leading to visible scarring or hairline distortion must be discussed openly with the patient preoperatively.

Scars

Undesirable scarring is often a matter of poor technique and a failure to handle tissue gently during an endoscopic browlift. Fortunately, keloid scars have not been observed, and hypertrophic scarring is almost nonexistent. Wide scars are more likely the result of incisional alopecia than excessive cicatrix formation. The use of trichophytic incisions is advisable when the surgeon is excising skin in the forehead-shortening modification. If an endoscopic browlift is undertaken in male patients with pattern baldness, there are special considerations. First, the surgeon should discuss with the patient the reason for selecting an endoscopic browlift rather than performing a browlift that respects the hairline (e.g., a mid-forehead browlift). Patients with Norwood Class I, II, or III pattern baldness need to understand that placement of their hairline will be aggravated with an endoscopic browlift and that a forehead-shortening modification cannot be performed due to the inability to hide resultant scarring. Such patients should be informed that hair restoration surgery would allow the browlift to be achieved and the hairline to be lowered, thereby keeping the incisions hidden. If patients with a more advanced Norwood classification (IV, V, or VI) elect to undergo an endoscopic browlift, incisions can be made in the transverse orientation if the surgeon feels these scars would be more acceptable to the patient.

Inadequate or Inappropriate Brow Correction

Unfortunately, inadequate or inappropriate brow correction is not uncommon after a browlift, although no studies documenting an accepted rate of incidence

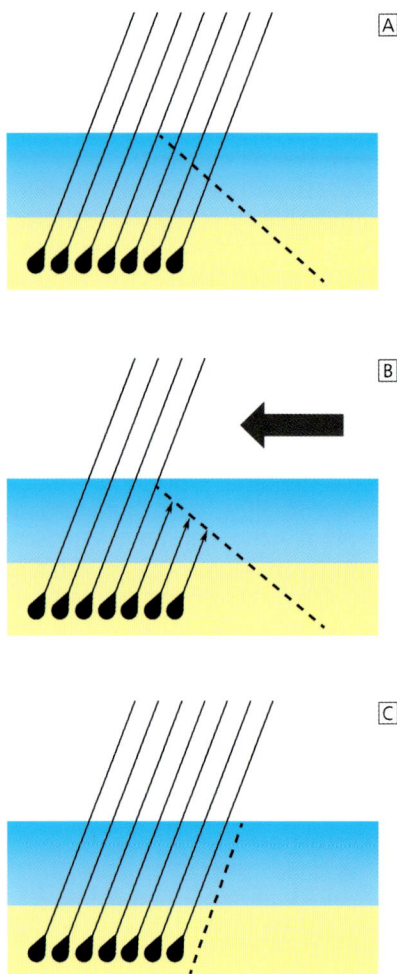

Fig. 9.8 Rendition of trichophytic versus pretrichial incision. **(A)** The dotted line denotes a trichophytic skin incision, placed 4–5 mm posterior to the hairline and beveled to include the most anterior 2–3 follicular units. **(B)** After excision of excess skin, the forehead flap is advanced superiorly to match the bevel of the scalp flap. This allows hair growth through the forehead flap from preserved hair follicles. **(C)** A pretrichial incision is made parallel to the hair shafts.

are available. The term inadequate refers to a deficient amount of correction, usually resulting from failure to release the firm periosteal attachments at the lateral orbital rim, thereby hampering flap mobility. Care should be taken to elevate the entire brow widely in a symmetric fashion, with conjoined tendon release, arcus marginalis release, and lateral brow release. Preoperative botulinum toxin injections to weaken the brow depressor muscles can aid the surgeon by decreasing the baseline tone of these muscles at the time of surgery to favor superior flap movement. In addition, continued botulinum toxin injections at regular intervals after surgery are strongly recommended by most surgeons despite surgical disruption of the brow depressors.

Inappropriate brow correction refers to a browlift with an unanatomic result, such as seen with excessive elevation of the medial brow.[22] This causes a surprised, shocked, or quizzical appearance, and contributes to an operated look instead of a rejuvenated one. Occasionally, inappropriate browlifting causes the patient to appear to have an unnatural stare. It is paramount to realize that the focus of the browlift is on achieving lateral instead of medial brow elevation. Iatrogenic asymmetry is also a possible cause of inappropriate brow correction and occurs if one brow is elevated more than the other. The surgeon should attempt to compensate for any preoperative brow asymmetry, restoring as much symmetry as possible. Obviously, it should be remembered that native brow position should be documented independent of the brow position achieved after botulinum injections have taken effect.

If either inadequate or inappropriate brow correction occurs, watchful waiting is the first and best step. Staples or sutures must be out, edema must be resolved, and adequate time allowed for the resolution of any frontotemporal branch weakness before action is taken. Furthermore, the effects of preoperative botulinum toxin will be present for three to four months, and these effects may be a contributory factor until the normal brow depressor activity has resumed. Once the surgeon is convinced there are no other factors at play, improvement may obtained with corrective botulinum toxin injections, reoperation, or both.

Hardware Failure

Complications related to browlift fixation are not uncommon and may include fixation failure, fixative exposure through the skin flap, patient intolerance of the fixation device, device inabsorbability, and even brain injury. Although titanium screws inserted into the skull's outer table provide a stable method for browlift fixation, the screw can loosen and fail to osseointegrate and thus become painfully palpable or even exposed through the overlying skin flap (**Fig. 9.9**).

In addition, suture materials used to fixate the flap can shear on the screw, with complete loss of unilateral

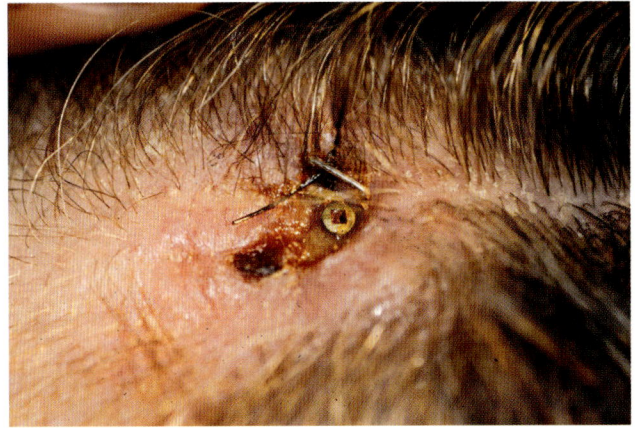

Fig. 9.9 Incision dehiscence and exposed titanium screw after browlift.

fixation. Other fixation techniques have evolved that use absorbable screws or barbed devices (Lactosorb, Biomet Fixation, Jacksonville, FL; or Endotine, MicroAire, Charlottesville, VA). Although these devices are purportedly temporary, there is a small rate of inabsorbability and formation of a foreign body granuloma that can necessitate incision and debridement of the implant remnant and any associated scar tissue or granuloma (**Figs. 9.10, 9.11, 9.12**).

Another fixation method obviates the need for any implant and simply relies on the creation of a bony tunnel or bone bridge to secure the lift. Although elegant, this fixation method is not immune to either suture shear or bone tunnel breakage, and it can be challenging because of the oblique nature of the drilling and necessity to protect the hair from getting wound around the drill.

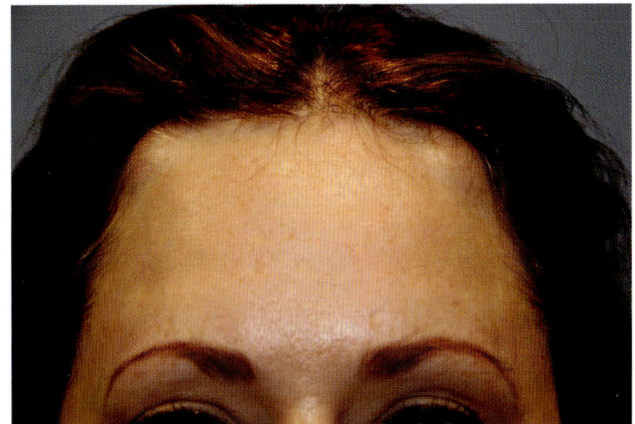

Fig. 9.10 Patient with inflammatory nodules at the site of absorbable browlift devices.

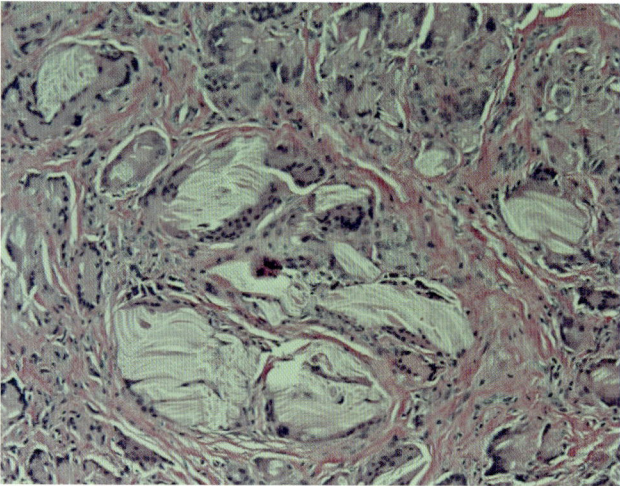

Fig. 9.11 High resolution H&E stain showing diffuse foreign body giant cell granulomatous response after a browlift using an absorbable fixation device.

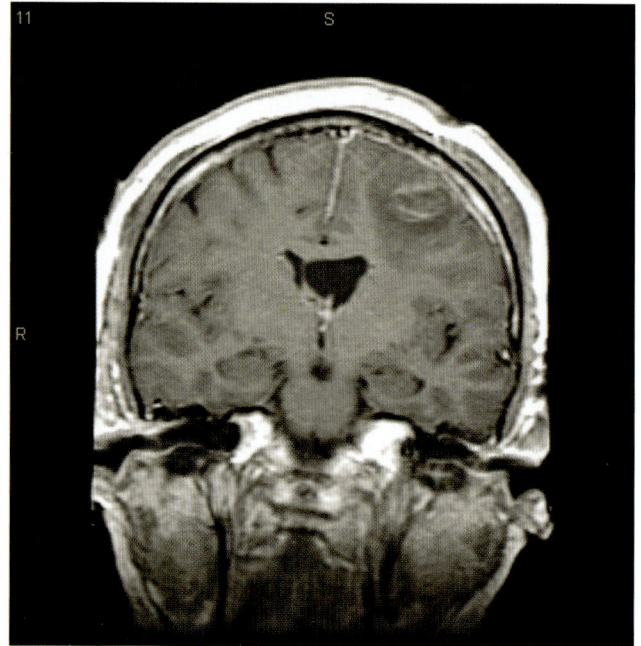

Fig. 9.13 Coronal T1-weighted MRI of the brain showing a left cortical injury with edema after endoscopic browlift.

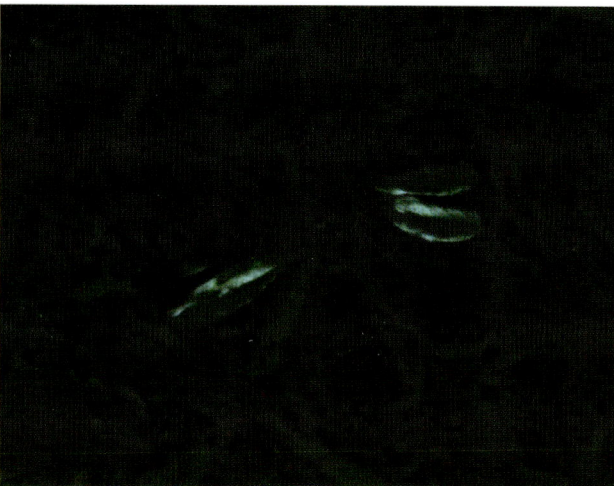

Fig. 9.12 Accompanying light micrograph showing polarizable material.

The most dread complication of browlift fixation is brain injury; although vanishingly rare, it can occur if the drilling associated with fixation traverses the skull and penetrates the dura mater. Subdural or epidural hematoma, meningitis, intracranial hemorrhage, or cortical brain injury can result (**Figs. 9.13, 9.14**). Great care must be taken, therefore, to limit the depth of drilling to the outer table of the skull only. If injury is suspected, MRI or CT brain imaging, close observation, and an expedited neurosurgical consultation are imperative.

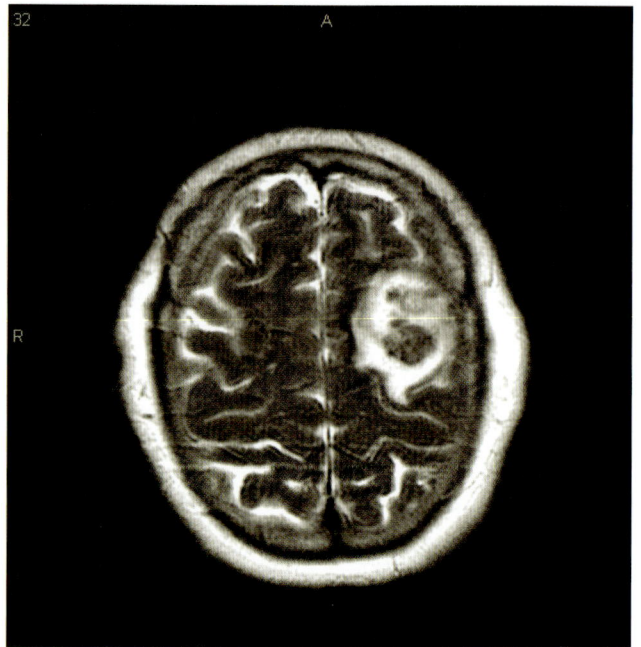

Fig. 9.14 Axial T2-weighted MRI of the same patient's brain showing left cortical bleed.

◆ Conclusion

In recent years, the endoscopic approach to browlifting has proven successful in upper facial rejuvenation by safely capitalizing on minimal access through hidden incisions with dissection using contemporary optics to achieve youthful brow repositioning. Successful outcomes depend upon (1) complete release of the brow at the supraorbital rim and arcus marginalis, (2) brow depressor muscle resection and disruption, (3) adequate and appropriate fixation of the new brow position, and (4) ideal patient selection, education, and preparation. Adherence to these general guidelines will protect patients from adverse outcomes that can be associated with contemporary brow rejuvenation.

PEARLS OF WISDOM

A thorough examination with careful documentation of preoperative brow and eyelid position will help prevent browlift complications.

Limiting flap traction during takedown of the arcus marginalis and lateral brow periosteum will reduce the incidence of frontotemporal branch weakness.

It is important to consider the hairline shortening modification with trichophytic incisions whenever a patient with brow ptosis is bothered by an accompanying high hairline.

Be wary of patients with true ptosis and understand Herring's Law.

Preoperative use of botulinum toxin, intraoperative release of the lateral brow attachments, and use of appropriate vectors of elevation will help the surgeon achieve an anatomic browlift that avoids the operated look.

Because there is no clear evidence for the best browlift fixation technique, surgeons should use the technique they feel most comfortable performing that yields the best outcomes.

References

1. Knoll BI, Attkiss KJ, Persing JA. The influence of forehead, brow, and periorbital aesthetics on perceived expression in the youthful face. Plast Reconstr Surg 2008;121(5): 1793–1802
2. Passot R. La churgerie esthetique des rides du visage. Presse Med 1919;27:258
3. Isse NG. Endoscopic forehead lift. Presented at the Annual Meeting of the Los Angeles County Society of Plastic Surgeons; September 12, 1992, Los Angeles, CA
4. Vasconez LO. The use of the endoscope in brow lifting (video). Presented at the Annual Meeting of the American Society of Plastic and Reconstructive Surgeons; September 1992. Washington, DC.
5. Core GB, Vasconez LO, Graham HD III. Endoscopic browlift. Clin Plast Surg 1995;22(4):619–631
6. Chiu ES, Baker DC. Endoscopic brow lift: a retrospective review of 628 consecutive cases over 5 years. Plast Reconstr Surg 2003;112(2):628–633, discussion 634–635
7. Cilento BW, Johnson CM Jr. The case for open forehead rejuvenation: a review of 1004 procedures. Arch Facial Plast Surg 2009;11(1):13–17
8. Chadwell JB, Mangat DS. The endoscopic forehead-lift. Facial Plast Surg Clin North Am 2006;14(3):195–201
9. Dayan SH, Perkins SW, Vartanian AJ, Wiesman IM. The forehead lift: endoscopic versus coronal approaches. Aesthetic Plast Surg 2001;25(1):35–39
10. Puig CM, LaFerriere KA. A retrospective comparison of open and endoscopic brow-lifts. Arch Facial Plast Surg 2002;4(4):221–225
11. De Cordier BC, de la Torre JI, Al-Hakeem MS, et al. Endoscopic forehead lift: review of technique, cases, and complications. Plast Reconstr Surg 2002;110(6):1558–1568, discussion 1569–1570
12. Ramirez AL, Ende KH, Kabaker SS. Correction of the high female hairline. Arch Facial Plast Surg 2009;11(2):84–90
13. Norwood OT. Male pattern baldness: classification and incidence. South Med J 1975;68(11):1359–1365
14. Withey S, Witherow H, Waterhouse N. One hundred cases of endoscopic brow lift. Br J Plast Surg 2002;55(1):20–24
15. Kern EB. The preoperative discussion as a prelude to managing a complication. Arch Otolaryngol Head Neck Surg 2003;129(11):1163–1165
16. Stuzin JM, Wagstrom L, Kawamoto HK, Wolfe SA. Anatomy of the frontal branch of the facial nerve: the significance of the temporal fat pad. Plast Reconstr Surg 1989;83(2): 265–271
17. Bernstein L, Nelson RH. Surgical anatomy of the extraparotid distribution of the facial nerve. Arch Otolaryngol 1984;110(3):177–183
18. Sabini P, Wayne I, Quatela VC. Anatomical guides to precisely localize the frontal branch of the facial nerve. Arch Facial Plast Surg 2003;5(2):150–152
19. Gosain AK, Sewall SR, Yousif NJ. The temporal branch of the facial nerve: how reliably can we predict its path? Plast Reconstr Surg 1997;99(5):1224–1233, discussion 1234–1236
20. Liebman, EP, Webster RC, Berger AS, Della Vecchia M. The frontalis nerve in the temporal brow lift. Arch Otolaryngol Head Neck Surg 1982;108(4):232–235
21. Trinei FA, Januszkiewicz J, Nahai F. The sentinel vein: an important reference point for surgery in the temporal region. Plast Reconstr Surg 1998;101(1):27–32
22. Freund RM, Nolan WB III. Correlation between brow lift outcomes and aesthetic ideals for eyebrow height and shape in females. Plast Reconstr Surg 1996;97(7):1343–1348

10

Rhinoplasty Complications

Jaimie DeRosa, Ryan M. Greene, and Dean M. Toriumi

Most plastic surgeons consider rhinoplasty one of the most complex facial plastic operations. Precise preoperative diagnosis and meticulous surgical technique are required to produce a favorable outcome and avoid complications. As anatomies differ and patient expectations vary, no single technique is appropriate for all patients. Rhinoplasty complications not only encompass those common to most surgeries, such as infection and hematoma, but also are frequently associated with functional and aesthetic problems. Traditional rhinoplasty techniques involve reductive, excisional methods, which may be associated with many untoward long-term changes. Grafting in rhinoplasty may also result in problems, such as graft visibility, mobilization, and extrusion. Methods to prevent or correct common rhinoplasty complications are detailed below.

◆ Preoperative Evaluation

The preoperative consultation is a critical step to avoid complications after rhinoplasty. It is essential that both the surgeon and patient have realistic expectations. If they cannot achieve common goals, due to either patient limitations (e.g., damaged soft-tissue skin envelope) or a surgeon's inexperience with or lack of comfort in performing the proposed procedure, the surgery should not proceed. This is especially true in patients seeking secondary rhinoplasty.

Computer imaging of the proposed changes can facilitate communication between the surgeon and patient. Perhaps more importantly, it can also provide a visual explanation of the proposed outcome. Patients often have difficulty expressing the changes they desire, or they may be unaware of what results are realistic and surgically attainable. Computer imaging may help overcome this problem. In fact, one study demonstrated that patient satisfaction was significantly improved when the procedure included preoperative imaging versus no imaging.[1] If computer imaging is used, the image shown should realistically represent what the surgeon can achieve. In fact, under-imaging, or showing less than ideal outcomes that the surgeon can generally achieve, is the most effective means of using computer imaging. The surgeon is warned against trying to sell the operation with unrealistic or idealized imaging.

The surgeon must assess the quality and thickness of the skin/soft tissue envelope (SSTE) preoperatively. In fact, a damaged SSTE may be the deciding factor as to whether or not a revision rhinoplasty can be undertaken. In some cases, significant scar tissue may be present from a previous surgery in which aggressive thinning of the subcutaneous tissue and/or dissection in the incorrect plane took place. If patients have an immobile SSTE that adheres tightly to the underlying cartilaginous framework, surgery is postponed until the SSTE loosens. In cases of severely damaged SSTE, surgery may not be offered at all. At times, the SSTE will be thin or devascularized from prior surgery. Visible irregularities, cutaneous telangiectasias, and purple discoloration of the skin are signs of SSTE damage (**Fig. 10.1**). It is important that these skin changes are recognized, because in such cases extensive soft-tissue elevation may lead to ischemia and skin necrosis. Moreover, revision surgery should be postponed until changes in skin color resolve, which may take years. Any irregularities or skin damage should documented in the chart and by close-up photography before surgery. Finally, the patient with a damaged SSTE needs to be counseled preoperatively about the risk of further skin damage, even necrosis, with surgery.[2]

During the preoperative evaluation for secondary rhinoplasty, the surgeon should assess the patient for the presence of alloplastic implants. These implants may result in SSTE damage and significant scar tissue (**Fig. 10.2**). The surgeon should be prepared to replace the alloplastic implants with alternative grafting materials, such as cartilage.

The surgeon should discuss the postoperative healing process candidly at the initial consultation. The patient should be aware that postoperative nasal edema

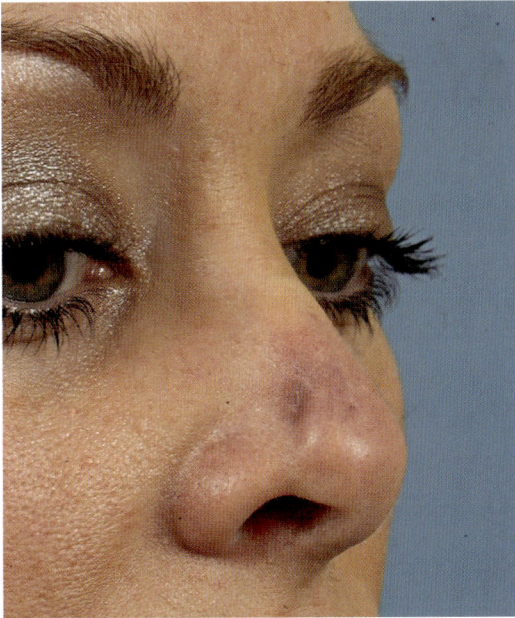

Fig. 10.1 Patient who underwent previous rhinoplasty with excessive thinning of the supratip skin that resulted in permanent damage.

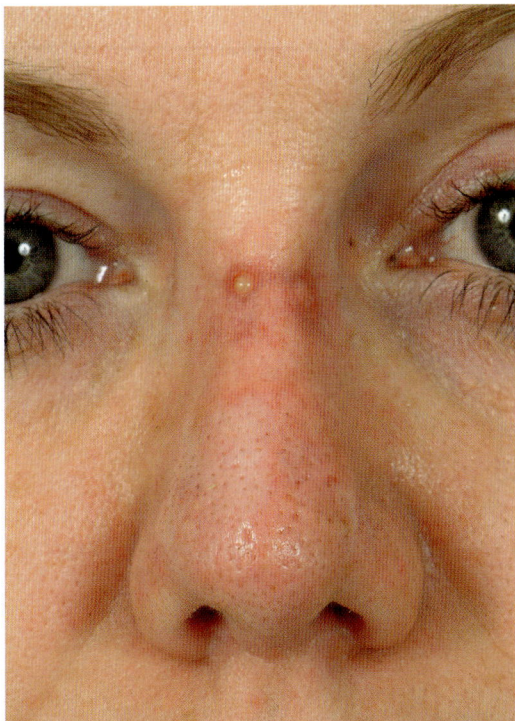

Fig. 10.2 Patient with an infected MEDPOR dorsal implant. The dorsal skin is severely damaged and scarred from the infection. Treatment required removal of the implant and resolution of the infection prior to reconstruction.

is normal in the healing period and may be significant, especially in patients with thick skin. Patients should be made aware that the healing process will continue throughout their lifetime as wound contracture continues; therefore, aesthetic changes will occur over a period of many years. Risks and possible complications should also be discussed.

A thorough medical history should be taken, and physical examination should be performed. All prior nasal surgery should be documented, and any accessible reports of these operations should be reviewed. Preoperative laboratory and other diagnostic studies need to be obtained. The specific panel of studies ordered is chosen according to the patient's age and overall health.

A complete blood count and coagulation studies are performed on every patient. Any history of unusual bleeding or excessive bruising, as well as any family history of abnormal bleeding, should lead to further investigation. This may involve coagulation studies or a more extensive hematologic workup. In fact, one study found that 9 of 1000 (0.9%) plastic surgery patients were diagnosed with von Willebrand's disease.[3] Patients should also be told to stop aspirin, ibuprofen, vitamin E, and herbal supplements at least three weeks before surgery to reduce the risk of excessive perioperative bleeding. In summary, a careful preoperative evaluation and good communication with a potential rhinoplasty patient may help to avoid some unwanted surgical complications.

◆ Intraoperative Complications

Unfortunately, many intraoperative errors made in rhinoplasty are either unrecognized or not revealed until the postoperative time period. Therefore, the surgeon must be meticulous to avoid untoward complications. A few specific problems that the surgeon may encounter intraoperatively are described below.

As the face is so well vascularized, bleeding is to be expected during rhinoplasty. Excessive bleeding can impair visibility and the surgeon's ability to execute the desired maneuvers. The use of a topical vasoconstrictive agent and deliberate injection of a local anesthetic containing epinephrine can help to reduce the amount of bleeding. Dissection in the correct plane (just superficial to the perichondrium) can also decrease the degree of bleeding. Bipolar electrocautery is used for hemostasis and should be specifically targeted to reduce the risk of vascular compromise to the SSTE.

During dissection, damage to the SSTE or the underlying cartilaginous structural framework may occur. It is preferable to avoid such complications (by careful dissection in the correct tissue plane), but once such problems are encountered, the surgeon must try to correct them. Violation of the SSTE should be treated either by local wound care or (if large) suture reapproximation. If the surgeon recognizes that he is dissecting too superficially (potentially damaging the SSTE), then he should return to the correct tissue plane, take care not to apply a tight nasal dorsal dressing (to avoid compromising the vascular supply to the skin), and monitor the skin closely postoperatively for any signs of damage or necrosis.

Another intraoperative complication that warrants discussion is the inadvertent disarticulation of the cartilaginous septal strut from the perpendicular plate of the septum. When this occurs, the strut must be reattached to prevent postoperative saddling. One method of stabilizing the septal strut is to suture it to the nasal bones via holes that are made along the caudal aspect of each nasal bone. Destabilization of the caudal aspect of the septal strut can also occur, which can be repaired by securing the caudal septum to the nasal spine (or its periosteum) with a permanent suture, such as a 5–0 clear nylon suture.

Manipulation of the nasal dorsum can lead to middle vault collapse. It is imperative that the surgeon identify preoperatively those patients who may be at risk of middle vault collapse. These include patients with short nasal bones, long weak upper lateral cartilages, thin skin, and a narrow projecting nose (**Fig. 10.3**).[4,5] In patients at high risk for middle vault collapse, several precautions can be taken. Attempts should be made to preserve the middle vault structures, and in many cases augmentation with spreader grafts is recommended. Additionally, osteotomies should be conservative. Pres-

ervation of the middle vault mucosa by the formation of precise pockets for spreader grafts will help minimize posterior displacement of the upper lateral cartilages following hump removal.[4]

One of the more common reasons that patients seek rhinoplasty is correction of a crooked nose. This is one of the most difficult problems encountered in rhinoplasty. Deviated segments of the nose are shifted back to the midline by fracturing bone or manipulating and realigning the cartilage framework. Absolute correction can be difficult to achieve, and there may be residual convexities or concavities along the dorsal nasal subunit that produce contour defects. Ideally, a contour line should be created by shadows that extend from the brow and dorsal nasal subunit to the tip-defining point.

Deviation in the upper third of the nose can be addressed with medial or lateral osteotomies. However, inadequate osteotomies may result in a greenstick fracture, which can result in a deviated bony nasal vault postoperatively. In some cases, double lateral osteotomies can be performed to mobilize the bony vault completely and decrease the likelihood of this deformity. However, the surgeon must take care to avoid comminution of the nasal bones, which may lead to their displacement.

In many crooked noses, there is also deviation in the lower two-thirds of the nose. It is essential that the cartilaginous structures are reoriented to the midline. If this realignment is not achieved after osteotomies, the nose may shift back to its preoperative position due to the memory of the deviated cartilaginous structures.[6] In instances where the nose cannot be shifted back to midline or where a residual concavity exists (as may be seen in a C-shaped deformity), an onlay cartilage graft can be placed lateral to the upper lateral cartilages to camouflage the defect.[7,8]

A fairly common complication following rhinoplasty is the collapse in the supra-alar region (**Fig. 10.4**). In patients with a weakened lateral wall, alar batten grafts can be placed prophylactically to prevent the development of any supra-alar pinching. They can also be used to correct preexisting external valve compromise, lateral wall collapse, or supra-alar pinching. An alar batten graft is placed into a precise pocket at the point of maximal lateral wall collapse or supra-alar pinching (**Fig. 10.5**).[9,10] A common tendency is to place the grafts too far cephalically along the upper lateral cartilage, which can result in a persistent fullness in the lateral wall. The surgeon should also avoid dissecting too far laterally, as this may cause bleeding and damage to the lateral nasal arteries that supply the nasal tip.

Excessive alar width or flaring may be corrected with alar base reduction. If not done properly, this procedure can lead to significant complications, including unsightly scarring and distorted nostrils (**Fig. 10.6**). To reduce the risk of visible scars, the skin edges should be everted on closure, which can be achieved by creating a favorable bevel with the excision.[11] This bevel should

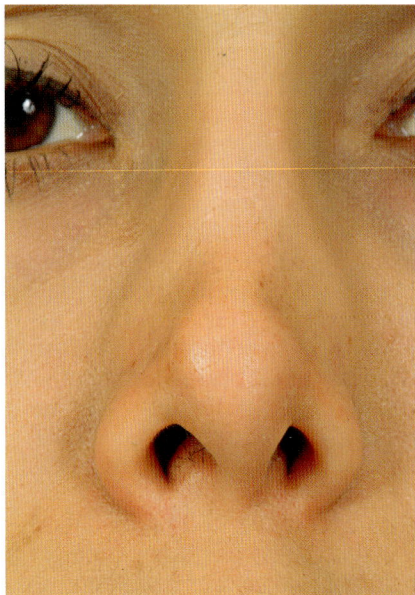

Fig. 10.3 Patient with short nasal bones and long upper lateral cartilages. Note the collapse of the upper lateral cartilages, resulting in an inverted-V deformity.

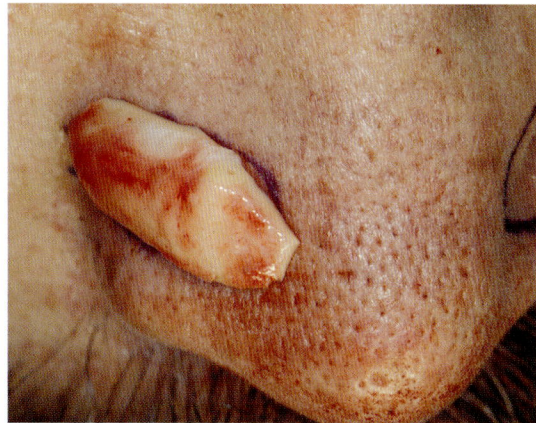

Fig. 10.5 Alar batten grafts can be placed into a pocket at the site of maximal supra-alar pinching. This auricular cartilage graft is placed with its concave surface placed medially.

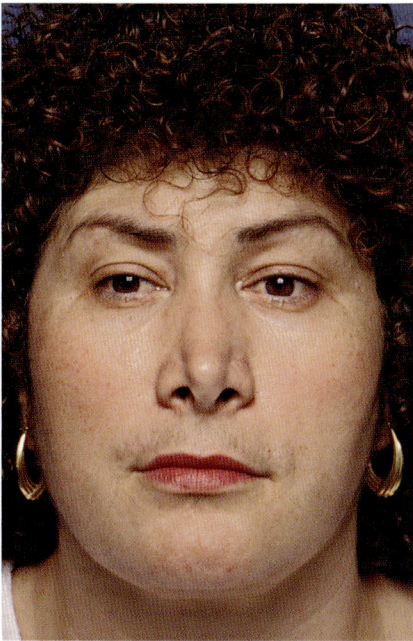

Fig. 10.4 Patient with severe supra-alar pinching due to over-resection of the lateral crura.

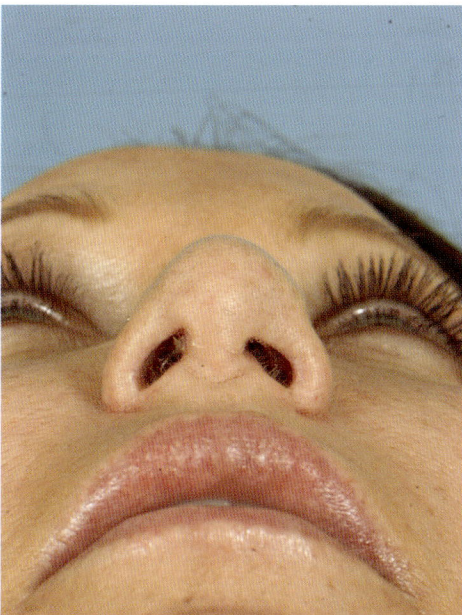

Fig. 10.6 Patient who underwent over-reduction of nasal base, leaving the patient with very small nostrils and airway obstruction.

be subtle, with an angle no greater than 10 to 15 degrees. Cautery should be avoided in this area as well, for necrosis or atrophy of the underlying subcutaneous tissue can lead to a depressed scar. Special care should be taken when approximating the subcutaneous tissues to ensure precise alignment. Any time base reduction is performed, conservative removal of tissue is recommended to reduce the risk of nostril distortion or excessive narrowing.

It is critical to avoid visible scars whenever external rhinoplasty is performed. Scarring can be minimized by both careful incisional technique and meticulous closure. Precise reapproximation of the incisions can vastly reduce the visibility of these scars. If the incisions do not align correctly during closure, the surgeon should remove the sutures and try to correct the closure. A subcutaneous suture and multiple 7–0 vertical mattress nylon sutures can be used to close the midcolumellar and alar base reduction incisions. Moreover, careful closure of the mucosal incisions is important to reduce the risk of internal nasal scarring, which can lead to vestibular stenosis and nasal airway compromise.

Whenever costal cartilage is harvested for grafting purposes in rhinoplasty, there is a risk of pneumothorax. To ensure that the pleura is intact, the wound cavity is filled with antibiotic solution after the costal cartilage has been taken, and the anesthesiologist creates a positive ventilatory pressure for the patient (a Valsalva maneuver). Air bubbles in the wound should alert the surgeon to a possible rent in the pleura, which should be repaired if identified. The wound is closed over a red rubber catheter placed on suction. With the chest expanded, the catheter can be removed. A postoperative chest X-ray can confirm full expansion of the lungs.

The key to repairing any intraoperative complication is the surgeon's ability to recognize the problem intraoperatively and then to try to remedy it promptly. Ignoring such problems intraoperatively will lead to a greater number of postoperative complications and unhappy patients.

◆ Postoperative Complications and Their Prevention

In the immediate postoperative period, the patient is expected to have nasal edema. This is especially true if the patient has thick sebaceous skin. Elevation of the head, reduction in sodium consumption to less than 1200 mg daily, and avoidance of overheating can help reduce the degree and persistence of nasal swelling. Although some surgeons advocate early injection of steroids to help reduce postoperative nasal edema, the senior author prefers to avoid steroid injections during the early postoperative period. The patient should be reassured that the swelling is normal and that it should begin to subside by four to six weeks postoperatively.

Nasal Tip

Many problems seen after rhinoplasty can be attributed to loss of nasal tip projection. Without intraoperative control of tip projection, the surgeon is forced to try to anticipate where the tip will eventually settle. When surgeons leave such an important component of the overall result to chance, they are likely to have patients with postoperative loss of tip projection. A critical factor in controlling the nasal tip is stabilization of the nasal base.[12] Methods to stabilize the nasal base include suturing the medial crura onto the septum or placing a columellar strut graft, a caudal extension graft, or an extended columellar strut graft. The indications and technical aspects of each method are beyond the scope of this chapter. For an in-depth discussion of nasal tip surgery, the reader is referred to alternate resources.[11,13]

A favorable tip-supratip relationship is essential. Postoperative loss of nasal tip projection can result in a supratip pollybeak, as the nasal tip drops below the supratip (**Fig. 10.7**). This leads to a rounded appearance of the tip, with the absence of a supratip break or a favorable columellar-lobule relationship. Pollybeak deformity may also result from a failure to reduce an overly elevated middle vault and supratip dorsum. Excessive excision of the dorsal septal cartilage may also result in a pollybeak deformity. This is especially true in patients with thick nasal skin, because the overlying SSTE may not redrape appropriately over the underlying structural framework if it is overly reduced. Scar and fibrosis then may develop within this tissue void, causing a supratip fullness and a soft-tissue pollybeak.

In general, correction (or avoidance) of a pollybeak deformity may be addressed in one of several ways, depending on the etiology of the problem.[2,14] When the pollybeak deformity arises from over-reduction of the underlying cartilaginous framework in a patient with thick, sebaceous skin, correction involves projecting the tip into the thick SSTE, sometimes with the addition of dorsal augmentation. If there was loss of tip projection with resultant pollybeak deformity, reestablishing tip support and projection is necessary for correction. Less

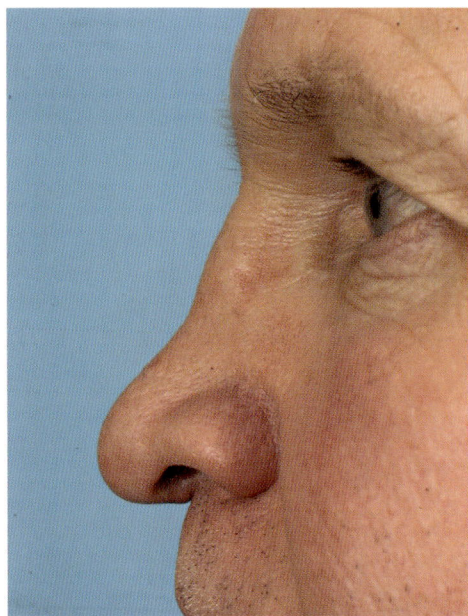

Fig. 10.7 Postoperative supratip pollybeak deformity from over-reduction of the nose and postoperative loss of nasal tip projection.

commonly, a pollybeak deformity may be improved by reducing an excessively high anterior septal angle.

The use of grafting in rhinoplasty enables the surgeon to accomplish not only structural stabilization but also aesthetic refinements. However, without proper camouflage, grafts are at risk of postoperative visibility and contour irregularity. Tip grafts are a good example of a graft that is at risk for postoperative visibility if camouflage is not adequately performed intraoperatively (**Fig. 10.8**). Often a graft becomes visible only after many years of scar contracture and gradual thinning of the nasal skin. Tip grafts should be avoided in patients with thin skin.

For any graft at risk for postoperative visibility, the surgeon can employ several techniques to decrease the risk of this complication. Every graft should be carved so that there is a smooth transition between it and its surrounding structures. The edges of a shield-like tip graft should be beveled (**Fig. 10.9**). A buttress graft can be placed behind the superior edge of a shield-like tip graft to help smooth the transition between the graft and its surrounding structures (**Fig. 10.10**). It also helps to prevent cephalic rotation of the tip graft. Any tip graft that sits 3 mm or more above the surrounding cartilage should be camouflaged with lateral crural grafts. These grafts are positioned at 45 degree angles from the posterior margin of the superior edge of the shield-like tip graft (**Fig. 10.11**).

The surgeon can achieve additional camouflage over grafts at risk of becoming visible postoperatively by covering the leading edge of the graft with crushed cartilage or perichondrium. Cephalic trims are an ideal

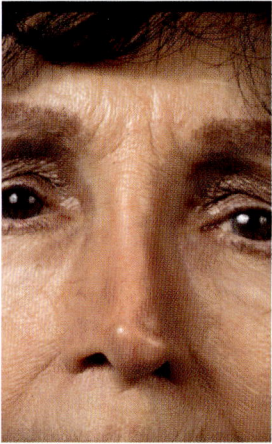

Fig. 10.8 Thin skin has contracted over the tip graft, leaving a visible deformity.

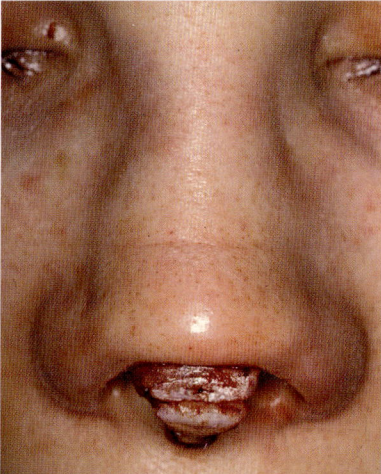

Fig. 10.9 Shield tip graft with beveled edges to help avoid visibility.

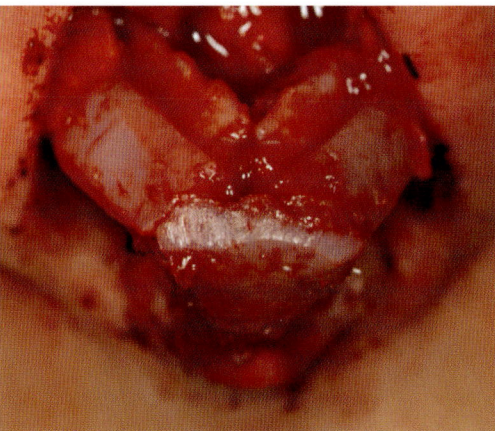

Fig. 10.10 Tip graft with buttress graft to stabilize and camouflage.

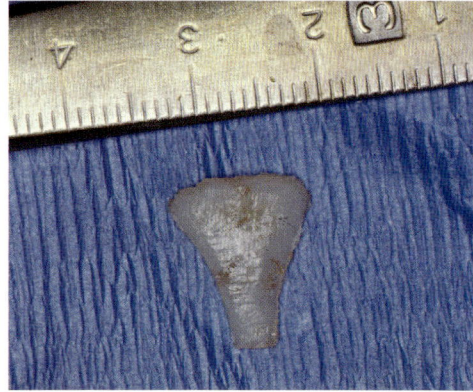

Fig. 10.11 Tip graft with lateral crural grafts to stabilize and camouflage.

source of soft cartilage for this purpose, as is the thick perichondrium from costal cartilage. The cartilage or perichondrium should be placed in a horizontal fashion, with complete coverage of the lateral aspect of the tip graft (**Fig. 10.12**).

Nasal tip bossae may result from unequal excision of the lower lateral cartilages, suturing asymmetries, or structural grafting. Bossae may also form due to knuckling and weakening of the lower lateral cartilages or tip grafts as SSTE contracture occurs. These bossae may be more pronounced in patients with thin nasal skin, intralobular bifidity, or strong cartilages.[15] Many of these irregularities may not be apparent for several months (until postoperative edema resolves), and they have been known to develop as late as 10 years after surgery.[16] Avoidance of tip irregularities involves smooth contouring of the domal regions, maintaining the strength of the lower lateral cartilages (without weakening their cephalic margin), and performing adequate camouflage.

Bulbosity of the nasal tip is often addressed with a cephalic trim of the lateral crura. However, overly aggressive resection of the lateral crus of the lower lateral

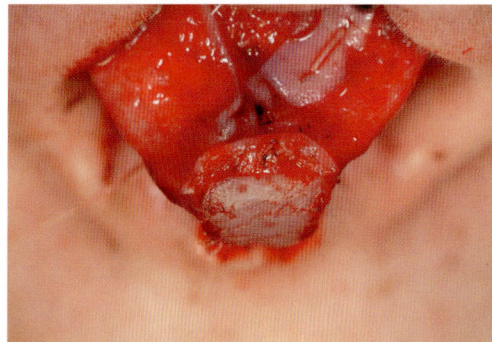

Fig. 10.12 Tip graft camouflaged with the cephalic trim of the lateral crura.

cartilage may lead to cephalic retraction of the alar margin. If a cephalic trim is performed, 8 mm to 12 mm of the vertical height of the lateral crus should be preserved to reduce the risk of alar retraction. Alar retraction occurs as scar contracture moves the tissue in a direction away from lesser support (the free alar margin) to an area of greater support (the bony-cartilaginous pyramid).

Correction of alar retraction can be challenging.[17] Sometimes the placement of alar rim grafts corrects the problem. In other patients, repositioning the lateral crura more caudally helps to push down the alar margin and correct the retraction (**Fig. 10.13**). In these cases, lateral crural strut grafts are placed on the undersurface of the cartilage (between the lateral crura and the ves-

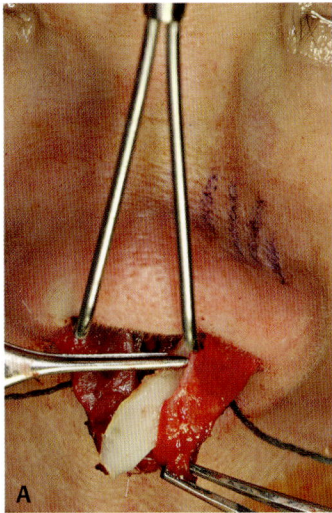

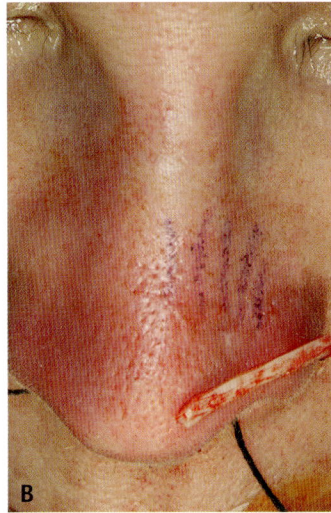

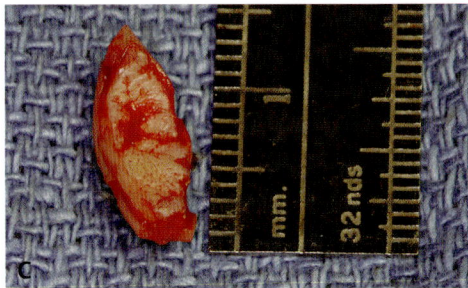

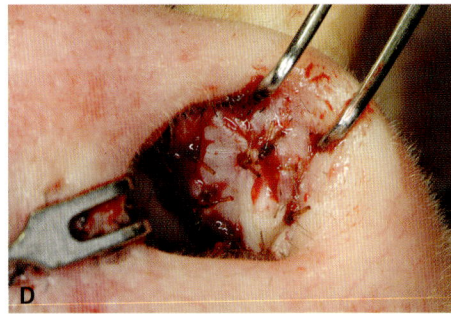

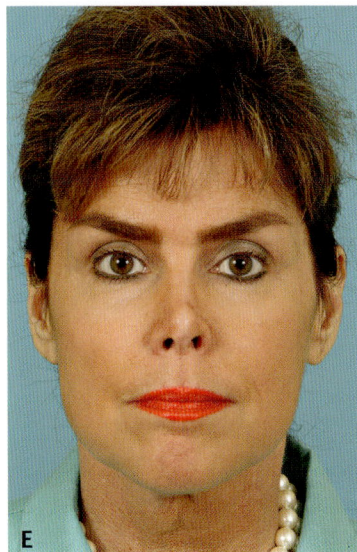

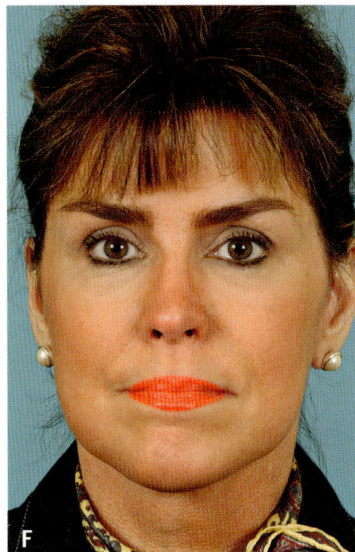

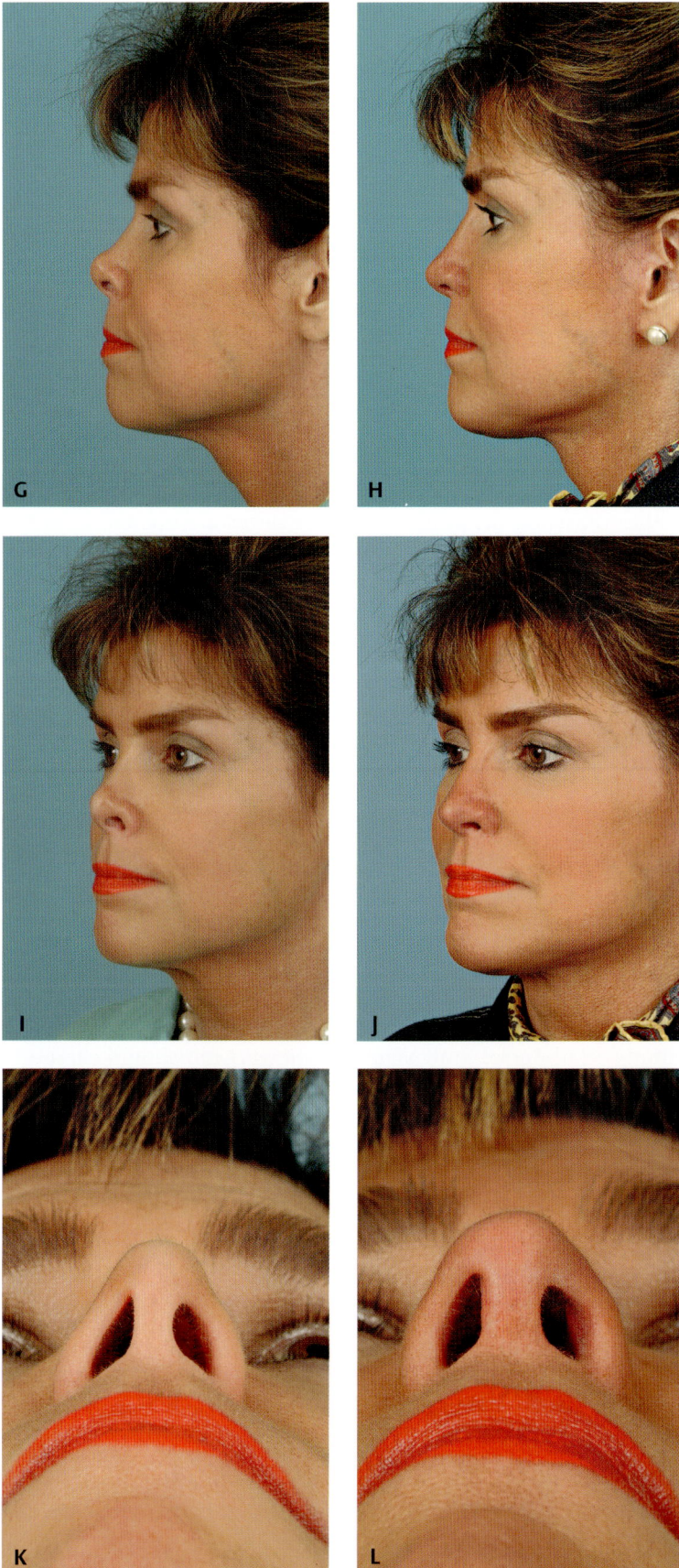

Fig. 10.13 Patient with severe retraction of left alar margin. Treatment required placement of a left lateral crural strut graft, alar rim graft and composite skin cartilage graft from auricle. **(A)** Placement of lateral crural strut graft that is sutured to undersurface of lateral crura. The lateral crura is then repositioned into a caudally positioned pocket to push the alar margin down. **(B)** Alar rim graft along left alar margin. **(C)** Composite auricular skin cartilage graft. **(D)** Composite graft positioned into pocket along left marginal incision. **(E,G,I,K)** Preoperative views. **(F,H,J,L)** Postoperative views.

tibular skin).[11,18] These grafts must be strong, so costal cartilage is a good choice for grafting material. Composite auricular cartilage and skin grafts also may be placed at the marginal incision to help correct both alar retraction and a deficiency in the vestibular skin (which may be seen with caudal repositioning of the ala).

Deficient columellar show may be the result of hanging alar lobules or columellar retraction. A retracted columella may result from excessive resection of the caudal septum. This may be corrected with either a caudal extension graft or an extended columellar strut graft.

Nasal Dorsum

One common complication arising from any rhinoplasty that involves the dorsum is irregularity. This complication may be created following osseous hump reduction and osteotomies. Dorsal irregularities also may arise along the cartilaginous dorsum due to asymmetric collapse or migration of the upper lateral cartilages relative to the septum. If adequate smoothing of the bony dorsum is not performed, palpable or visible edges may result. Another troublesome complication is the open roof deformity, which follows bony hump removal with osteotomies that do not adequately medialize the nasal bones. It is possible to avoid these complications with close inspection and palpation of the nasal dorsum intraoperatively. Any irregularities may require smoothing or camouflaging while stabilizing the dorsum and middle vault.

A more dramatic deformity results from the improper positioning of the height of the upper or middle third of the nasal dorsum. This complication may be seen in patients who have a low radix preoperatively. An inexperienced surgeon who fails to recognize this preoperatively may adjust the dorsal alignment by reducing a relative convexity at the upper and middle vaults. This reduction may lead to a scooped appearance of the nasal dorsum. This problem can be prevented by augmenting the radix to an appropriate level, with less removal of the dorsal hump instead. Correction of this complication may require dorsal or radix grafting.

An overly reduced nasal dorsum at the middle vault may also lead to a saddle nose deformity. Collapse of the mid-dorsum will create less shadowing on a frontal view and an illusion of increased width. This undesirable result can be avoided by maintaining an ideal dorsal profile with an adequately projected nasal tip. In patients with a saddle nose deformity, the dorsal height may be augmented with cartilaginous grafts. A graft from the nasal septum or auricular concha can be used for dorsal augmentation, although when significant dorsal height is needed, a costal cartilage graft may be required.

A saddle nose deformity can also result from a loss of septal support. This may occur following removal of septal cartilage if there is a failure to preserve an adequate (at least 1.5 cm) L-shaped dorsal and caudal strut. The deformity may also be seen as a consequence

of a septal hematoma, abscess, or subtotal perforation. These disastrous complications may be prevented by having a high index of suspicion for septal hematoma and by careful reapproximation of the septal mucosal flaps intraoperatively. Any signs of a septal hematoma or abscess should be emergently addressed. Patients with inflammatory disorders, such as Wegener's granulomatosis, may also be susceptible to a saddle nose deformity, and one should consider maintaining increased septal support (or not disrupting the septum at all) in affected patients.

Excessive narrowing of the middle vault is common after rhinoplasty and often manifests postoperatively as an inverted-V deformity.[19,20] Over time, scar contracture and negative pressure from airflow will tend to increase inferomedial collapse of the upper lateral cartilages. Inferomedial collapse of the caudal margin of the upper lateral cartilage can result in a collapse of the middle vault that compromises the nasal valve. This may occur when the upper lateral cartilages are divided from the nasal septum during hump removal. Loss of support of the upper lateral cartilages may also occur whenever a cephalic trim of the lateral crura is performed or with lateral osteotomies and medialization of the upper lateral cartilages. In most patients, these maneuvers will not result in middle vault collapse; however, a combination of these maneuvers in a high-risk patient may result in excessive narrowing of the middle vault, with internal nasal valve collapse.[4,5,21]

Residual nasal deviation may be seen postoperatively. This can be due to incomplete osteotomies, in which case revision that completes the osteotomies is indicated. However, in cases in which the surgeon is confident that the nose was fully mobile intraoperatively, a residual, subtle nasal deviation may be corrected by the use of nasal exercises.

Complications secondary to dorsal augmentation can be seen postoperatively as well. These include graft visibility, misplacement, and migration. To reduce the risk of dorsal graft visibility, the surgeon should carve the graft into a canoe-like shape, with all edges beveled (**Fig. 10.14**). For further camouflage, the edges can be covered with perichondrium. If the graft is noted to be visible postoperatively, correction can be done in a similar fashion.

To reduce the risk of dorsal graft mobility, the surgeon should place the graft into a tight dorsal pocket. Care should be taken not to make the pocket too large or high, because this graft is usually used to set the nasal starting point. Another error that may occur is setting the nasal starting point in a rhinoplasty for an Asian patient at the same location as for a Caucasian patient (at the level of the upper eyelid crease). For Asians the nasal starting point is lower, at the level of the mid-pupillary line.

Movement of the dorsal graft after placement can be problematic. To try to prevent this complication, the

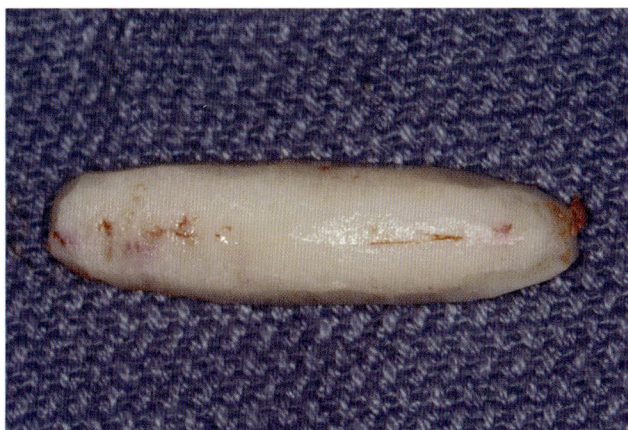

Fig. 10.14 Canoe-shaped costal cartilage dorsal graft. The shape of the dorsal graft will create a natural appearing dorsum.

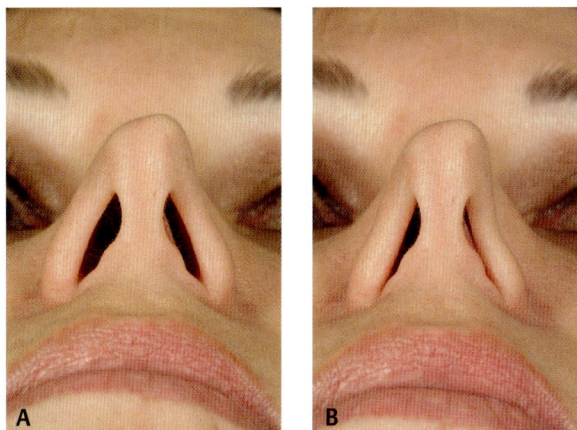

Fig. 10.15 Patient with weakened lateral walls. **(A)** Narrowing of nostrils. **(B)** External nasal valve collapse noted on moderate inspiration through the nostrils

dorsal graft should be fixated by sutures in at least two points (to the upper lateral cartilages). An additional fixation point is established by having a tight dorsal pocket cephalically. If the graft appears to sit off of the midline postoperatively, the surgeon can direct the patient to perform specific nasal exercises to help reposition the graft properly.

Persistent Nasal Airway Obstruction

A common complaint in patients undergoing rhinoplasty is that of worsening or persistent nasal airway obstruction. This can be subdivided into either a dynamic obstruction (e.g., nasal valve collapse) or a fixed one (e.g., deviated septum). Dynamic forms of nasal obstruction are influenced by nasal airflow and are usually secondary to a deficiency in structural support of the lateral nasal wall. This collapse of the nasal wall occurs because negative airway pressure is generated during inspiration. Examination of a patient who complains of nasal airway obstruction should include examination of the internal and external nasal valves, the nasal septum and turbinates along the lateral nasal wall, and the nasal airway during quiet nasal breathing. The technique used to correct the problem should be selected carefully, based on the likely causes of the obstruction. If the cause of the obstruction is not identified and addressed correctly, there may be persistent airway obstruction postoperatively.

Nasal breathing can also be compromised by external nasal valve collapse, with collapse of the nostril margin on moderate to deep inspiration through the nose (**Fig. 10.15**).[5,22] This is often seen in patients with narrow, slit-like nostrils, a projecting nasal tip, and thin alar sidewalls.[9,10,23] Cephalic positioning of the lateral crura, which results in a lack of support of the alar lobule, may predispose patients to this phenomenon. External na-

sal valve collapse may be addressed by deprojecting an overly projected nasal tip to increase the width of slit-like nostrils, realigning cephalically positioned lateral crura into a more caudal location, and placing structural grafts (alar batten grafts and alar rim grafts) to provide lateral wall and external valve support that will help prevent collapse.

Nasal airway obstruction may also occur because of a fixed obstruction, such as a deviated septum. This may be addressed with removal of the deviated septal cartilage, with preservation of a 1.5 cm L-shaped septal strut to maintain adequate support and prevent saddling of the dorsum. Any cartilaginous or bony septal spurs present on the maxillary bone should be removed as well. In cases of dorsal or caudal septal deviation, subtotal septal reconstruction may be indicated to correct the obstruction.

Infection

After rhinoplasty, infection in the patient can range from a mild cellulitis to septicemia or cavernous sinus thrombosis. Despite the presence of potentially pathogenic commensals within the nasal cavities, the reported rate of perioperative infection has been low, usually less than 3.0 percent.[24–26] A rarely reported serious complication is toxic shock syndrome after rhinoplasty with the insertion of nasal packing.[27] Because it has a rapid onset, patients should be counseled to return to the hospital or the office if they have any suggestive signs or symptoms, such as high fever, weakness, and tachycardia.

The use of perioperative antibiotics in rhinoplasty has been controversial. Recent studies have demonstrated benefit from the prophylactic use of antibiotics at the time of surgery but no decreased infection rate with postoperative antibiotic use.[28,29] However, most would recommend their use in the setting of active infection or septal hematoma, or if nasal packing or alloplastic implants are present. We continue to use perioperative antibiotics on all rhinoplasty patients.

Hemorrhage

Postoperative bleeding is one of the more common complications following nasal surgery. Multiple series have reported a rate below 4 percent.[26,30-32] Teichgraeber et al. found that postoperative bleeding was more frequent in patients who also underwent a septoplasty or turbinectomy.[32] Bleeding is most often seen after packing or splints have been removed. Persistent bleeding can be common at osteotomy sites or along the maxillary crest. If there is no success from conservative measures, such as topical vasoconstriction, silver nitrate cautery, or anterior packing, a return to the operating room may be warranted to localize and control the site of bleeding. As discussed previously, the most effective way to manage postoperative epistaxis is preoperative identification of patients who may be at higher risk of bleeding. A personal and family history of bleeding should be elicited, and the patient should be instructed to refrain from aspirin, nonsteroidal anti-inflammatory medications, vitamin E, and herbal supplements for at least three weeks before and two to four weeks after surgery. A preoperative laboratory workup should also be completed, with a complete blood count and coagulation profile.

Necrosis

Necrosis of various tissue components may occur after rhinoplasty, and it can lead to septal perforation, saddle-nose deformity, skin necrosis, and cartilage lysis.[20] Skin necrosis may be seen following the insertion of an alloplastic implant or after aggressive thinning and electrocautery of the SSTE. Initially, the overlying skin will become erythematous, with subsequent blanching and necrosis. If this process is suspected, any underlying inciting factors, such as an alloplastic implant, should be removed immediately. Certain patients may be at greater risk for postoperative necrosis because of preexisting medical conditions. Patients with diabetes, vascular disorders, connective tissue diseases, or epithelial disorders may have small vessel disease that can compromise healing. These patients are often not good candidates for rhinoplasty, but if surgery is performed, these patients must be monitored closely for any signs or symptoms of impending complication(s).

Septal Perforation

Septal perforation can occur from damage of the mucoperichondrial flaps during septoplasty and also may result from a compromised blood supply to the muco-sa. If opposing tears in the septal mucosa are created, they may be sutured, and crushed cartilage, costal cartilage perichondrium, or acellular dermis (Alloderm, LifeCell Corp.) may be placed between the flaps to facilitate mucosal coverage. Although most perforations will heal spontaneously, persistent small defects may be repaired through the use of grafts or local flaps. Any patient with a septal perforation should be instructed to keep the nasal mucosa moist and free of crusts with the use of aggressive saline irrigation, ointments, and humidification.

◆ Conclusion

Many aesthetic and functional abnormalities seen after rhinoplasty can be avoided by identifying those patients who are at risk of developing such complications. To prevent these secondary deformities, establish a surgical plan based on the patient's specific anatomy and anticipated postoperative healing. Intraoperatively, identify any maneuvers that may predispose to the development of complications and undertake appropriate measures to minimize the risk of a resulting deformity. Finally, patients should be followed closely during the postoperative period to identify any developing complications that may need to be addressed in the office setting or revision surgery.

PEARLS OF WISDOM

Complications from rhinoplasty arise from errors in analysis, technique, and surgical judgment.

Careful preoperative evaluation is essential to reduce the number of postoperative complications.

Computer imaging is a useful tool for communication between the surgeon and patient and helps to ensure that they have similar expectations and goals for any surgery.

In any revision rhinoplasty, the surgeon must carefully evaluate the patient for any additional factors that may increase the risk of complications. These include a damaged SSTE, the presence of alloplastic implant(s), and a compromised nasal vascular supply.

To reduce the number of postoperative problems, the surgeon must be vigilant intraoperatively to maintain meticulous technique, to take the time to correct any potential errors, and to camouflage all potentially visible grafts intraoperatively.

Frequent and long-term examination of the postoperative rhinoplasty patient will help the surgeon to identify complications in a timely manner.

Every complication in rhinoplasty should be seen as an opportunity for the surgeon to improve his or her preoperative assessment, intraoperative techniques, and postoperative care.

References

1. Sharp HR, Tingay RS, Coman S, Mills V, Roberts DN. Computer imaging and patient satisfaction in rhinoplasty surgery. J Laryngol Otol 2002;116(12):1009–1013

2. Kim DW, Toriumi DM. Nasal analysis for secondary rhinoplasty. Facial Plast Surg Clin North Am 2003;11(3):399–419

3. Guyuron B, Zarandy S, Tirgan A. von Willebrand's disease and plastic surgery. Ann Plast Surg 1994;32(4):351–355

4. Toriumi DM, Johnson CM. Open structure rhinoplasty: featured technical points and long-term follow-up. Facial Plast Surg Clin North Am 1993;1:1–22

5. Toriumi DM. Management of the middle nasal vault in rhinoplasty. Op Tech Plast Reconstr Surg 1995;2:16–30

6. Anderson JR. Straightening the crooked nose. Trans Am Acad Ophthalmol Otolaryngol 1972;76(4):938–945

7. Toriumi DM, Ries WR. Innovative surgical management of the crooked nose. Facial Plast Surg Clin North Am 1993;1:63–78

8. Kim DW, Toriumi DM. Management of posttraumatic nasal deformities: the crooked nose and the saddle nose. Facial Plast Surg Clin North Am 2004;12(1):111–132

9. Tardy ME, Garner ET. Inspiratory nasal obstruction secondary to alar and nasal valve collapse: technique for repair using autologous cartilage. Oper Tech Otolaryngol--Head Neck Surg 1990;1:215–218

10. Toriumi DM, Josen J, Weinberger M, Tardy ME Jr. Use of alar batten grafts for correction of nasal valve collapse. Arch Otolaryngol Head Neck Surg 1997;123(8):802–808

11. Toriumi DM. New concepts in nasal tip contouring. Arch Facial Plast Surg 2006;8(3):156–185

12. Johnson CM, Toriumi DM. Open Structure Rhinoplasty. Philadelphia: WB Saunders; 1990

13. Toriumi DM. Structure concept in nasal tip surgery. Op Tech Plast Reconstr Surg 2000;7:175–186

14. Tardy ME Jr, Kron TK, Younger R, Key M. The cartilaginous pollybeak: etiology, prevention, and treatment. Facial Plast Surg 1989;6(2):113–120

15. Kridel RW, Yoon PJ, Koch RJ. Prevention and correction of nasal tip bossae in rhinoplasty. Arch Facial Plast Surg 2003;5(5):416–422

16. Gillman GS, Simons RL, Lee DJ. Nasal tip bossae in rhinoplasty. Etiology, predisposing factors, and management techniques. Arch Facial Plast Surg 1999;1(2):83–89

17. Tardy ME Jr, Toriumi D. Alar retraction: composite graft correction. Facial Plast Surg 1989;6(2):101–107

18. Gunter JP, Friedman RM. Lateral crural strut graft: technique and clinical applications in rhinoplasty. Plast Reconstr Surg 1997;99(4):943–952, discussion 953–955

19. Perkins SW, Tardy ME. External columellar incisional approach to revision of the lower third of the nose. Facial Plast Surg Clin North Am 1993;1:79–98

20. Holt GR, Garner ET, McLarey D. Postoperative sequelae and complications of rhinoplasty. Otolaryngol Clin North Am 1987;20(4):853–876

21. Zijlker TD, Vuyk HD. Nasal valve surgery: spreader grafts. In: Trenite GJN, ed. Rhinoplasty: A Practical Guide to Functional and Aesthetic Surgery of the Nose. Amsterdam: Kugler; 1993:67–73

22. Constantian MB. The incompetent external nasal valve: pathophysiology and treatment in primary and secondary rhinoplasty. Plast Reconstr Surg 1994;93(5):919–931, discussion 932–933

23. Sheen JH. Spreader graft: a method of reconstructing the roof of the middle nasal vault following rhinoplasty. Plast Reconstr Surg 1984;73(2):230–239

24. Weimert TA, Yoder MG. Antibiotics and nasal surgery. Laryngoscope 1980;90(4):667–672

25. Lawson W, Kessler S, Biller HF. Unusual and fatal complications of rhinoplasty. Arch Otolaryngol 1983;109(3):164–169

26. Foda HMT. External rhinoplasty: a critical analysis of 500 cases. J Laryngol Otol 2003;117(6):473–477

27. Tobin G, Shaw RC, Goodpasture HC. Toxic shock syndrome following breast and nasal surgery. Plast Reconstr Surg 1987;80(1):111–114

28. Rajan GP, Fergie N, Fischer U, Romer M, Radivojevic V, Hee GK. Antibiotic prophylaxis in septorhinoplasty? A prospective, randomized study. Plast Reconstr Surg 2005;116(7):1995–1998

29. Andrews PJ, East CA, Jayaraj SM, Badia L, Panagamuwa C, Harding L. Prophylactic vs postoperative antibiotic use in complex septorhinoplasty surgery: a prospective, randomized, single-blind trial comparing efficacy. Arch Facial Plast Surg 2006;8(2):84–87

30. Goldwyn RM. Unexpected bleeding after elective nasal surgery. Ann Plast Surg 1979;2(3):201–204

31. McKinney P, Cook JQ. A critical evaluation of 200 rhinoplasties. Ann Plast Surg 1981;7(5):357–361

32. Teichgraeber JF, Riley WB, Parks DH. Nasal surgery complications. Plast Reconstr Surg 1990;85(4):527–531

11

Facelift Complications

Jonathan M. Sykes, Ji-Eon Kim, and Ira D. Papel

Rejuvenation procedures of the aging face are increasing in frequency. Numerous techniques have been described since the first facelift was performed by Lexer in 1906.[1] In 1968 Skoog performed the facelift procedure in a subfascial plane, improving the surgical results in the lower face.[2] This led to Mitz and Peyronie's contribution in 1976, defining the superficial fascia enveloping the face.[3] They termed this fascia the superficial musculoaponeurotic system (SMAS). Identifying and defining the SMAS layer has led to a better understanding of facial anatomy and has spurred a variety of surgical facelift techniques.

The facelift procedure remains the gold standard for surgical rejuvenation of the midface and lower face. Although numerous technical variations of the facelift have been described, the basic premise involves elevation of a facial skin flap with tightening of the underlying superficial fascia. After this is accomplished, the overlying excess skin is trimmed and reapproximated. When executed correctly, the rhytidectomy (facelift) procedure provides significant improvement in the appearance of the lower two-thirds of the face. This chapter identifies the common complications associated with this procedure and describes ways to prevent and treat these complications. The discussion covers prevention and management of preoperative, intraoperative, and postoperative problems.

◆ Preoperative Considerations

To prevent complications such as bleeding and skin necrosis, the surgeon must perform a careful preoperative work-up. This includes obtaining a detailed medical history and performing a thorough physical examination. The history should include the identification of all medical conditions that can cause poor wound healing, such as tobacco use, hypertension, peripheral artery disease, diabetes mellitus, and prior radiation therapy. The history should also identify any medications that can cause perioperative bleeding or delayed wound healing.

Informed Consent

Informed consent must be obtained before any medical intervention or surgical procedure. The informed choice process is even more important in elective cosmetic surgery, such as rhytidectomy. This process is defined as a two-way communication between the practitioner and patient, during which the goals of therapy are discussed, along with all therapeutic options, their associated risks, and potential complications. Informed consent involves full disclosure and must be presented in a clear and understandable manner.

Adequate informed consent in cosmetic surgery requires both the patient and surgeon to have good communication skills. The surgeon must thoroughly explain the procedure, the attendant risks, the incisions, preoperative and postoperative care, and expected healing times. The surgeon should assess the patient's ability to withstand the aesthetic surgery, both physically and psychologically. The patient should be able to process this information, ask questions, and avoid the temptation to have preconceived ideas and expectations related to the surgical procedures.

Informed consent fails when there is a lack of communication. This occurs when the surgeon does not take the time or have the skills to explain the procedure adequately. Informed consent is also unsuccessful when the patient has preconceived ideas about surgery and unrealistic expectations relating to the cosmetic outcome. Poor communication between practitioners and patients is more likely if the patient has underlying psychological issues, such as anxiety, depression, body dysmorphic disorder (BDD), or significant problems with self-image.[4] Inadequately performed informed consent in cosmetic surgery is common. Poor communication can lead to anger, frustration, and litigation; for these reasons, the number of malpractice suits filed against cosmetic surgeons is relatively high in relation to other specialties.[5]

Medical Conditions

Many systemic medicines, both prescribed and over-the-counter, can increase the risk of intraoperative and postoperative bleeding. The list includes well-known anticoagulants such as oral warfarin, platelet function inhibitors such as aspirin, and nonsteroidal anti-inflammatory medications. Other less commonly recognized oral remedies that can increase the risk of perioperative bleeding include vitamins such as vitamin E, herbal supplements such as *Gingko biloba*, fish oil, and antioxidants (**Table 11.1**).[6] It is important to provide patients with a thorough list of medicines and supplements to avoid.

A comprehensive medical history should be obtained from the patient. This is often facilitated by providing a detailed questionnaire before the initial consultation. All preoperative medical conditions and prior surgeries should be known and discussed. In particular, any conditions that may impact flap vascularity or postoperative healing should be identified. Some medical conditions, such as hypertension, may increase the risk of postoperative bleeding. For this reason, medical conditions should be evaluated and treated preoperatively to minimize postoperative risks.

Certain medical conditions predispose the aesthetic surgery patient to postoperative complications. These include cardiac disease, peripheral vascular disease, and associated hypertension. Pulmonary disease, such as emphysema or chronic obstructive pulmonary disease, can increase the incidence of diminished flap vascularity and associated flap necrosis. In addition, patients with pulmonary diseases have a greater chance of postoperative coughing and straining, which can increase the risk of postoperative hematoma.

Although it is very uncommon to experience impairment in facelift flap vascularity or even frank necrosis

of facelift flaps, some medical conditions can predispose patients to these complications. Diabetes mellitus increases the risk of postoperative bruising, delayed healing, and infection. Although perioperative control of serum glucose should be obtained, patients with diabetes mellitus continue to have small-vessel peripheral artery disease, which may compromise vascular supply to the skin flaps. Cigarette smoking also decreases vascularity to skin flaps and therefore increases the risk of wound-healing issues and flap necrosis.[7] For this reason, many surgeons refuse to perform facelift surgery on active smokers. Smokers should be encouraged to cease cigarette use for four weeks before and at least two weeks after the facelift procedure. If facelifts are performed on active smokers or on patients with diabetes mellitus, flap length should be decreased to minimize the potential for flap compromise.

◆ Hematoma

Subcutaneous hematoma is one of the most common complications of facelift surgery. The incidence ranges from 2 to 15% of cases, depending on the published reports.[7,8] The occurrence of a hematoma requires urgent treatment, and even if the hematoma is successfully evacuated, the sequelae may be long lasting.

The prevention of facelift hematoma should be the surgeon's highest priority. This demands that the surgeon take a careful preoperative history and as much as possible eliminate or reduce known risk factors. For example, all rhytidectomy patients should discontinue medications containing aspirin for at least two weeks before surgery. Many patients are not aware that common over-the-counter preparations contain aspirin. Patients should be asked to read the labels of all medications in the two weeks prior to surgery. If patients are on anticoagulants such as warfarin sodium, the surgeon should consult with their primary physician to determine if it is safe to discontinue anticoagulation for elective aesthetic surgery. Other risk factors include the chronic use of nonsteroidal anti-inflammatory medications, platelet inhibitors, and high doses of vitamin E.

Tobacco smoking has been linked to an increased risk of complications in facelift surgery, including hematoma. All smokers must be required to stop smoking for at least four weeks before surgery. Some patients will not be fully truthful in reporting their progress in smoking cessation, but the tobacco smell can be easily detected in the preoperative area. The surgeon must be willing to cancel surgery in this situation. Smokers also have a much higher incidence of flap necrosis.

Hypertension is also a significant risk factor. Labile blood pressure in the postoperative period may predispose a patient to bleeding and hematoma.[9] Preoperative screening should be performed to identify uncontrolled hypertension. Patients should be encouraged to con-

Table 11.1

Medicines to Avoid Prior to Rhytidectomy (Not Comprehensive)	
Aspirin/NSAID products	Aleve, aspirin, BC powder, Bufferin, Diclofenac, Excedrin, Florinal, Goody's headache powder, ibuprofen, ketolarac, Midol, Motrin, Naprosyn, Norgesic, salicylic acid, Soma, Toradol
Herbal/natural products	Ginger, *Gingko biloba*, garlic, ginseng, echinacea, fish oils (omega-3 fatty acids), dong quai, feverfew, licorice root, pine bark extract, St. John's wort, yohimbine
Vitamins	Vitamin E
Anticoagulants	Heparin, warfarin

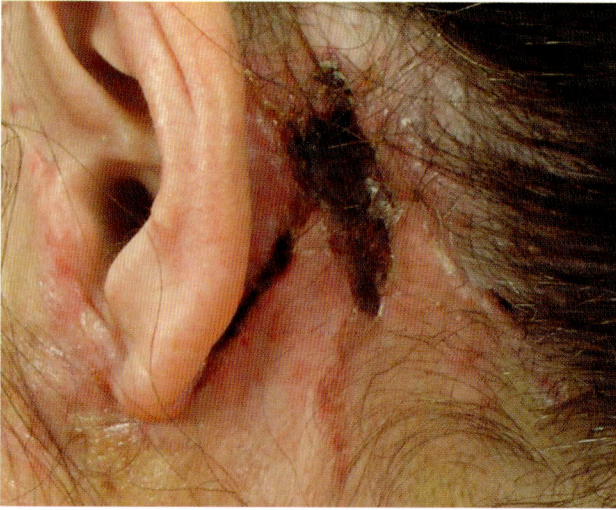

Fig. 11.1 Postauricular skin flap necrosis.

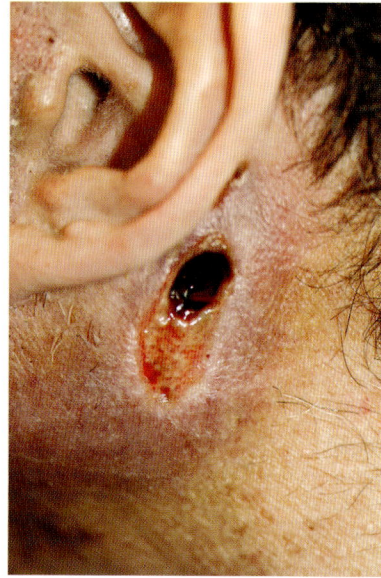

Fig. 11.2 Posterolateral neck skin flap necrosis.

tinue their antihypertensive medication throughout the preoperative period. If hypertension is not well controlled, patients should be referred to their primary care physicians to adjust their antihypertensive medication. Meticulous surgical technique with care to dissect in proper tissue planes, combined with careful hemostasis, is essential for successful rhytidectomy surgery.

The clinical presentation of a hematoma includes pressure and pain beyond the postoperative discomfort usually expected. Because bulky dressings may hide a hematoma, the surgeon must be suspicious of a hematoma if the patient has unilateral or severe pain. If a hematoma is suspected, the dressings should be removed for close inspection. Once a hematoma is diagnosed, treatment should begin immediately to drain the collection and prevent further complications. Since the skin flaps receive blood supply from the subdermal plexus, the pressure of a hematoma may reduce blood flow to the skin flap and lead to later skin necrosis (**Figs. 11.1, 11.2**). Large collections of blood and serum usually require opening of the incisions, evacuation and irrigation of the subcutaneous cavity, identification of the site of the bleeding, and reclosure of the incisions. This may require general anesthesia to ensure an adequate airway and patient comfort. In most circumstances, however, this procedure can be accomplished with local anesthesia if the patient is cooperative.

Smaller collections may require only a rolling of the flaps using gauze, combined with removal of a few sutures, to evacuate the fluid. Even small organized clots can be extruded with this method. At times, aspiration with a #16 or #18 gauge needle may be all that is necessary, if the area is still liquid. Aspiration of small amounts of serum is common on the day after surgery and usually causes minimal discomfort for the patient.

Failure to recognize a hematoma may lead to significant postoperative complications (**Fig. 11.3**). Skin necrosis with soft tissue loss is the most significant complication, and this may take many weeks to heal. There will usually be some permanent scars, but most superficial necrosis heals in a surprisingly acceptable manner. In many patients with even minor hematomas, subcutaneous edema and irregularity may persist for many months before subsiding. At times, this can lead to permanent subcutaneous irregularities (**Fig. 11.4**).

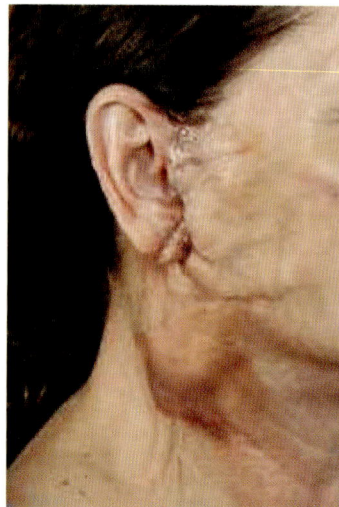

Fig. 11.3 Neck hematoma after facelift surgery.

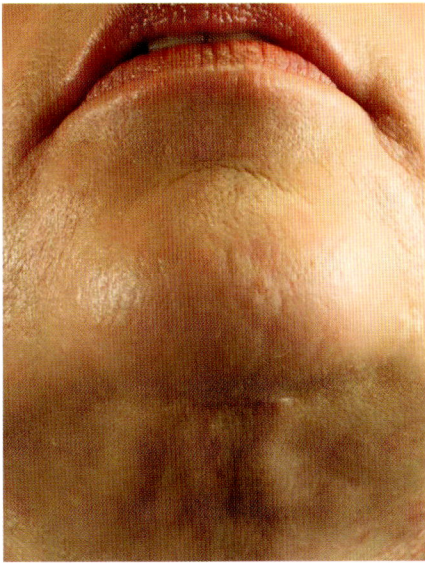

Fig. 11.4 Skin and soft-tissue irregularity after facelift surgery.

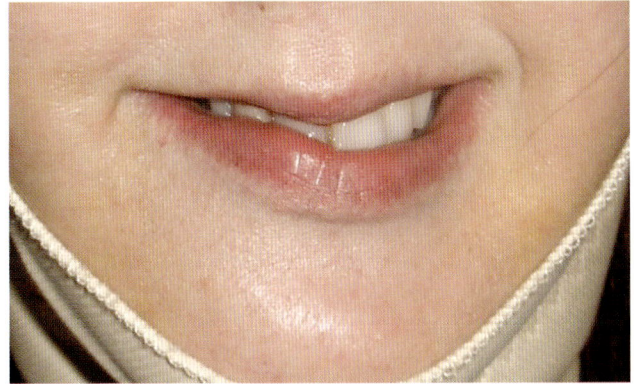

Fig. 11.5 Injury to the right marginal mandibular branch of the facial nerve after facelift surgery.

◆ Motor Nerve Injuries

Facial nerve injuries in rhytidectomy are rare. The incidence is thought to be in the area of 1 to 3%.[10] The most common facial nerve branches injured are the temporal and marginal mandibular nerves. This type of injury is very symptomatic for the patient and is best avoided by careful surgical technique and thorough knowledge of anatomy. Careful dissection in the subcutaneous plane in the temporal region will avoid the facial nerve.[11] Avoiding aggressive cautery in this thin tissue will also help prevent inadvertent thermal injury to the nerve.

The facial nerve branches are deep to the facial muscles in most of the face. In the temporal region, the motor nerves run superficial over the zygomatic arch within the temporoparietal fascia, where the temporal branch is vulnerable to aggressive dissection. The cervical and marginal branches are vulnerable as they course about one centimeter anterior to the posterior border of the platysma muscle (**Fig. 11.5**). If the posterior edge of the platysma is elevated too far for suspension to the mastoid periosteum, the nerves may be damaged.[12] Injuries to the main trunk of the facial nerve should be very rare in the usual rhytidectomy dissection area, because the thickness of the parotid gland protects the nerve.

With the use of deep plane rhytidectomy techniques, the buccal and zygomatic branches of the facial nerve are more exposed than in subcutaneous short flap techniques. Dissection below the platysma just above the parotidomasseteric fascia exposes the nerves just beneath the thin fascia. Careless use of cautery or scissors in this area can harm the nerves and cause facial asymmetry.

Facial nerve injuries may recover spontaneously if the nerve injury is not complete. Reinnervation may occur if multiple branches are present in one area. In the temporal area, botulinum toxin can be used to paralyze the normal (uninjured) side for a short period and simulate facial symmetry.[13] Fortunately, a high percentage of these nerve injuries usually recover.

◆ Hairline Distortion

The surgeon can easily prevent alteration of the natural hairline after rhytidectomy. The position and amount of the temporal hair tuft should be maintained, and the natural line of the postauricular hair must also be preserved.

The primary vector of elevation of the skin-SMAS complex in the midface is vertical. If the temporal skin incision is made vertically (as a coronal extension of the preauricular incision) and the skin is closed according to the deep suspension sutures, the temporal hair tuft will be unnaturally elevated (**Fig. 11.6**). There are two simple methods to avoid temporal hairline elevation. The first is to make the temporal incision at the hairline (tricophytic). If the tricophytic incision is used, it is important to bevel the incision (leaving follicles on the temporal flap), to allow hair to grow through the eventual scar later. The second method to avoid temporal tuft elevation is to advance the temporal hair flap inferiorly before closing the incision. This will ensure that the first closure suture (or staple) recreates the original hairline position.

In the postauricular region, it is also important to avoid changing the natural position of the hairline. The usual vector of pull of the neck skin is directly posterior. If the entire flap is moved in this direction (without attention to the hairline), an unnatural step-off is produced in the postauricular hairline. A postauricular step-off can be avoided by aligning the hairline first, before placing any other closure sutures (staples). If the hairline align-

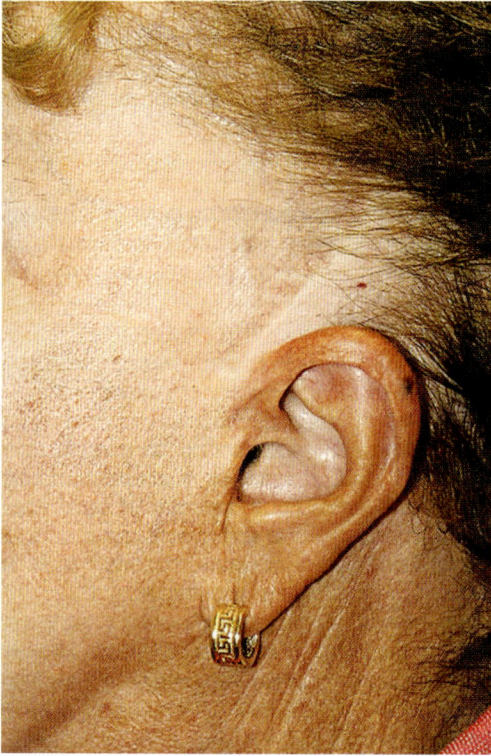

Fig. 11.6 Unnaturally elevated temporal hair tuft after facelift surgery. Used with permission from Clevens RA. "Avoiding Patient Dissatisfaction and Complications in Facelift Surgery." Facial Plastic Surgery Clinics of North America. Nov 2009. 17(4). p. 519., Fig. 4.

ment suture is accomplished first, all other closure can then be performed, with Burow's triangles occurring to match flaps. Alternatively, the postauricular incision can be made at the hairline so that it does not cause hairline elevation or an unsightly step-off. However, a posterior hairline incision can be noticeable, particularly if the patient wears short hair or if the hair color is dark.

◆ Sensory Nerve Injury

Elevation of a cervicofacial skin flap always causes transient hypesthesia or anesthesia. This change in sensation is most noticeable in the periauricular region and usually exists for three to six months. It is important for the facial plastic surgeon to inform the patient preoperatively about the expected numbness and the variable nature of the return of sensation. The patient should understand that postoperative numbness is an expectation, not a complication.

The most commonly injured nerve in rhytidectomy surgery is the great auricular nerve, which is a cervical sensory branch from C_2 and C_3. Injury to this nerve oc-

curs in 1 to 7% of patients.[14] The great auricular nerve provides sensation to the lower half of the ear, the periauricular skin, and the skin over the angle of the mandible. The nerve is located in the fascia overlying the sternocleidomastoid (SCM) muscle at the anterior border of this muscle. The surgeon should take care to raise the postauricular skin flap in a very superficial plane, as the SCM muscle becomes very superficial in this area. This will avoid injury to the great auricular nerve. If the nerve is transected, reapproximation with #9–0 or #10–0 nylon suture should be performed at the time of injury. If a transected nerve is not repaired, a painful neuroma may occur.

◆ Alopecia

Hair loss after rhytidectomy causes emotional distress to most patients. Hair loss occurs from injury to the hair follicles, either from traction or from actual follicle transection. The reported incidence of alopecia is approximately 2.8%.[15]

Transection of hair follicles is uncommon and can be avoided by careful flap elevation and visualization of the undersurface of the follicles.[16] Injury to the hair follicles from either traction or from electrocautery is more common than actual follicle transection. Hair regrowth usually occurs in 45 to 90 days. If sufficient hair regrowth does not occur, areas of alopecia may be treated with microfollicular hair grafts or with advancement of temporal scalp flaps.

◆ Parotid Fistula

Parotid fistula after rhytidectomy is a rare complication and can be avoided by a careful knowledge of the applied anatomy. The parotid fascia is typically a dense connective tissue that protects the parotid gland on its lateral (superficial) surface. The SMAS layer is often fused with the true parotid fascia immediately in front of the ear; for this reason, elevation of a SMAS flap is usually not initiated in the immediate preauricular region.

Careful subcutaneous elevation in the preauricular and infraauricular regions will avoid injury to the parotid fascia and underlying parotid gland. This will prevent the complication of parotid fistula. If injury to the gland does occur, intraoperative repair of the gland and the overlying fascia can usually prevent postoperative fistula. If parotid fistula occurs, botulinum toxin may be used to minimize symptoms.

◆ Infection

Perioperative infection following rhytidectomy is rare. The incidence of infection is less than 1%, and this low frequency is due to the very rich vascular supply of the cervicofacial skin and soft tissues.[17] Although postoperative facelift infection is uncommon, its risk increases in diabetic patients, smokers, and patients who are immunocompromised. Unevacuated hematomas may also predispose patients to infection.

The symptoms and signs associated with postoperative facelift infection include pain, swelling, and tenderness greater than that typically encountered after facelift. The wounds may be locally tender or erythemtous, and the patient will often develop a fever.

Infection is often prevented with the use of perioperative prophylactic antibiotics. Antibiotics should be administered between 30 minutes and 2 hours before the initial skin incision and stopped within 48 hours after surgery. If infection does occur, management includes (1) local wound care, (2) aspiration or incision and drainage if an abscess is suspected, (3) removal of infected sutures, (4) culture and sensitivity of the wound, and (5) initiation of appropriate systemic antibiotics.

Local wound care after facelift infection is essential. Proper care increases the chances that the infection will not spread. Local wound care includes the use of one-half strength hydrogen peroxide topically, often followed by a thin topical application of antibiotic ointment. In cases of progressive infection, it is appropriate to obtain an infectious disease consultation.

◆ Skin Flap Necrosis

The viability of skin flaps after a facelift is based on a variety of factors related to the patient's preoperative condition and the surgeon's intraoperative technique. The vascular supply to the facial skin is typically very rich. Conditions that affect the microcirculation to the skin can increase the risk of the flap necrosis after a facelift. These conditions include diabetes mellitus, atherosclerosis, a prior history of radiation therapy, chronic pulmonary disease (such as COPD or emphysema), and smoking.

The effects of smoking on skin flap survival have been well documented both clinically and experimentally. Nicotine releases catecholamines, which impair epithelialization and decrease inflammation. According to Rees, 80% of patients with skin slough after facelift smoked more than one package of cigarettes per day at the time of their surgery. He estimated the risk of skin slough in active smokers to be 12 to 13 times the risk of necrosis in the nonsmoking patient.[18] For this reason, it is advised that smokers cease smoking for at least two weeks preoperatively and three weeks postoperatively. Many surgeons refuse to operate on active smokers.

Intraoperative causes of flap necrosis after facelift are related to the length and thickness of the skin flap. Other intraoperative causes of flap compromise include increased tension on the skin wound (and flap edges). When the skin flap is longer and thinner, the risk of com-

promise to the distal edges of the flap increases. Similarly, if too much skin is excised during flap advancement, the risk of flap necrosis increases. In patients with an increased preoperative risk of flap compromise (e.g., smokers, diabetics, patients with prior history of radiation therapy), a shorter, thicker skin flap decreases the risk of flap necrosis.

Postoperative causes of facelift skin flap compromise include excessively tight dressings and lack of recognition of seromas, hematomas, or infection. Untreated hematomas or seromas may compromise distal skin vascularity, resulting in epidermolysis and full-thickness skin loss. For this reason, early recognition and treatment of hematomas and seromas are advised.

◆ Hypertrophic Scarring

The preauricular scars created during rhytidectomy usually heal in a relatively unnoticeable manner. However, in some instances scars may become hypertrophic, or keloid scars may develop.

Unsightly scars are occasionally unpreventable. These usually occur in thick-skinned, darkly pigmented individuals who may have a history of poor wound healing of scars from prior surgeries. In most cases, however, perioperative circumstances contribute to the poor scar formation. Scars may thicken or widen as a side effect of increased wound tension. If the deep-layer closure does not adequately decrease tension on the skin closure, the cutaneous scars may become hypertrophic and widen. For this reason, it is important that the facelift surgeon place an adequate amount of deep sutures to reduce cutaneous wound tension sufficiently. Additionally, the surgeon should not resect skin too much, to help prevent increased incisional tension during closure.

Other perioperative conditions can contribute to poor wound healing and increased scarring. These include bleeding, hematoma, infection, and poor vascularity to the skin flaps. Compromised vascularity to facelift skin flaps is more common in patients who smoke, have had prior radiation therapy, or have a history of diabetes mellitus. In cases in which flap vascularity is in question, a thicker, shorter flap minimizes the chance of facelift flap compromise.

Hypertrophic scars occur most frequently in the postauricular region. Keloid scars are less common. Treatment includes early recognition and the topical application of steroid or silicone-impregnated tape. Intralesional steroid injections (triamcinolone 10 to 40 mg/ml) can be injected directly intradermally. These injections can be repeated (approximately every four weeks) and help to soften and flatten hypertrophic scars. In rare instances, scar revision is necessary. Of course, the basic principle of minimizing skin wound tension is crucial if improvement is to be achieved with postauricular scar revision. Again, repeated intralesional steroid injections are to be expected after scar revision.

◆ Conclusion

The facelift procedure is the gold standard for rejuvenation of the midface and lower face. The surgeon must consider several factors to minimize the risk of complications associated with facelift surgery. Obtaining proper informed consent prior to surgery requires good communication between the surgeon and patient. Medical conditions that may predispose the patient to excessive bleeding or flap necrosis should be identified, and medications that predispose the patient to postoperative bleeding must be avoided if possible.

Subcutaneous hematomas are one of the most common complications after facelift surgery and can result in serious adverse consequences. Injury to a branch of the facial nerve can often be avoided by thorough knowledge of the facial anatomy and careful dissection technique. Hairline distortions of the temporal and postauricular area can occur because of the vector of lift, but they can be avoided with careful planning. Less common complications of facelift surgery include alopecia, parotid fistula, and wound infection. Skin flap necrosis, when large, can have devastating consequences. Therefore, careful preoperative screening is recommended. When skin flap necrosis is encountered after surgery, early detection and management are essential. Hypertrophic scarring can often be minimized or managed by taking care to avoid some of the previously mentioned potential complications and by using intralesional steroid injections. With careful attention to detail and sound technique, the surgeon can minimize many of the complications of facelift surgery.

PEARLS OF WISDOM

A detailed informed consent explaining the proposed procedure, potential complications, risks, and possible limitations of the surgery should be obtained.

It is important to select the patient carefully and to determine if the patient has reasonable expectations.

A comprehensive medical history should be obtained. The patient should be given a list of medicines to avoid perioperatively to minimize the chance of postoperative bleeding.

Existing medical conditions, such as hypertension, should be well controlled prior to surgery.

A thorough knowledge of facial anatomy minimizes the risk of sensory or motor nerve injury.

Meticulous postoperative care, including psychological support, is crucial to ensure optimal physical and mental healing from surgery.

References

1. Fomon S. The surgery of injury and plastic repair. Baltimore: Williams and Wilkins; 1939:1344
2. Skoog T. Plastic Surgery: New Methods and Refinements. Philadephia, PA: WB Sauders Co; 1974
3. Mitz V, Peyronie M. The superficial musculo-aponeurotic system (SMAS) in the parotid and cheek area. Plast Reconstr Surg 1976;58(1):80–88
4. Shridharani SM, Magarakis M, Manson PN, Rodriguez ED. Psychology of plastic and reconstructive surgery: a systematic clinical review. Plast Reconstr Surg 2010;126(6):2243–2251
5. Kaplan JL, Hammert WC, Zin JE. Lawsuits against plastic surgeons: Does locale affect incidence of claims? Can J Plast Surg 2007;15(3):155–157
6. Destro MW, Speranzini MB, Cavalheiro Filho C, Destro T, Destro C. Bilateral haematoma after rhytidoplasty and blepharoplasty following chronic use of *Ginkgo biloba*. Br J Plast Surg 2005;58(1):100–101
7. Grover R, Jones BM, Waterhouse N. The prevention of haematoma following rhytidectomy: a review of 1078 consecutive facelifts. Br J Plast Surg 2001;54(6):481–486
8. Baker DC, Stefani WA, Chiu ES. Reducing the incidence of hematoma requiring surgical evacuation following male rhytidectomy: a 30-year review of 985 cases. Plast Reconstr Surg 2005;116(7):1973–1985, discussion 1986–1987
9. Berner RE, Morain WD, Noe JM. Postoperative hypertension as an etiological factor in hematoma after rhytidectomy. Prevention with chlorpromazine. Plast Reconstr Surg 1976; 57(3):314–319
10. Payne DL. Facial nerve deficits following face lift surgery. Am J Otol 1992;13(1):91–92
11. Baker DC, Conley J. Avoiding facial nerve injuries in rhytidectomy. Anatomical variations and pitfalls. Plast Reconstr Surg 1979;64(6):781–795
12. Daane SP, Owsley JQ. Incidence of cervical branch injury with "marginal mandibular nerve pseudo-paralysis" in patients undergoing face lift. Plast Reconstr Surg 2003;111(7): 2414–2418
13. Clark RP, Berris CE. Botulinum toxin: a treatment for facial asymmetry caused by facial nerve paralysis. Plast Reconstr Surg 1989;84(2):353–355
14. McKinney P, Katrana DJ. Prevention of injury to the great auricular nerve during rhytidectomy. Plast Reconstr Surg 1980;66(5):675–679
15. Webster RC, Davidson TM, White MF, Bush JE, Smith RC. Conservative face lift surgery. Arch Otolaryngol 1976;102(11): 657–662
16. Kridel RW, Liu ES. Techniques for creating inconspicuous facelift scars: avoiding visible incisions and loss of temporal hair. Arch Facial Plast Surg 2003;5(4):325–333
17. LeRoy JL Jr, Rees TD, Nolan WB III. Infections requiring hospital readmission following face lift surgery: incidence, treatment, and sequelae. Plast Reconstr Surg 1994;93(3): 533–536
18. Rees TD, Aston SJ. Complications of rhytidectomy. Clin Plast Surg 1978;5(1):109–119

12

Complications with Facial Implantation

Edwin F. Williams III and Srinivasan Krishna

Contemporary care in facial plastic surgery mandates familiarity and facility with facial implants. Over the past few decades, trends have stressed the restoration of facial volume and the importance of enhancing skeletal facial proportions. One has only to look at the success of facial fillers to see this. Like injectable fillers, facial implantation has also become an increasingly popular way to replenish lost volume and to correct contour abnormalities that result from developmental, traumatic or age-related etiologies. When it is possible, most surgeons prefer the implantation of autologous tissue; however, the additional morbidity associated with the harvest of donor tissue, the limitation of tissue availability, and the risk of graft distortion or resorption are potential drawbacks. Alternatives to autologous tissue include allografts, xenografts, and alloplastic materials. The use of allograft tissue tends to have similar limitations to the use of autologous tissue in terms of resorption and distortion (perhaps more so), in addition to the remote possibility of disease transmission. Their more predictable long-term outcomes and limitless availability make alloplastic implants particularly attractive; however, the use of alloplastic implants is not without its own set of risks (including elevated risk of infection), and the search for the optimal implant material continues.[1]

The Ideal Facial Implant

Table 12.1 outlines the commonly used facial implant materials and their characteristics.

Most alloplastic implants used today for facial enhancement are synthetic polymers. These are macromolecules of repeating monomeric units. They may be solid polymers, such as polydimethylsiloxane or solid silicone (Silastic, Dow Corning, Midland, MI) and polymethylmethacrylate; porous polymers, such as high density porous polyethylene (MEDPOR, Porex Surgical, Newman, GA) and fibrillated expanded polytetrafluoroethylene (ePTFE) (Gore-Tex, WL Gore, Flagstaff, AZ); or meshed polymers such as polyethylene terephthalate (Mersilene, Ethicon, Somerville, NJ). In addition, certain metals such as gold (Au-79) and titanium (Ti-22) are used as implants, primarily for reconstructive purposes.[2] Ceramics such as hydroxyapatite are also useful, particularly in craniofacial reconstructive procedures.

The biocompatibility or interaction between implant and host is influenced by many factors, including the chemical composition of the implant material, host reaction, and surgical technique. The ideal implant material is nontoxic, nonantigenic, noncarcinogenic, acceptable to the host, durable, and resistant to infection. It is cost-effective, easy to sculpt or customize without compromising its integrity, easy to insert, and able to withstand mechanical strain without changing its shape. It has few surface imperfections, is able to conform to irregular surfaces, and is easily removable without causing significant tissue injury.[3] Although a multitude of implant materials are available in the market, currently none satisfy all these criteria. Each implant material has its own risks and benefits, and there is presently no ideal permanent implant.

Implant Complications

Understanding the complications associated with facial implantation from study of the literature has its limitations. Some surgeons are reluctant to report complications or poor results, and patients with adverse outcomes often seek alternative opinions and are lost to follow-up.[4] In any event, complications from facial implantation do occur and result from a combination of factors related to the patient (host), the implant material, and the surgeon's technique. The following discussion will treat each of these areas separately.

Patient-Related Complications

Patient-related complications are typically from mismanaged expectations that lead the patient to be dissatisfied with the outcome. These complications are largely preventable with open and frank communication between patient and surgeon. Prevention begins with a comprehensive evaluation of the patient, includ-

Table 12.1

Facial Implant Characteristics						
Material	Polydimethyl-siloxane	Expanded polytetra-fluoroethylene (ePTFE)	High density polyethylene	Polyester fiber	Polymethyl-methacrylate	Hydroxyapatite/carbonated apatite cement
Trade name	Silastic (silicone rubber)	Gore-Tex	MEDPOR Marlex mesh	Mersilene/Dacron	Cranioplast	Bone Source/Norian CRS
Tissue interface	fibrous capsule	limited tissue in-growth	fibrovascular and osseous in-growth	tissue in-growth	tissue in-growth	osseointegration
Advantages	easy to contour and remove	comes in sheet or tubular forms, can be layered, easily removed	versatile, stable, resists infection	easy to contour, can be layered	can be molded in situ	paste—can be molded easily
Disadvantages	bone resorp-tion, exposure	palpable, expensive	difficult to remove	difficult to remove	exothermic reaction, expo-sure	exposure or infection
Complications	malposition. extrusion, infection	malposition. extrusion, infection	malposition. extrusion, infection	infection, extru-sion	malposition, infection	exposure, infection
Common sites for use	chin, malar, cranioplasty	chin, malar, lips, nose, nasolabial folds	malar, orbit, chin, mandible	chin, malar, nose	orbital, cranial, malar recon-struction	craniofacial

Adapted from Sykes JM, Tollefson TT, Frodel Jr, JL. In: Cummings CW, ed. Cummings Otolaryngology—Head & Neck Surgery. Philadelphia: Elsevier Mosby Publishers; 2005:801–821.

Trade names include Silastic (Dow Corning, Midland, MI), Gore-Tex (WL Gore, Flagstaff, AZ), MEDPOR (Porex Surgical, Newnan, GA), Cranioplast (Advanced Biomaterial Systems, Passaic, NJ), Norian CRS (Synthes-Stratec, Paoli, PA), BoneSource (Stryker Leibinger, Flint, MI).

ing careful analysis of standardized digital photographs. Consistent photographic techniques with appropriate views are essential for accurate preoperative and post-operative comparisons. Inadequate preoperative analysis can lead to selection of the improper implant and an unhappy patient. Computerized morphing techniques may be used to manage patient expectations and demonstrate the need for appropriate additional interventions to achieve the best possible aesthetic outcome. One must be careful to emphasize that such morphing is an approximation and by no means a guarantee of a surgical result. Having the patient sign a waiver to this effect is helpful from a legal standpoint.[5]

Although they are designed to be inert, specific implant materials can cause hypersensitivity reactions in some patients and therefore produce adverse outcomes. Hypersensitivity tends to be more common with filler materials such as bovine collagen, which has a 2–3% incidence of an allergic or hypersensitivity reaction and requires double skin testing prior to usage.

Complications Related to Surgical Technique

Complications from surgical technique are somewhat generic to any implantation procedure, but the risk varies with specific sites and the implant material(s) used. Most surgical complications are fortunately minor and self limiting. Major complications must be dealt with expeditiously to avoid long-term sequelae. A thorough knowledge of the anatomy and meticulous attention to surgical technique are critical to avoid adverse surgical outcomes. The surgical complications commonly encountered with facial implants are discussed below.

Hematoma

Blood that accumulates in a tight pocket can lead to pressure necrosis of the overlying skin and soft tissue, resulting in implant exposure and extrusion. Hematomata need to be drained and the bleeding controlled in a timely fashion.[6]

Nerve Injury

Depending on the site of implantation, nerve injury can manifest as paresthesias or dysesthesias involving the infraorbital or mental nerve. Occasionally, weakness involving the frontotemporal or marginal mandibular branches of the facial nerve (VII) can also occur. Nerve injuries are commonly neurapraxias resulting from aggressive retraction or transmitted thermal injury, and they typically resolve in less than three weeks. Should they persist beyond that time period, one must have a low threshold for exploring the area and ruling out malposition of the implant and induced neurapraxia.[7] Very rarely, nerve injuries can be permanent.[6]

Prolonged Edema

Postoperative facial edema after implantation typically resolves in three weeks or less. Occasionally edema can last several months and can be caused by chronic inflammation. Discrete areas may be treated with intralesional triamcinolone.[6] Patients commonly need reassurance.

Implant Migration and Extrusion

Displacement of the implant from its intended position is a well-known complication of facial implant surgery. Malposition itself is problematic (e.g., a chin implant that lies obliquely to or off the midline), but it also can cause problematic asymmetry when paired implants are employed (e.g., malar implants may be differently positioned). Malposition can result from an improperly sized pocket or inadequately secured implant[3] (**Fig. 12.1**). Pocket inadequacy or an excessively sized implant may cause pressure necrosis of the overlying skin/soft tissue envelope, resulting in exposure and eventual extrusion. A displaced implant needs to be repositioned expeditiously. Extrusion can also occur from an infected implant. Extrusion warrants implant removal, with possible reinsertion once the extrusion site is completely healed.[6]

Persistent Seromas

Persistent seromas tend to occur most often with Silastic (silicone) implants and may need to be drained repeatedly.[8] The exact pathophysiology of seroma formation after silicone implantation is unclear.

Infection

Infection can occur with any implantation procedure but may be more common with intraoral approaches. Some studies suggest that soaking the implant in an antibiotic solution (Bacitracin 50,000 units in 1 liter of normal saline) and using perioperative antibiotics may decrease the incidence of implant-related infections.[3] Should an infection occur, aggressive antibiotic therapy with gram-

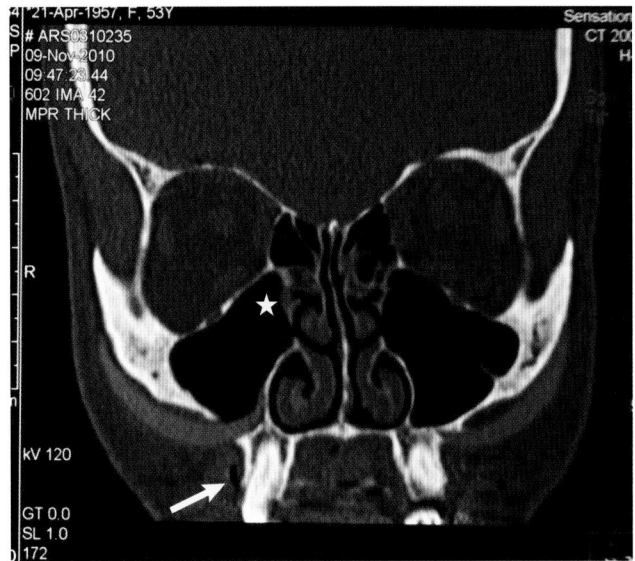

Fig. 12.1 Coronal CT of the face revealing significant displacement of a 10-year-old Silastic malar implant. The patient was experiencing right facial swelling, discomfort, and other symptoms consistent with unilateral maxillary sinusitis. Physical examination also revealed a 3 mm oroantral fistula on the affected side. In addition to the displaced implant, the CT also illustrates soft tissue near the right maxillary ostium (*star*), which was consistent with polypoid degeneration seen on nasal endoscopy. The fistula tract is also partially visualized on CT (*arrow*).

positive and anaerobic coverage is indicated. Commonly cultured organisms include staphylococcal and streptoccoccal species and anaerobes. Certain implants with good vascular ingrowth may be salvageable (such as Gore-Tex and MEDPOR) with antibacterial therapy, but infection frequently requires removal of the implant.

Preventive measures to help reduce the incidence of such complications include timely cessation of aspirin, anticoagulants, nonsteroidal anti-inflammatory medications (NSAIDs), vitamins (especially vitamin E), and herbal medications. As long as it is cleared with the patient's primary physician, patients should be off these medications long enough to return the blood clotting cascade or platelet function to normal. Most commonly, two weeks before surgery is sufficient. Steroids are commonly administered intraoperatively, and continued for 24 hours perioperatively to decrease postoperative edema. Similarly, an appropriate intravenous dose of a first-generation cephalosporin or clindamycin should be administered (ideally 30 minutes before the initial incision), and perioperative antibiotics (again, with good gram-positive and anaerobic coverage) are prescribed for five days. A pressure dressing can be helpful for the first 24–48 hours after any implantation procedure to decrease the risk of a hematoma and limit edema. Patients are additionally instructed to elevate their heads and to use cold compresses on the surgical site for the first 48 hours after surgery.

Implant-Related Complications

Implant-related complications tend to vary with the implant material used and site of implantation. As previously indicated, implant and host factors are inter-related. Common implant-related problems include inflammation, edema, displacement, infection, exposure, extrusion and bone resorption. Rare complications include the potential risk of carcinogenicity, but the level of this risk is ill-defined in the literature. Silicone, in particular, has been implicated as an etiologic factor in certain connective tissue diseases, yet several large series show no increased risk in women following silicone breast augmentation.[4] A link to anaplastic large cell lymphoma occurring in the fibrous capsule around silicone breast implants, however, is presently under FDA investigation.[9] It is unknown if this would have any implications for facial implantation.

Many of the implant materials used today have a long track record of safety. For example, ePTFE (Gore-Tex) has been used for more than 20 years, especially in vascular surgery, with excellent biocompatibility and long-term success. Gore-Tex and other porous polymers have a variable degree of tissue in-growth, making them relatively stable.[3] The tubular form of ePTFE (Softform, Ultrasoft, Advanta) has been used for subcutaneous augmentation of nasolabial folds, the perioral area, facial scars, soft-tissue defects, and lip augmentation. Over the long term, Softform (Collagen Corporation, Palo Alto, CA) becomes firmer, more palpable, and tends to shorten due to fibrous in-growth into the interstices of the material. Ultrasoft (Tissue Technologies Inc., San Francisco, CA), which has thinner walls, was developed to circumvent some of these problems and has been more acceptable.[10] A dual porosity ePTFE implant, Advanta (Atrium Medical Corporation, Hudson, NH) is softer, has better biointegration and less risk of shrinkage and migration.[11] Because the risk of palpability and extrusion (**Fig. 12.2**) is higher when the implant is placed closer to the surface, it is advisable to be very conservative with the use of ePTFE for soft-tissue augmentation. Additionally, there is a higher risk of infection, particularly with using ePTFE in the lips. The nasolabial fold is one area where its use has been found to be favorable. Currently, with the availability of semipermanent soft-tissue injectable fillers with excellent long-term safety profiles, many practioners have essentially abandoned the use of ePTFE implants in the perioral area in favor of these injectable fillers that can be used in the office.

Solid silicone (Silastic) implants have also been in use for many years. Silastic implants are enveloped by a thin organized capsule with a mild chronic inflammatory reaction. There is, however, no bonding between the silicone and the capsule, and hence it is more prone to be

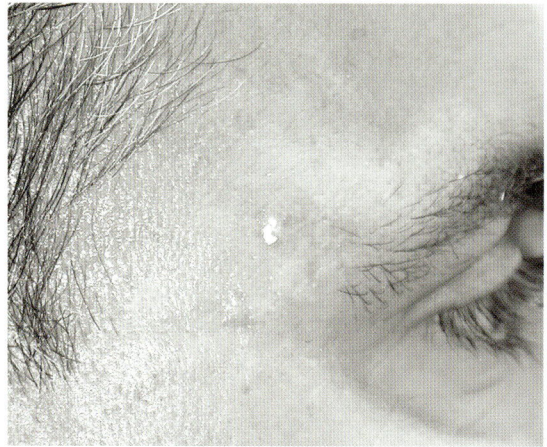

Fig. 12.2 Extrusion of Gore-Tex implant, 2.5 months after subcutaneous implantation for depressed acne scarring in right temporal area.

dislodged. It is also prone to extrude when the overlying soft-tissue coverage is thin, as in nasal or auricular applications.[8]

One of the most comprehensive reviews of implant complications was published in 1997 by Rubin and Yaremchuk.[4] Based on a review of nearly 200 clinical studies, they reported on complication rates related to specific implant materials and sites. Their findings, along with additional data from more recent studies, are summarized in **Table 12.2**.

◆ Facial Enhancement with Implants

The study of facial anatomy has led to a greater understanding of the ideal facial proportions that contribute to attractiveness. Certain convex facial features (e.g., the malar eminence or the chin) can be either masculinizing or feminizing, depending on their size and contour, independent of traditional facial proportions. Furthermore, the aging face characteristically changes in a relatively consistent fashion according to skeletal and soft-tissue alterations, and it can be rejuvenated with implants that act to mitigate these changes. As a result, procedures have evolved for certain anatomic areas that are particularly amenable to augmentation in the human face, including the chin (menton), the malar eminences, the lateral mandible, the nasolabial folds, the lips, and the nose.

Chin and Mandibular Implants

The authors prefer ePTFE (Gore-Tex) for mentoplasty, even though it is significantly more expensive than alternative materials. The main reason for this preference

Table 12.2

Complication Rates with Various Implants and Sites

Implant Site	Chin			Nasal			Malar	
Implant material	Silicone	Surgical mesh	ePTFE	Silicone	Surgical mesh	ePTFE	Silicone	Porous polyethylene
Patients	1220	1245	324	229	266	484	404	9
Number of studies	6	5	1	4	3	6	7	1
Follow-up time	Up to 3 Y	Up to 2 Y	5M–10 Y	6 M–15 Y	11 M–5 Y	1–6 Y	1.5–4 Y	Up to 4 Y
Mean rate of infection, %	0.7	1.6	0.6	<0.5	5.3	1.7	1.2	0
Mean rate of displacement, %	<0.5	1.0	0	0.9	0	0.8	2	0

Adapted from Rubin JP, Yaremchuk MJ. Complications and toxicities of implantable biomaterials used in facial reconstructive and aesthetic surgery: a comprehensive review of the literature. Plast Reconstr Surg 1997;100:1336–1353, and from Godin MD, Costa L, Romo T, et al. Gore-Tex chin implants, a review of 324 cases. Arch Facial Plast Surg 2003;5:224–227.

Abbreviations: M: months; Y: years

is the ease of removability. Gore-Tex also lends itself to easy sculpting and does not cause the significant bone erosion seen with other materials (**Fig. 12.3**). A popular technique uses a submental approach with placement of the implant in subperiosteal pockets laterally, while ensuring that the central portion of the implant, at the symphysis, is placed superficial to the periosteum. Mersilene mesh tends to have much more fibrovascular in-growth, which makes removal quite challenging and leads to significant morbidity if removal ever becomes necessary.[3] The patient in **Fig. 12.4** required removal of her Mersilene chin implant seven months after her initial procedure. This removal resulted in extensive bruising and inflammation in the perioral area. She subsequently had a second procedure to insert a Gore-Tex chin implant and had a satisfactory outcome.

Two surgical approaches are commonly used for mentoplasty. In the authors' experience, the submental approach is more favorable than the transoral approach. In the transoral approach, the mentalis muscle is disinserted from the mandibular symphysis, which can result in problems with implant positioning, often leading to inferior displacement of the implant and alteration in the location and appearance of the labiomental sulcus. Downward displacement of the overlying soft tissue and muscle can result in a "witch's chin" deformity.[7] This observation has been supported by Zide et al., who reviewed over 100 postoperative problems with chin augmentation and reported a higher incidence of complications with the transoral approach, specifically pertaining to implant position.[12]

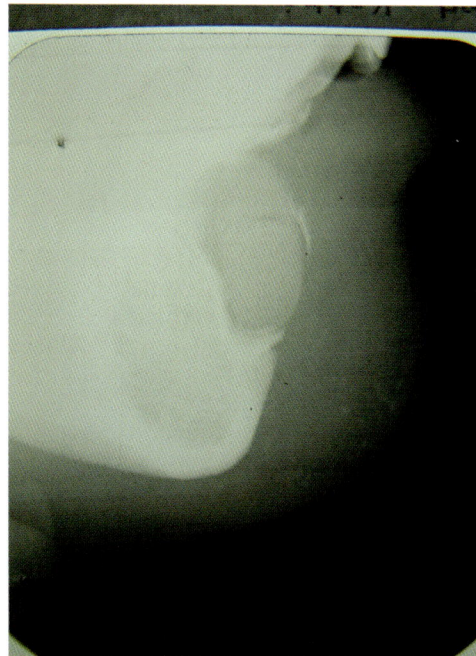

Fig. 12.3 Lateral skull X-ray illustrating mandibular bone erosion associated with a chin implant performed 20 years earlier.

Godin et al. published a retrospective review of 324 Gore-Tex chin implants performed by six different surgeons.[13] The submental approach was used in 95% of the cases. Only two implants (0.6%) required removal for

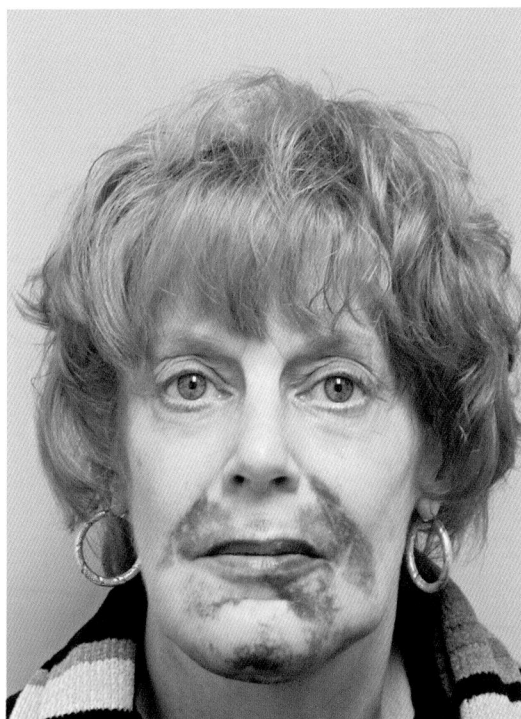

Fig. 12.4 Extensive bruising and inflammation following removal of a Mersilene chin implant.

persistent infection after multiple courses of antibiotics were tried. Four patients (1.2%) requested implant removal due to dissatisfaction with their appearance. Soaking the implant preoperatively in antibiotic solution produced no significant difference in infection rates. It must be remembered that chin implants can get infected up to 10 years later, which is typically secondary to seeding from a dental source.[7] Ongoing research in biofilms may elucidate some of the mechanisms for such infections and their best therapy.

Gross et al. published a review of their senior author's 14 years of experience with Mersilene mesh augmentation mentoplasty in 264 patients.[14] The submental approach was used more commonly, and all implants were placed subperiosteally. Mean follow-up was five years. The overall complication rate was 2.3%, with an infection rate of 0.8% and displacement rate of 1.5%. Temporary paresthesias were noted in 5.3% of patients. There was no difference in the complication rate based on the approach (transoral versus submental). They concluded that Mersilene mesh was a safe, inexpensive, and well-tolerated implant.

Bone resorption has been noted with mandibular augmentation, particularly of the anterior mandible, more so than with any other alloplastic implantation (**Fig. 12.3**). This tends to occur more often with some implant materials such as Silastic, acrylic, and MEDPOR.[14] It typically occurs with subperiosteal implant placement and can be prevented by placing the implant in a supraperiosteal plane.[15,16]

As with mentoplasty, complications of midlateral and posterolateral mandibular augmentation also include malposition, infection, extrusion and nerve damage. These can be minimized by paying careful attention to technique, specifically to subperiosteal elevation, staying away from the mental foramen, and double-layered closure of the wound.[7]

Malar Implants

Several approaches to midfacial augmentation have been described, including transoral, subciliary, rhytidectomy, transconjunctival, transtemporal, and transcoronal. The transoral approach is the most common. Avoidance of complications in malar (and submalar) implantation is largely technique dependent. Injury to the infraorbital nerve is avoided by passing the retractor lateral and parallel to the nerve. Care is taken to avoid transecting the zygomaticus muscle to prevent permanent muscle weakness that can affect lip elevation and change smile configuration. Patients are evaluated within 48–72 hours, with special attention to ensure symmetry. An appropriate cavity and adequate fixation are critical to avoiding displacement of malar implants. Implant malposition can lead to revisional surgery. Fixation is easily achieved using a transoral screw to the maxilla or a percutaneous suture fixation over a bolster.[3,7]

The authors prefer the transoral approach for malar augmentation and use Gore-Tex implants secured with a screw. In our experience, infections are uncommon, but may lead to implant extrusion when they occur. The patient in **Figs. 12.5A,B** underwent malar augmentation with Gore-Tex implants. She developed an infection about a month later (**Fig. 12.5A**) and was treated aggressively with antibiotics. Her clinical response was not satisfactory and implant removal was offered. The patient refused and wanted to continue with conservative measures. With time, she developed skin necrosis and exposure of the implant (**Fig. 12.5B**), which was eventually removed.

Metzinger et al. published a five-year review of malar augmentation with Silastic implants in 60 patients, the majority of which were performed through a transoral approach.[16] Their average follow-up was 41 months. They had no infections, hematomas, seromas, measurable bone resorption, extrusions, or facial nerve injuries. They had four cases of superior displacement, one misalignment, three transient trigeminal hypesthesias, and one case of persistent edema. Although they had no infections, their overall complication rate was 16.7%, but only 3.4% required a revision procedure.

Binder et al. described the successful use of customized Silastic midfacial and submalar implants through an intraoral approach in 22 patients who had facial wasting syndrome associated with HIV.[17] In their se-

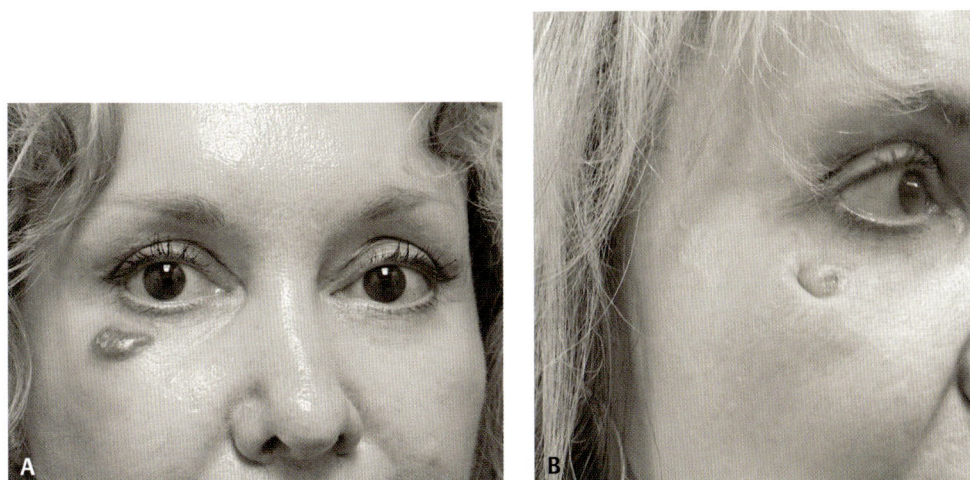

Fig. 12.5 (A) Infected malar implant approximately one month after transoral placement. Notice thinning and impending skin erosion. **(B)** Skin ulceration and exposure of infected malar implant.

ries, there were no serious complications. Two patients required implant removal for an infection. In one case, the implant was replaced successfully after antibiotic therapy.

Nasal Implants

The thin skin/soft-tissue envelope of the nasal dorsum puts dorsal nasal implants at high risk for extrusion. In Ruben and Yaremchuk's review,[4] extrusion rates were close to 23% for silicone, but were negligible with surgical mesh and ePTFE. However, infection rates were 5.3% for mesh and 1.7% for ePTFE. Therefore, autologous tissue is most advisable for nasal grafting. Of the alloplastic implants, Gore-Tex is favored over other alternatives. Infections are uncommon but may require implant removal when they occur. The patient in **Fig. 12.6** developed erythema and induration four months after dorsal augmentation rhinoplasty with Gore-Tex. She did not respond to aggressive antibiotic therapy with cephalexin and ciprofloxacin, resulting in implant removal a month later. Cultures grew *Staphylococcus aureus*. She was subsequently offered a revision procedure with autologous rib grafting but has been reluctant to undergo further surgery.

Godin et al. published a retrospective review of 309 patients who underwent rhinoplasty with Gore-Tex implantation. The average follow up was 40.4 months. The overall infection rate requiring graft removal was 3.2%, with a significant difference between primary (1.2%) and revision rhinoplasties (5.4%). The average time period between placement and removal of the implant was 16 months. The only predisposing factor identified in this study was nasal septal perforation, which was present in 30% of the patients requiring implant removal for infection.[18]

Schoenrock et al. reported on their series of 750 Gore-Tex facial implants.[19] They had two infections requiring

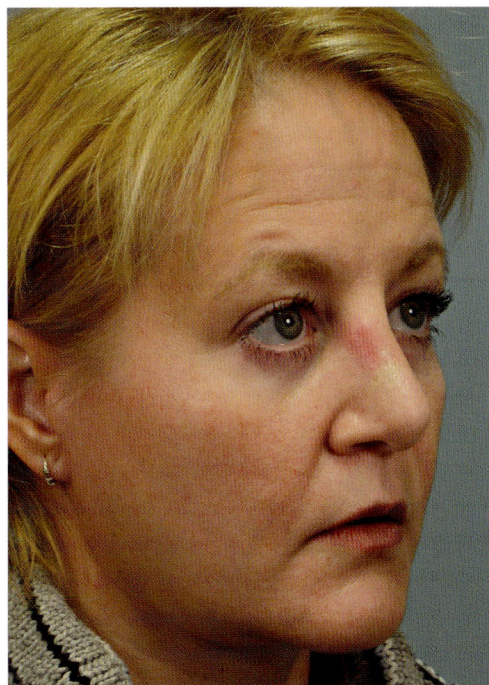

Fig. 12.6 Oblique view of a patient with erythema and induration after placement of Gore-Tex implant for nasal dorsal augmentation. Antibiotic therapy failed and implant was removed a month later. Culture grew coagulase-negative *Staphylococcus aureus* and *Streptococcus viridans*.

implant removal, both of which were in the nasal area. In both cases, *Staphylococcus aureus* was cultured and treated successfully with antibiotics. The authors caution against the use of Gore-Tex in cases of revision rhinoplasty, where the soft-tissue envelope tends to be quite thin.[19]

◆ Autologous Fat

Transfer of autologous fat is rapidly gaining in popularity, due in part to its ease of harvest, persistence, and usefulness in nearly all anatomic areas commonly enhanced with volume. Thus any discussion of facial implantation must include lipotransfer. Complications from lipotransfer tend to be technique dependent but not universally so. The commonly encountered complications include prolonged edema, induration, bruising, and asymmetry. The lower eyelid and lateral canthal area tend to be less forgiving, and contour irregularities are more noticeable[20] (**Fig. 12.7**). Occasionally, persistent inflammation can lead to granulomatous nodules (**Fig. 12.8**) or hyperpigmentation (**Fig. 12.9**). Infections are rare with strict aseptic technique.[20]

Although significant complications with fat transfer have been described, they are quite rare and can largely be avoided by the use of appropriate techniques and precautions.[21-24]

Specifically, fat embolism can be a devastating complication of facial lipotransfer, and adherence to the contemporary tenets of injecting fat in minuscule amounts, using multiple passes with a 0.9–1.2 mm blunt cannula, for example, has reduced the incidence of complications significantly. Injections are performed as the cannula is withdrawn and with minimal force.[20] Granulomatous inflammation may be treated successfully with intralesional triamcinolone, and there may also be a role for 5-fluoro-

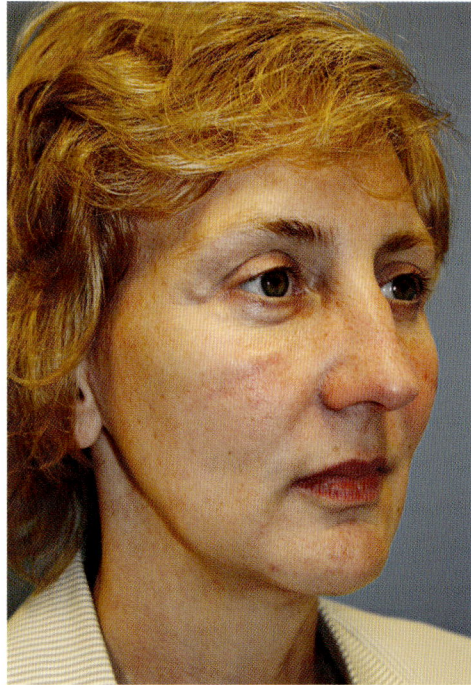

Fig. 12.7 Visible nodularity of the lateral canthal area and malar crescent, 6 months after autologous lipotransfer.

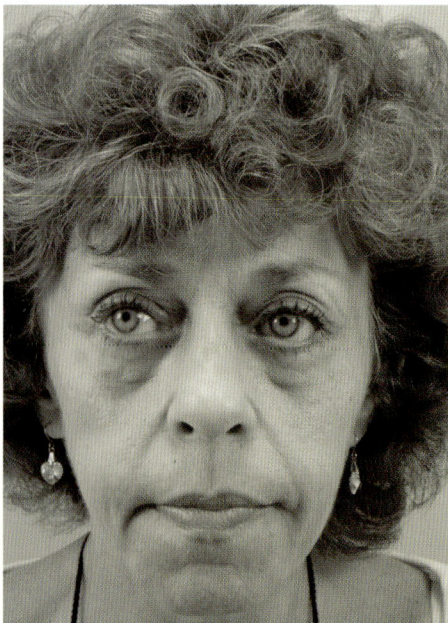

Fig. 12.9 Brownish hyperpigmentation in lower eyelid area following autologous lipotransfer.

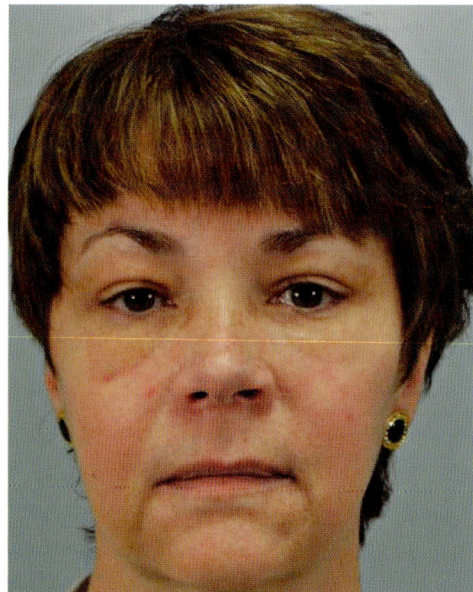

Fig. 12.8 Granulomatous inflammation in tear trough area following autologous lipotransfer.

uracil injections for problematic cicatricial nodularity after fat transfer, although this latter option is not well elucidated in the literature. If persistent nodularity remains despite conservative measures or if the problem is simply one of too much injected fat, surgical excision probably remains the best option. Hyperpigmentation typically responds to topical applications of hydroquinone.

◆ Conclusion

Alloplastic implantation is a readily available and durable option for aesthetic and functional facial enhancement. As with all facial plastic surgery interventions, careful patient selection and risk-benefit assessment are critical to a successful outcome. When the procedure is performed correctly in appropriate individuals, enhanced facial proportions and rejuvenation are safe and achievable with facial implants. Such complications as implant malposition, asymmetry, or infection are ultimately treatable with implant removal and replacement if necessary. Semipermanent implants, such as autologous fat, are an excellent alternative to permanent filler materials and are rapidly gaining in popularity.

PEARLS OF WISDOM

There is no ideal implant material, although autologous tissue is often best.

Comprehensive preoperative evaluation, consistent photography, and open communication to manage the expectations of the patient are essential for successful facial implant outcomes.

Facial implants placed on bone or the periosteum are less likely to extrude.

Ease of removal is an important consideration in the choice of facial implant material.

Implant-associated infection typically requires implant removal.

Autologous fat transfer is an excellent soft-tissue volume enhancement technique, with minimal morbidity and favorable long-term results.

References

1. Quatela VC, Sabini P. Synthetic Implants. In: Papel ID, ed. Facial Plastic and Reconstructive Surgery. New York: Thieme Medical Publishing; 2002:61–72

2. Silver FH, Maas CS. Biology of synthetic facial implant materials. Facial Plast Surg Clin North Am 1994;2:241–253

3. Binder WJ, Moelleken B, Tobias GW. Aesthetic Facial Implants. In: Papel ID, ed. Facial Plastic and Reconstructive Surgery. New York: Thieme Medical Publishing; 2002:276–298

4. Rubin JP, Yaremchuk MJ. Complications and toxicities of implantable biomaterials used in facial reconstructive and aesthetic surgery: a comprehensive review of the literature. Plast Reconstr Surg 1997;100(5):1336–1353

5. Buckingham ED, Lam SL, Williams EF III. In: Williams III EF, Lam SM, eds. Comprehensive Facial Rejuvenation. Philadelphia: Lippincott Williams and Wilkins; 2004:28.

6. Roy DB, Mangat DS. Facial implants. Dermatol Clin 2005; 23(3):541–547, vii–viii

7. Terino EO. Complications of chin and malar augmentation. In: Peck G, ed. Complications and Problems in Aesthetic Plastic Surgery. New York: Gower Medical Publishers; 1991

8. Davis PKB, Jones SM. The complications of Silastic implants. Experience with 137 consecutive cases. Br J Plast Surg 1971; 24(4):405–411

9. FDA Medical Device Safety Communication: Reports of Anaplastic Large Cell Lymphoma (ALCL) in Women with Breast Implants. The U.S. Food and Drug Administration. January 26, 2011.

10. Monhian N, Ahn MS, Maas CS. Injectable and Implantable Materials for Facial Wrinkles. In: Papel ID, ed. Facial Plastic and Reconstructive Surgery. New York: Thieme Medical Publishing; 2002:247–261

11. Truswell WH. Dual-porosity expanded polytetrafluoroethylene soft tissue implant: a new implant for facial soft tissue augmentation. Arch Facial Plast Surg 2002;4(2): 92–97

12. Zide BM, Pfeifer TM, Longaker MT. Chin surgery: I. Augmentation—the allures and the alerts. Plast Reconstr Surg 1999;104(6):1843–1853, discussion 1861–1862

13. Godin MD, Costa L, Romo T, Truswell W, Wang T, Williams E. Gore-Tex chin implants: a review of 324 cases. Arch Facial Plast Surg 2003;5(3):224–227

14. Gross EJ, Hamilton MM, Ackermann K, Perkins SW. Mersilene mesh chin augmentation. A 14-year experience. Arch Facial Plast Surg 1999;1(3):183–189, discussion 190

15. Li KK, Cheney ML. The use of sliding genioplasty for treatment of failed chin implants. Laryngoscope 1996;106(3 Pt 1): 363–366

16. Metzinger SE, McCollough EG, Campbell JP, Rousso DE. Malar augmentation: a 5-year retrospective review of the Silastic midfacial malar implant. Arch Otolaryngol Head Neck Surg 1999;125(9):980–987

17. Binder WJ, Bloom DC. The use of custom-designed midfacial and submalar implants in the treatment of facial wasting syndrome. Arch Facial Plast Surg 2004;6(6):394–397

18. Godin MS, Waldman SR, Johnson CM Jr. Nasal augmentation using Gore-Tex. A 10-year experience. Arch Facial Plast Surg 1999;1(2):118–121, discussion 122

19. Schoenrock LD, Repucci AD. Correction of subcutaneous facial defects using Gore-Tex. Facial Plast Surg Clin North Am 1994;2:373–387

20. Krishna S, Williams EF III. Lipocontouring in conjunction with the minimal incision brow and subperiosteal midface lift: the next dimension in midface rejuvenation. Facial Plast Surg Clin North Am 2006;14(3):221–228

21. Feinendegen DL, Baumgartner RW, Schroth G, Mattle HP, Tschopp H. Middle cerebral artery occlusion and ocular fat embolism after autologous fat injection in the face. J Neurol 1998;245(1):53–54

22. Ricaurte JC, Murali R, Mandell W. Uncomplicated postoperative lipoid meningitis secondary to autologous fat graft necrosis. Clin Infect Dis 2000;30(3):613–615

23. Yoon SS, Chang DI, Chung KC. Acute fatal stroke immediately following autologous fat injection into the face. Neurology 2003;61(8):1151–1152

24. Miller JJ, Popp JC. Fat hypertrophy after autologous fat transfer. Ophthal Plast Reconstr Surg 2002;18(3):228–231

13

Complications of Facial Trauma Repair

Sydney C. Butts and Robert M. Kellman

Facial trauma patients suffer injuries to complex soft-tissue structures as well as to components of the facial skeleton. Proper healing depends upon principles common to the management of facial trauma—that is, strict attention to soft-tissue closure techniques, patient health factors, meticulous wound care, and adequate reduction and fixation of fractures. The individual anatomic and functional features of each facial subsite, however, must be appreciated more fully to understand the development and management of complications. This chapter will address each of the major regions of the craniofacial skeleton separately—the mandible, orbit and zygoma, maxilla, naso-orbital ethmoid complex, and frontal sinus—as well as important facial soft-tissue structures.

◆ Mandibular Fractures

Infection is the most common adverse event following the treatment of mandibular fractures, with reported rates from 2.9% to 30% of cases.[1–6] Reported rates of infection must be interpreted within the context of trends in treatment modalities. Rigid fixation techniques have assumed a primary role in fracture treatment in many medical centers in the United States over the past 20 years.[3,7] Improved bone stability and reliability of healing with correct application of the techniques have resulted in significant improvements in the clinical outcomes in facial trauma. Thus, it is generally expected that rates of infection in the era of rigid fixation are less compared with rates in years past. Infection rates in clinical reports must also be judged based on the site of the mandibular fracture, the length of any prophylactic antibiotic course, patient compliance factors, and surgical technique.[3,8,9]

Infection may develop in instances of delayed treatment, patient comorbidities that result in immunocompromise, technical errors resulting in improper reduction or stabilization (or both), and bacterial seeding of the fracture site, particularly in the presence of preexisting caries or dental infection.[1,2,9–11] Infection in the fractured mandible often starts to develop when there is excessive movement of the ends of the fracture.[1]

Successful bone healing occurs two different ways, depending upon the mobility and interval distance of the fractured segments: healing and indirect bone healing. Complete immobilization with exact approximation of the fractured ends allows direct bone healing with minimal development of an intervening callus.[1,12] When these conditions are not completely satisfied but the fractured ends are not distracted, the bone edges will experience some movement in the initial postinjury phase.[1,12] Indirect bone healing commences in this situation. This process involves a cascade of events marked by the differentiation of hematoma to fibrocartilage and ultimately to bone. The formation of a callus occurs early in the process of indirect bone healing and serves as an early stabilizer of the bone segments and also as a foundation for the ingrowth of more specialized tissues.[1,7,12] If there is a wide gap between the fracture segments, interfragmentary motion may be excessive, so a callus will not form.[7,11] Excessive motion, which is often seen in delayed patient presentations or with the use of inappropriate stabilization techniques, promotes seeding of bacteria into the fracture[1] and the ingrowth of fibrous tissue instead of cartilaginous and bone precursor cells.[11,13]

The initial choice of fracture treatment must be tailored to the fracture. Once biomechanical forces acting on the mandible were elucidated by pioneers such as Champy, Michelet, Luhr, and Spiessl, techniques for proper plate application followed.[7,14] The ideal osteosynthesis line (**Fig. 13.1**) described by Champy is based on an understanding of the three forces that act on the mandible during function: tensional, compressive, and torsional.[7,14–16] When occlusal force is applied anteriorly, tensional forces are generated at the alveolar ridge and follow a line posteriorly along the oblique line. Tension tends to distract a fracture. Generally, compression occurs at the inferior border of the mandible during function, although forces applied in proximity to the fracture will often tend to compress the alveolar border and distract the inferior border.[15,16] The suprahyoid muscles (digastric m., mylohyoid m., stylohyoid m., and geniohyoid m.) exert a torsional force on the anterior mandible (symphysis and parasymphyseal region), which requires

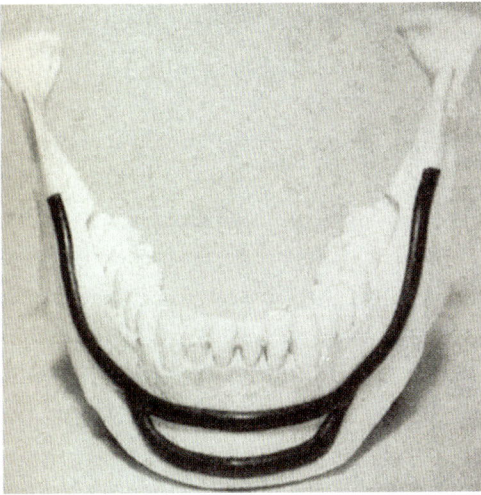

Fig. 13.1 The ideal mandibular osteosynthesis line. This line, defined by Champy, marks the optimal location for the application of rigid fixation. Used with permission from Costantino PD and Wolpe M. Facial Plating Systems. In Papel ID, ed. Facial Plastic and Reconstructive Surgery. New York: Thieme; 2002:769–781.

that both the tension zone and the compression zone along the inferior border of the mandible be stabilized.[15] Although the ideal osteosynthesis line originally described by Champy does not mandate the use of superior and inferior border plates for fixation of the body and angle, there is debate among surgeons regarding the ideal arrangement of fixation in these regions, given higher rates of infection in these areas of the mandible despite rigid fixation.[3,17]

It is clear from historical outcomes that if the biomechanical forces and principles of osteosynthesis are respected, the application of rigid fixation will be successful most of the time. If, however, the hardware fails to achieve its goals, it becomes a foreign body and therefore an additional catalyst for infection. The physical findings in a patient with an infected mandible fracture include edema over the fracture site, pain, mobility of the fracture segments on palpation, purulent drainage, or hardware exposure.[1] When we recall that most infected mandible fractures arise in the setting of fragmentary motion, it follows that treatment of this complication requires proper fixation of the mobile segments.[1,18] Treatment calls for incision and drainage of abscess collections, removal of ineffective hardware, and the establishment of fracture immobility. Maxillomandibular fixation, stronger internal fixation, or an external fixator are all ways this can be achieved. Teeth in the fracture line are often extracted once an infection or healing delay has developed.[1] Any devitalized tissue must also be debrided. Although it may seem counterintuitive to place hardware into an infected field, it must

be remembered that the infection is not likely to resolve unless rigid fixation is established and that bone healing is jeopardized until stabilization is achieved.[1,18] The use of antibiotics and minimization of patient comorbidities (e.g., malnutrition) certainly play adjunctive roles.

Incidence of posttraumatic osteomyelitis is related to fracture infection. Whereas an infected fracture is considered a soft-tissue reaction to the stimulus of fracture mobility, posttraumatic osteomyelitis (PTOM) is a true bone infection. The clinical presentation includes severe pain and commonly an orocutaneous fistula with purulent discharge.[19] These two entities will be distinguished radiographically by nuclear scans showing both an active inflammatory process in the bone as well as increased bone turnover.[19] The treatment of PTOM has evolved in response to the availability of improved rigid fixation systems. PTOM may be managed in single or multiple stages. An open approach to the fracture allows the wide exposure required. Any failed hardware is removed. Wide bone debridement to healthy bleeding bone is undertaken. Load-bearing osteosynthesis is then applied in the form of a reconstruction plate. It is essential that the screws be placed in healthy bone. A suction drain is placed in the wound. If the amount of debridement required has resulted in a segmental defect, the decision must be made as to whether primary cancellous bone grafting will be performed. Alternatively, the patient may be placed on intravenous antibiotics and brought back for the bone graft after the infection has cleared. Kellman[19] reported results of primary bone grafting and rigid fixation in 14 patients with PTOM. Initially, bone grafting was performed as a secondary procedure. Later in the clinical experience, primary plating and bone grafting were instituted. All of the patients went on to union with no further complications, confirming the safety of this approach.

One factor that differentiates bone from many other tissues in the body is its ability to replace small gaps in tissue with bone instead of scar. As described earlier, bone ingrowth into the fracture site occurs by two processes, depending on the degree of movement at the fracture site. The growth factors and early cellular infiltrates that characterize a fracture hematoma are similar to those involved in soft-tissue wound healing. It is not surprising, then, that if osteogenesis is hampered in the early wound (increased fragmentary motion, infection, necrosis), bone healing is delayed and fibrous tissue ingrowth occurs by default. Certain conditions at the fracture site promote fibrous ingrowth over osteogenesis.[13] The duration until bony union under optimal repair conditions has been defined as four weeks in children, six weeks in adults, and eight weeks in the elderly.[12,13] These time frames were more clinically relevant when closed reduction was the primary modality for treating mandible fractures, because the time to healing determined the length of treatment. However, in the age of rigid fixation, the concept of delayed union takes more of a historical place. Delayed union results from incomplete healing caused by motion. When maxillary-mandibular fixation (MMF) is applied, incomplete healing due to motion can often be corrected by further stabilization.[13] However, in the presence of a rigid fixation appliance, motion generally indicates failure of the fixation. Rather than MMF, correction generally requires removal of loose hardware, usually with the application of new, stronger fixation.[1,3,12,20]

Nonunion, in which the bone edges are in proximity but fibrous tissue has grown between the edges, can often be corrected by excising the intervening fibrous tissue that has bridged the bone gap and inserting proper rigid fixation, using a load-bearing repair.[12,13,21] As mentioned previously, bone grafting may be necessary to bridge any gaps. Large volumes of cancellous bone can be harvested from the iliac crest or tibia.[1,15]

Rates of bone healing disturbance described as nonunion have been reported in 1–3% of treated mandible fractures.[12,18] Most patients in a review by Haug and Schwimmer[18] had improper fracture stabilization, either because of flawed application of rigid fixation or loosening of closed fixation devices. Over half of their patient group developed infections. In Mathog's series, 9 of 25 patients were identified as having poor fracture fixation.[12] In both studies, the body of the mandible had the highest rate of nonunion or fibrous union, which confirms the role that weak stabilization plays, as this region of the mandible is subject to strong forces from the muscles of mastication.

Malunion results when the bone fragments heal in a way that does not restore the premorbid occlusion. Although fractures of the parasymphyseal region are readily approached intraorally, the application of plates and screws to fractures in the posterior body and angle can be difficult transorally.[15] If intraoral repair poses difficulty for the surgeon, there should be no hesitation about employing extraoral approaches to avoid compromising treatment. The surgeon must be meticulous about attaining adequate occlusion and must use information from the patient, past dental radiographs, dental models, photographs, and the patient's wear facets to restore premorbid occlusion. Seemingly minor bony discrepancies can result in obvious changes in occlusion and thus an unsatisfactory outcome. Minor malocclusions can sometimes be treated with occlusal grinding,[18] but more significant problems require orthodontic intervention[22] and sometimes orthognathic surgery.[23–25]

The incidence and degree of sensory disturbance in the distribution of the inferior alveolar nerve (V3) can be related to the initial trauma or to subsequent surgical manipulation. The areas of the mandible through which the inferior alveolar nerve runs are most vulnerable and are the focus of most reports.[26–28] Preoperatively, the degree of displacement of the fractured bone ends has consistently been shown to be correlated with rates of sensory deficits. Iizuka and Lindqvist[27] reported that 73.5% of patients with greater than 5 mm of fragment displacement had hypesthesia based on pretreatment sensory testing, compared with 25.8% of patients in which the fracture was not displaced. Over all, 58% of their patients had hypesthesia immediately after the mandibular injury, with 46.6% reported to have some persistent sensory deficit after one year. In most of these cases, the residual deficit was mild, and many patients were subjectively unaware of significant hypesthesia. Patients who were edentulous had worse rates of recovery. Marchena et al.[28] also published long-term follow-up data. The incidence of immediate postinjury sensory disturbance was 56%. They also found that the degree of fracture displacement was related to increased rates of postinjury hypesthesia. Objective testing revealed that only ⅓ of patients experienced full sensory recovery, though just 55% had awareness of the deficit.

Widening of the lower face has been described as a complication after open reduction internal fixation of symphyseal fractures, particularly in the presence of subcondylar fracture(s) due to a failure to close the lingual cortical side of the fracture. This allows flaring of the mandibular angles, which results in the increased width. To prevent distraction of the lingual cortex, the plate should be slightly overbent at the line of the fracture to ensure compression of the lingual side. In the presence of bilateral subcondylar fractures, the angles should be pushed together to minimize this risk.[29]

◆ Condylar and Subcondylar Fractures

Fractures of the condylar process of the mandible deserve individual consideration, because treatment goals for such injuries differ from those of injuries to other areas of the mandible. Successful outcome of treatment is judged primarily by the presence of unimpaired function of the temporomandibular joint (TMJ), whether or not reduction of the fracture is attained.[1,30] With the high performance of titanium fixation plating systems and safer methods of approaching the TMJ,[31] stricter criteria for successful treatment outcomes can be expected in the future, including restoration of posterior facial height and symmetric jaw movements, in addition to the attainment of premorbid occlusion.[32,33]

Clinically, unilateral condylar fractures can present with premature contact of the posterior dentition on the side of the fracture due to shortened ramus height, which generally occurs due to the overlap of the fractured fragments.[34] The patient will therefore have a contralateral posterior open bite. The mandible deviates toward the fractured side because of unopposed action of the contralateral lateral pterygoid muscle (which is pulling the contralateral condylar process toward the midline).[35] Bilateral condylar process fractures result in an anterior open bite (premature contact of the posterior dentition bilaterally), as well as retrognathia.[30]

It is important to consider initial treatment options, for certain types of therapy and aftercare may decrease complication rates. First, it should be pointed out that though many have advocated closed reduction using MMF, it is in fact a misnomer, as MMF does not result in reduction of the fracture, although it can restore the occlusion. For many years, closed reduction of condylar fractures was used almost exclusively. The main factors guiding this preference were functional adaptation at the joint, reasonably good occlusal outcomes, and the high complication rates experienced with open reduction, particularly the unsavory complication of facial nerve paralysis.[18,30,34,36]

Functional adaptation is the ability of the masticatory muscles to continue to function despite imperfect reduction of the condylar process after fracture.[37] Since this in fact occurs, treatment of condylar fractures focuses on occlusal guidance.[30] Training elastics attached to arch bars are applied so that the teeth are guided into occlusion. In many centers the standard treatment of the majority of condylar fractures has been and continues to be MMF for a short period (seven to fourteen days) followed by elastic MMF for occlusal guidance until the patient can attain a reproducible occlusion.[18,34,36] The patient also begins jaw physiotherapy exercises after rigid MMF is released. This includes jaw-opening exercises and lateral excursive movements. Function, despite nonanatomical reduction, is critical to muscle adaptation and the prevention of TMJ ankylosis, trismus, and growth disturbances in pediatric patients.[30,35,37,38] In our institutions, we believe that a period of rigid MMF actually delays the initiation of physiotherapy, so we prefer to progress immediately to training elastics and physiotherapy.

Zide and Kent[39] provided a classically accepted list of absolute and relative indications for open reduction of condylar fractures. The absolute indications include fracture dislocation of the condyle into the middle cranial fossa, lateral extracapsular dislocation of the condyle, an inability to restore occlusion with closed techniques, a foreign body within the TMJ, an open or penetrating injury to the TMJ, and a fracture that results in mechanical obstruction of TMJ. Open approaches to the TMJ include the submandibular approach (Risdon), the preauricular approach, the retromandibular approach, and the intraoral approach, which may be performed with endoscopic guidance.[15,30,31,34] Stated advantages of open reduction and fixation include restoration of ramus height, avoidance of facial asymmetry, the possibility of immediate function and superior occlusal results found by some authors, even when absolute indications are not present.[31-34] Few surgeons open fractures of the condylar head, though this may become more common in the future as well.[34]

Several reports have evaluated the development of malocclusion in groups of patients treated with MMF versus open reduction and internal fixation. Worssae and Thorn[40] found that 8 of 24 (30%) of patients treated with MMF developed malocclusion, compared to 1 of 28 patients who had the joint opened. Ellis et al.[36] found that at one year follow-up, patients who had closed treatment were consistently rated to have significantly higher percentages of poor occlusions compared to cases treated with ORIF. Malocclusion may be the result of poor reduction of the fracture segments with persistent ipsilateral premature contact, or it may be the result of growth interference in a pediatric fracture. The condylar head can partially resorb over time as a response to the initial injury or from the surgical manipulation required during treatment.[37,41] The malocclusion in these instances is caused by a shortened vertical ramus height on the fractured side. For less severe malocclusions, orthodontics may be adequate treatment.[34] Orthognathic surgery can correct the malocclusion by using osteotomies to reposition the proximal ramus and restore the ramus height in more severe cases.[24,41] This is a successful approach for unilateral cases. A vertical ramus osteotomy allows the proximal segment to be positioned superiorly to equalize the ramus heights. If anterior or posterior repositioning is required, a sagittal split osteotomy is performed.[41]

When planning orthognathic surgery to correct traumatic dental-skeletal anomalies, the surgeon must use an approach that not only corrects malocclusion but also repositions the bone fragments in a stable manner to avoid relapse. This may mean performing osteotomies away from the site of the initial injury.[42] Superior movements and clockwise rotation of the mandibular ramus are stable, while inferior positioning of the ramus and counterclockwise rotation are unfavorable.[43] Although one option to correct an anterior open bite would involve bilateral mandibular ramus osteotomies, the resulting counterclockwise rotation of the distal segments required to restore occlusion is a situation prone to relapse. Alternatively, the anterior open bite may be corrected by a LeFort I osteotomy with posterior impaction of the maxilla.[23] This allows autorotation of the mandible superiorly with closure of the open bite.

When condylar/subcondylar fracture patients are treated with MMF, the premorbid condyle position is not always achieved. Often the condylar process is displaced in such a way that the fracture segments overlap, or the condyle may not be positioned upright. Either of these situations shortens the total height of the posterior mandible and may result in decreased posterior facial height and facial asymmetry.[32,34] In a study of posterior facial heights of patients undergoing closed or open reduction, Ellis[32] found a statistically significant difference between the fractured and nonfractured sides in patients treated with closed reduction (mean of 5 mm decreased posterior facial height at two years follow-up). Most patients achieved functional occlusion; however, their facial appearance was not commented upon, so it is not clear how directly the change in ramus height translated to obvious facial asymmetry.

TMJ ankylosis occurs when the joint space is partially or totally obliterated by fibrous or osseous tissue. Patients with unilateral ankylosis will have trismus and deviation to the affected side. Reviews of TMJ ankylosis implicate trauma as the cause in 30–98% of cases.[44–46] Although the pathophysiology of ankylosis is not completely understood, several factors are known to play a significant role. Bone growth is enhanced in the presence of hematomas and growth factors released by platelets within clots. This is felt to be particularly important in pediatric condylar fractures, because the condylar head is highly vascular.[30,37,47] In addition, damage to the meniscus and joint dislocation[37] have been correlated with increased rates of ankylosis. Prolonged joint immobilization during extended courses of rigid MMF, combined with inadequate adherence to a protocol of jaw motion exercises, results in decreased TMJ function during convalescence. These factors predispose the patient to the development of ankylosis, although ankylosis can still develop despite mobilization. When a patient with traumatic TMJ ankylosis is encountered, evaluation requires a maxillofacial CT scan to assess the full extent of the lesion (**Fig. 13.2**). As pointed out by Raveh,[47] the bony overgrowth can extend beyond the glenoid fossa to the adjacent middle cranial fossa and medially along the skull base.

Surgery is indicated to improve the maximal interincisal opening (MIO), restore joint function, and prevent future growth disturbance in pediatric patients.[44,45,47]

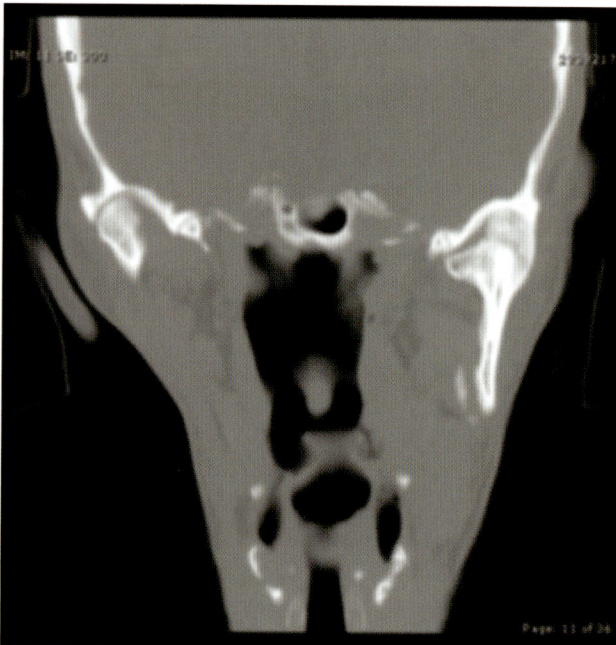

Fig.13.2 Coronal CT scan of left temporomandibular joint ankylosis.

Many surgical approaches have been described. All of the described protocols advocate safe but aggressive removal of the bony or fibrous lesion. In a series of 14 patients (both pediatric and adult), Kaban et al.[44] reported retrospective data with a treatment protocol that included resection of all abnormal bone, unilateral or bilateral coronoidectomy to augment mobility, an autologous costochondral graft to replace the condyle, and lining of the glenoid fossa with a turned-down temporalis muscle flap. All patients were placed in MMF for a brief time and then enrolled in jaw physiotherapy for one year. Other surgical approaches call for lining the TMJ with auricular cartilage or total joint replacement with an allopastic joint.[30,46,47]

Growth disturbance of the condyle highlights the importance of restoring normal joint function in the pediatric population.[35,47,48] It has been confirmed by human and animal studies that fractures heal more quickly in younger patients.[30] Although functional adaptation is the rule in restoration of joint function in adults, young children usually experience joint remodeling and recapitulation of the premorbid condyle and fossa anatomy after treatment.[44] The development of scar tissue can tether the downward growth of the condyle and ramus if early treatment and therapy are not instituted. Facial stigma include a shortened ramus on the fractured side, deviation of the chin toward the fractured side, and flattening of the face on the contralateral side.[30,48] Dental compensations lead to a posterior crossbite on the affected side. Condylar fractures can be difficult to diagnose in children if the evaluating physician does not have a high clinical suspicion. The examination may be limited, especially if the child is anxious. The condylar fracture may be difficult to detect by plain films (mandible series), since there is a higher percentage of greenstick fractures in children.[30] It is recommended that a condylar fracture be suspected in children with trauma to the chin and conclusively ruled out.[30] Distraction osteogenesis is being used successfully in the treatment of the hypoplastic ramus in these patients.[48]

◆ Orbit and Zygoma Fractures

Fractures of the facial bones around the eye can be associated with globe malpositions. Enophthalmos is defined as posterior displacement of the globe, while hypoglobus refers to inferior displacement of the globe.[49–51] Increased orbital volume caused by trauma is the most frequent cause of enophthalmos and hypophthalmos. Other factors contributing to the development of enophthalmos include tethering of orbital contents within an unrepaired fracture and fibrosis and scar contracture of intraorbital contents.[51–55] Atrophy of intraorbital fat has been, for the most part, discounted as a significant factor, although actual loss of orbital fat certainly can be.[54]

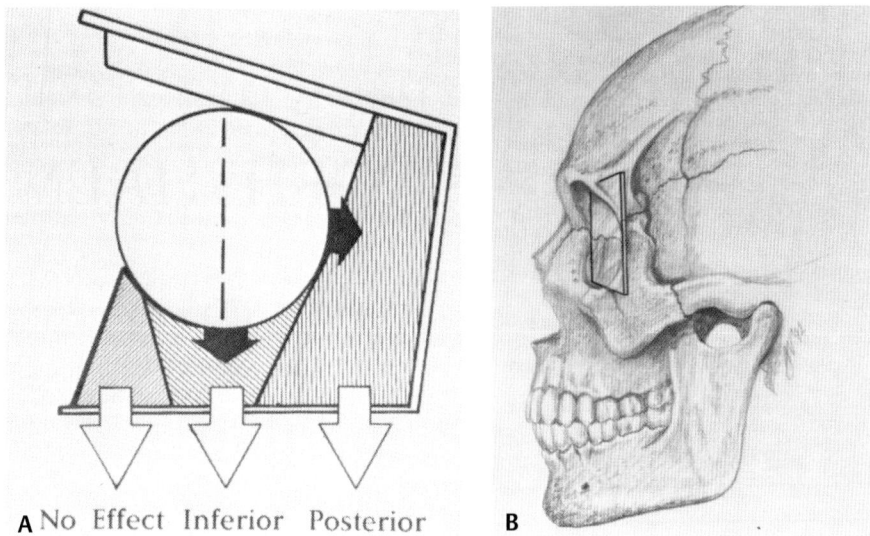

Fig. 13.3 Globe axis. **(A)** Bone loss at the axis can lead to changes in vertical globe position while posterior globe displacement occurs only with bone loss of the posterior orbital floor. **(B)** Section located at the axis of the orbit. Some of the floor is anterior to this plane but all of the lateral wall is posterior to it. Used with permission from Pearl RM. Treatment of Enophthalmos. Clinics in Plastic Surgery 1992;19(1):99–111.

Enophthalmos results from fractures of the orbital walls behind the axis of the globe (**Fig. 13.3**), which includes all of the lateral wall, most of the medial wall, and the posterior aspects of the inferior and superior walls.[54,56] Hypoglobus results from bone loss from the floor at the globe axis.[54,56] Bone loss anterior to the globe axis does not generally affect globe position[56] (**Fig. 13.3**). Facial trauma surgeons usually encounter enophthalmos as a delayed complication of orbital blowout and zygomatic fractures, since only rather severe fractures will present with acute enophthalmos.[49,52,57-59] Patients with unrepaired fractures and orbital volume increases will typically develop enophthalmos weeks after the injury, once edema has resolved.[57,59,60] With CT scan imaging now a routine part of the work-up in patients with facial trauma, large-volume fractures are detected immediately.[57,58] The goal of early fracture management is to predict, based on CT assessment of the fractures, which patients are likely to develop enophthalmos.[57] Many surgeons advocate treating high-risk fractures within one to two weeks of the injury, at a point when edema has resolved but before fibrosis has developed.[57-59,61] There have been strong advocates for a more expectant posture whose justification relied on a relatively low rate of postinjury enophathlmos and successful camouflage treatment when it did arise;[62] however, this management philosophy is not commonly accepted today. Currently, a large-volume fracture (50% or more of the orbital wall involved) is a clear indication for exploration and repair.[57]

Posttraumatic enophthalmos is due to orbital blowout fractures and displaced zygomatic fractures.[54] Patients presenting with late enophthalmos generally fall into two groups: those who were not treated primarily and those who have had prior surgical repair without full restoration of the orbital volume present before the injury.[49,54,60,61] Three to twelve percent of repaired zygomatico-maxillary complex (ZMC) fractures may be complicated by enophthalmos.[63-66] Hawes and Dortzbach found that while 7% of patients who had repair of the orbital fracture within two months of the injury developed enophthalmos, 88% of patients presenting for treatment two months after their injury had enophthalmos.[59] Catone et al. presented their data on 20 patients with unrepaired orbital blowout fractures, 15% of whom developed enophthalmos.[58]

Malar Flattening and Increased Facial Width

The zygoma makes up the inferolateral orbit through three of its five projections[67] (**Fig. 13.4**). Volume-enhancing vectors of movement include lateral displacement of the zygoma and inferior distraction exacerbated by the pull of the masseter muscle.[56,63] The zygoma contributes significantly to facial form, and its posterior displacement leads to a flattened malar prominence and increased facial width from outward bowing of the zygomatic arch[54,61] (**Fig. 13.4**).

Some important technical errors can lead to failures of primary repair of orbitozygomatic fractures. Adequate dissection into the posterior orbit is required to identify the posterior ledge of the fracture, which may extend 40 mm posterior to the infraorbital rim.[54,67] Exposure of the medial orbital wall must be addressed when required, and this wall is sometimes overlooked.[54,56,68] The key surgical principle in the treatment of zygomatico-maxillary complex (ZMC) fractures is three-point reduction of the zygoma and at least two-point fixation.[56,63,67] Two-point reduction does not ensure that the zygoma is not rotated at another articulation.[56,63,67]

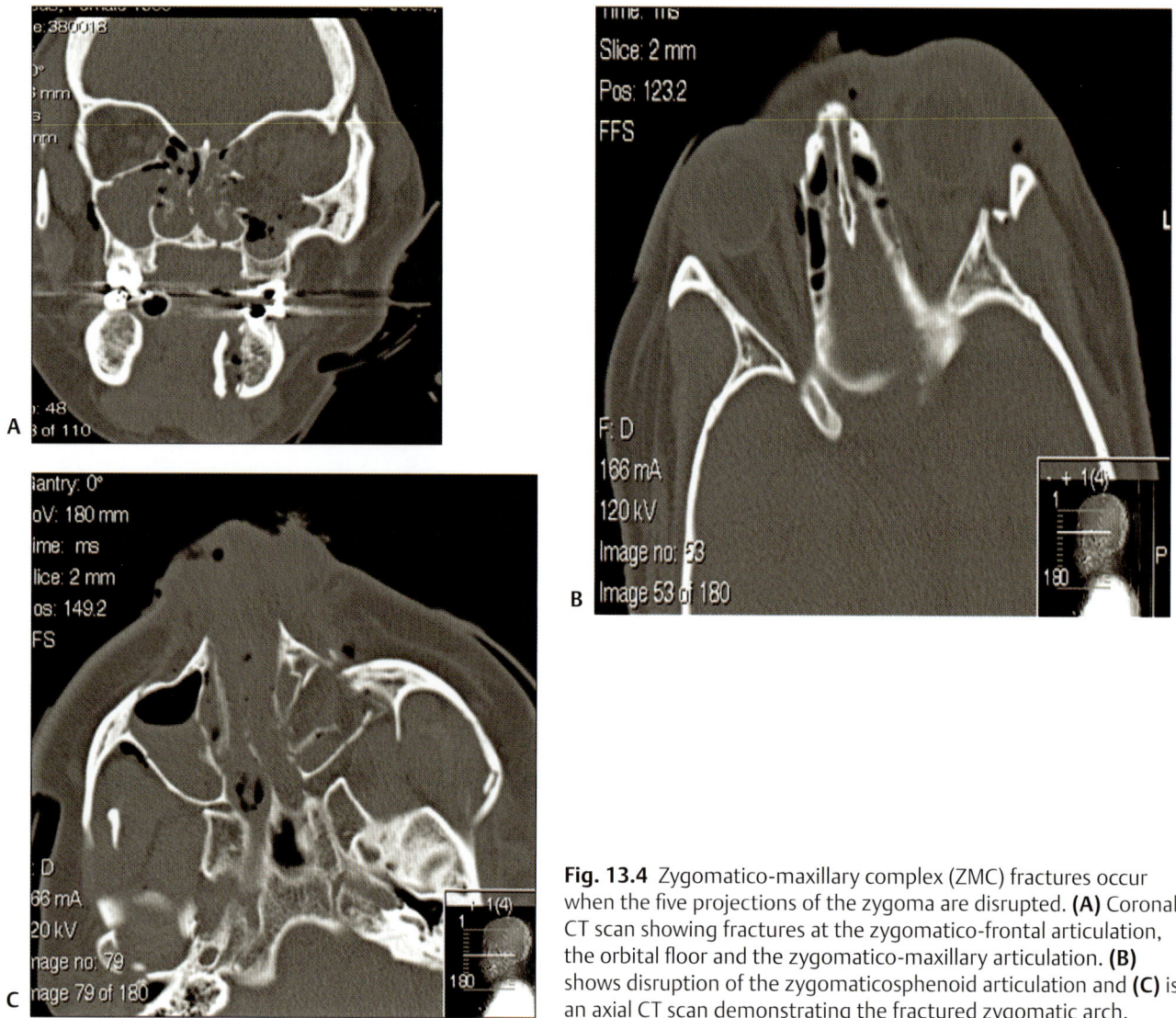

Fig. 13.4 Zygomatico-maxillary complex (ZMC) fractures occur when the five projections of the zygoma are disrupted. **(A)** Coronal CT scan showing fractures at the zygomatico-frontal articulation, the orbital floor and the zygomatico-maxillary articulation. **(B)** shows disruption of the zygomaticosphenoid articulation and **(C)** is an axial CT scan demonstrating the fractured zygomatic arch.

Diplopia

Persistent diplopia may occur in patients after timely primary fracture repairs. Diplopia in the acute setting has several causes, which can be broadly categorized as mechanical or neurogenic. Extraocular muscle entrapment, edema, or hemorrhage (either in combination or isolation) may contribute to mechanical restriction of globe motion. Injury to the motor nerve of an extraocular muscle represents a neurologic cause of diplopia after orbitozygomatic trauma.[58,68] As might be expected, postoperative resolution of diplopia is variable, depending on its cause. Edema should resolve with a gradual improvement of diplopia over one to two weeks.[57] The course of recovery of diplopia from a neurogenic cause

is harder to predict and depends on the degree of nerve injury. Prolapse of orbital contents can result in both enophthalmos (delayed) and diplopia and explain why these symptoms often coexist.[54,68] The goals of treatment in this instance are volume restoration with globe repositioning and improved extraocular muscle function after it is released from the constraint of the fracture.[54–56,60,68] The increased use of endoscopic approaches to the repair of orbital blow-out fractures offers several advantages in terms of visualization and avoidance of a lower lid incision. Application in the right cases and recognition of the limitations of this approach are important factors in adequate repair with the endoscopic technique. Endoscopy via the transantral route also has a role as an adjunct to standard eyelid approaches to confirm complete reduction of the orbital contents and proper placement of floor implants.[69]

Several aspects of the residual injury can be quantified. Zygomatic fractures may present with all of these secondary findings, while orbital blowout fractures are less often associated with the facial deformities outlined below. Posterior globe displacement is well visualized from the worm's eye or bird's eye view. A Hertel exophthalmometer quantifies globe projection by measuring the projection of the orbit relative to the lateral orbital rim.[49,54,60] Any difference greater than 3 mm between the globes is abnormal,[49,68] though differences of 1–2 mm may be noticeable on some people. When the lateral orbital rim is displaced (as may be the case in a ZMC fracture) a Naugle exophthalmometer is used—the reference point is the forehead.[54] From the worm's eye view, the distance between the brow and the upper lid may be revealing as well. Vertical globe dystopia from hypoglobus (hypophthalmos) can result in an inability to level the planes of the retinas, with splitting of images even in the primary gaze.[68] Superior sulcus deformity and pseudoptosis of the upper lid may also be seen (**Fig. 13.5**). The lateral canthus can be inferiorly displaced if the fracture of the lateral orbital wall is superior to Whitnall's tubercle (the attachment point of the lateral canthal tendon).[49,51,52,54] As the zygoma is pulled inferiorly, so too is the lateral attachment of the eyelids, giving a downward slant to the palpebral fissure. Malar flattening and increased facial width are common hallmarks of displacement of the zygoma.[61,63] Ptosis of cheek soft tissues with deepening of the nasolabial fold and an aged appearance may accompany the initial injury or result from failure to properly resuspend the soft tissues after surgery.[54,70] Descent of the cheek soft tissue can contribute to lower eyelid displacement.

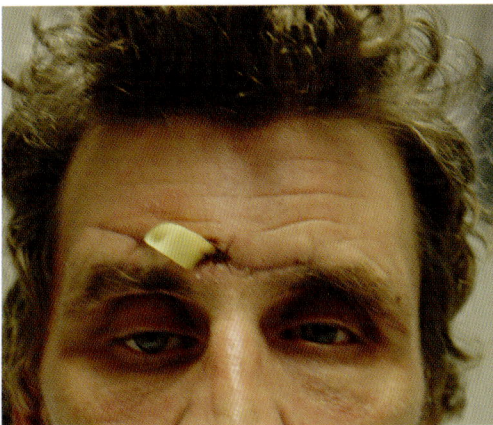

Fig. 13.5 Right superior sulcus deformity and hypoglobus. The patient had complex frontal sinus and orbital fractures. Titanium mesh used to reconstruct the anterior table of the frontal sinus became infected and was ultimately removed.

Vision Loss

Severe vision loss has been reported in 0.8–1.6% of cases in recent reports of facial fractures involving the orbit or trauma to the periorbital structures.[71-73] Incidences are higher when direct trauma to the globe is considered.[74] Visual loss may develop after the initial presentation but before any planned surgical intervention.[74] Because many orbitozygomatic fractures can be managed electively, patients must receive adequate counseling so they are familiar with the signs and symptoms of orbital pathology that should cause them to seek medical attention before the scheduled date for their operation.

Visual impairment is a rare complication of facial fracture surgery that has been reported in 0.3% of ZMC fracture repairs.[72,74] Girotto et al. reported a 0.24% incidence of blindness after repair of 1240 midfacial fractures over a 10-year period.[74] The most common reason for blindness after surgery to repair facial fractures in the orbital region is the development of a retrobulbar hemorrhage.[72,75-77] Blindness that develops in the absence of this finding is caused by traumatic optic neuropathy or other perioperative conditions that decrease end-organ perfusion.[72,74,78,79]

Retrobulbar Hemorrhage

Retrobulbar hemorrhage usually occurs secondary to an arterial bleed in the orbit, either from the infraorbital, anterior, or posterior ethmoid arteries.[76,77,80] The ensuing hematoma causes increased intraocular pressure, which leads to compression of the arteries that supply the optic nerve and results in ischemia.[76-78,80] Irreversible loss of ganglion cells in the optic nerve can occur within 90 minutes,[81] so the development of this complication is a true surgical emergency. The clinical findings associated with retrobulbar hemorrhage include proptosis, pain, subconjunctival hemorrhage, sluggish or absent afferent pupillary reflex, Marcus Gunn pupil, and loss of vision.[75-78,80] A CT scan should not be pursued if there are clear physical findings, because the time needed to acquire it will delay treatment and further threaten vision.[77,80]

Protocols for the management of retrobulbar hemorrhage have been outlined and are summarized in **Table 13.1**.[76-78,80] An immediate decrease in the intraocular pressure can be accomplished at the bedside by performing a lateral canthotomy and inferior cantholysis under local anesthesia. This allows the lower eyelid to be distracted from the orbital rim and may allow partial evacuation of the clot.[77,78] Orbital incisions used to gain access to the fracture may need to be opened (transconjunctival or subciliary) and the clot expressed through them.[77] Medical therapy can help reduce intraocular pressure (mannitol, acetazolamide, or timolol eye drops) and may be protective by decreasing the generation of the by-products of ischemia, such as oxygen free radicals (high doses of steroids); specific dosing regimens

Table 13.1

Management of Retrobulbar Hemorrhage
a. Perform immediate lateral canthotomy and inferior cantholysis at the bedside under local anesthesia with opening of surgical incisions (transconjunctival or subciliary).
b. Contact an ophthalmologist for urgent consultation.
c. Initiate medical decompression of intraorbital pressure (mannitol, acetazolamide, timolol eye drops).
d. Return the patient to the OR for surgical exploration, evacuation of any hematoma, control of hemorrhage, and orbital decompression.

have been outlined.[76–78,80] Generally, medical therapy is adjunctive and may allow the situation to be temporized until the patient can be brought to the operating room for formal exploration or decompression. Certain protocols suggest instituting medical therapy once the diagnosis has been made and using the stability of vision to determine whether formal decompression is required.[80] Orbital decompression may be accomplished through a variety of approaches.[77,78] It is essential to recognize a retrobulbar hemorrhage in the postoperative period to prevent significant visual loss. A clearly defined and strictly followed postoperative regimen of visual checks is the best way to ensure close monitoring of the patient's vision.[75] We use a regimen for monitoring that has also been described in the literature[75,80]: vision checks are performed every 15 minutes for the first hour, every 30 minutes for the second hour, and hourly until the next day.

Trigeminal Nerve Paresthesia

Alteration of sensation in the distribution of the infraorbital nerve branch of the fifth cranial nerve (V2) is one the most common complications of fracture treatment in this region. At initial presentation, 80–94% of patients with orbitozygomatic fractures have sensory disturbance of the V2.[82,83] Reports of 40–50% of patients with some persistent sensory disturbance, whether surgery or observation was chosen, confirm the high prevalence of this complication.[84–86] Rigid fixation of ZMC fractures has been shown to result in greater rates of sensory recovery compared with closed or open reduction without fixation.[85,86] Some patients may suffer from chronic pain in the V2 distribution, which is confirmed by an infraorbital nerve block.[87] Decompression of the nerve as it exits the infraorbital foramen at the time of fracture repair has a positive effect on sensory recovery.[87] Microsurgery of the infraorbital nerve has been discussed in the literature recently. Procedures include nerve de-

compression, removal of scarring, and excision of a neuroma if present, with neurorrhaphy and endoneurial or perineurial repair depending on the degree of injury. Specific indications for this procedure include worsening sensory deficit and dysesthesia or paresthesia that is intolerable to the patient.[87] Some patients may develop dysesthesia afterward, so careful patient selection and preoperative counseling are advised.

Anisocoria

Posterior exploration of the orbit to identify the edge of the orbital floor fracture may result in injury to the ciliary ganglion where the parasympathetic nerve fibers synapse en route to the sphincter of the iris. The action of the ciliary nerve results in pupillary constriction. Anisocoria is unequal size of the right and left pupils. In this case, mydriasis of the pupil of the operated eye is the cause. The pupil is reactive, but in certain instances a tonic pupil develops.[88] This condition results from an injury that directly involves the ciliary ganglion or the postganglionic fibers (short ciliary nerves) that innervate the sphincter of the iris. Preganglionic fibers run in close proximity to the inferior oblique and inferior rectus muscles. Elevation of these muscles out of the orbital floor fracture may traumatize these nerve fibers. Reported cases of postsurgical anisocoria show this condition to be self-limited.[88,89]

◆ Late Considerations of Orbitozygomatic Trauma

Implant-associated complications can be seen in the use of autogenous or alloplastic materials. Generally, autogenous materials are more resistant to infection and extrusion. Alloplastic implants differ in terms of permanence (resorbable vs. non-resorbable). However, alloplastic implants have a lifetime risk of infection, migration, and extrusion (**Fig. 13.6**). Porous implants allow some vascular ingrowth, which potentially imparts resistance to infection and improves fixation to the wound bed.

Ophthalmologic examination is a prerequisite to any corrective orbital surgery. CT scans in axial, coronal, and sagittal planes are routinely obtained. 3-D reconstructions can be obtained to assess posttraumatic (residual) deformities of the zygoma. CT-based navigation systems are now being used at several centers to simulate the osteotomies and movements required to restore the premorbid zygomatic position.[70,90,91] The final position of the bone is then registered, and markers are placed on the bone intraoperatively to transmit the position and movements in space until the predetermined position is reached.[70,90,91] Stereolithography is a more recent adjunct used for model surgery and planning.[70] Stereolithographic models reproduce the craniofacial skeleton

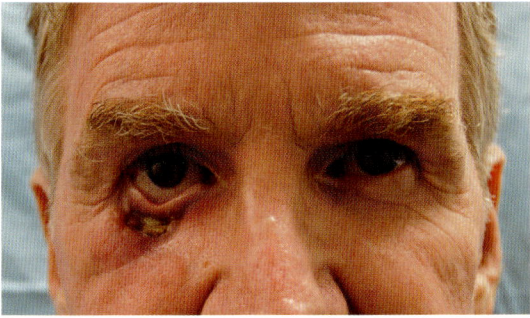

Fig. 13.6 Extruding orbital implant with ectropion.

and can then be sectioned so the zygoma is reduced to its premorbid position. This technology, while adding additional expense, has the advantage of improving precision and possibly decreasing the time of the operation.

Several approaches allow access to the orbit and zygoma, including the transconjunctival approach via a pre- or postseptal route.[14] The subciliary incision is perhaps more direct but has a higher rate of ectropion, and most surgeons have abandoned the direct infraorbital lower lid incision because of poor exposure and significant problems with lower lid edema. Additional incisions that can facilitate exposure of the orbit and malar complex include the medial canthal (Lynch), coronal, lateral brow, upper blepharoplasty, and the upper gingivobuccal sulcus incisions. Descriptions of their execution are detailed elsewhere.[14,25,53,54,56,92–94]

The benefits of late correction of orbitofacial deformity and diplopia must be explained to the patient in the context of both the surgical risks and the realistic outcomes of surgery. The risks include vision loss (including blindness), worsening of diplopia, hypesthesia of the maxillary nerve (V2), retrobulbar hemorrhage, implant extrusion, and lower lid shortening.[51,54,94,95] Although these risks are similar to those encountered when primary surgery is performed, they are heightened in the chronic orbit, where scarring has set in and anatomic landmarks may be distorted. Chronic diplopia may not completely resolve and occasionally worsens. The patient should also be informed that improvement may require several stages.[54,96–98] Patients with persistent diplopia after secondary reconstructive attempts should consider prisms or strabismus surgery, in consultation with an ophthalmologist.[52,99]

The volume enlargement that results after orbital blow-out fractures is corrected by onlay grafting.[54,68,95] Grafts are placed at the globe axis to correct hypoglobus and along the posterior orbital floor or medial orbital wall to address enophthalmos.[51,56] Using the same techniques that are employed in the acute setting, the surgeon explores the orbit, and the orbital contents are reduced. Traditionally a nearly circumferential elevation

of the periobita[53,60,68] has been advocated, but more recent surgical descriptions support directed dissections of the tethered areas.[54,55] Dissection must allow advancement of the orbit to correct the enophthalmos. The surgeon assesses the potential for orbital advancement intraoperatively by performing the forced traction test.[54]

Techniques to correct enophthalmos after chronic ZMC fractures use many of the techniques outlined above with some important differences. Surgical goals not only include correction of functional impairments (diplopia and lower lid dysfunction) but also must address malar and other periorbital deformities more commonly associated with zygomatic fractures. Displacement of the lateral wall is usually the main contributor to increased orbital volume in a ZMC fracture, with orbital floor disruption usually being a less significant source.[56] Both the volume enlargement and malar hypoplasia can be corrected by onlay grafting alone, as described by Freihofer.[94] For more severe displacement, the zygoma is osteotomized and repositioned. It is then placed back to a more anatomical position, restoring malar projection and decreasing intraorbital volume.[49,54–56] Despite this movement of the zygoma, the orbit often must be explored to repair any concomitant orbital floor fracture with an onlay graft.[56] Often the original fracture lines can be identified and osteotomized to free the bone. Intraorbital bone cuts begin at the inferior orbital fissure[63] and proceed anteromedially toward the infraorbital rim and superolaterally through the zygomatico-sphenoid suture to meet the osteotomy through the zygomaticofrontal suture.[55,56] An osteotomy along the anterior face of the maxilla and then through the zygomatico-maxillary suture is connected to the osteotomy along the temporal aspect of the zygoma. Finally, the zygomatic arch is osteotomized[63] (**Fig. 13.7**). Bone grafting may be required once the zygoma is reduced to span deficits created by the bone movement. Variations in surgical technique center on the type of exposure obtained, the amount of intraorbital dissection performed, and (more recently) the use of models and or CT navigation systems. Mathog et al. reported the results of surgical correction of enophthalmos, diplopia, or both in a series of 38 patients.[60] Only two of the thirty-eight patients had persistent enophthalmos greater than two millimeters postoperatively. Twenty patients suffered from diplopia, with 15 experiencing resolution and four patients improvement.[60] Surgical methods included multiple approaches to the orbit, 270 degree periorbital dissection, and directed placement of bone grafts at the sites of deficits. Other reports suggest less optimistic results when orbital blowout fractures are repaired after significant time delays.[59] This finding suggests the need for more aggressive orbital dissection to free scarred tissues and advance the globe and also suggests that the persistent posttraumatic diplopia seen in many patients may not be correctable.

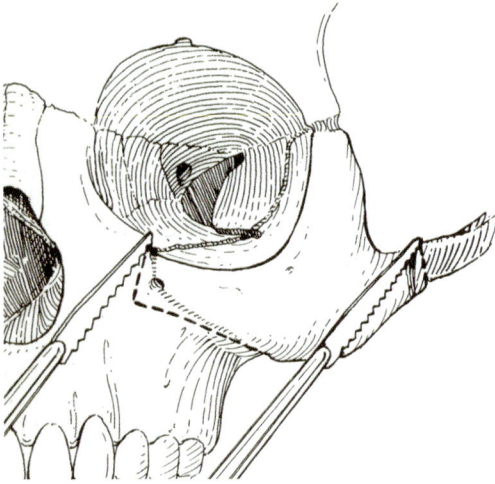

Fig. 13.7 Zygomatic osteotomies to mobilize the zygoma for correction of malunion. These include the suture lines at the zygomatic articulations and an osteotomy along the orbital floor. Used with permission from Longaker MT and Kawamoto HK. Evolving Thoughts on Correcting Posttraumatic Enophthalmos. Plast Reconstr Surg 1998;101(4):899–906.

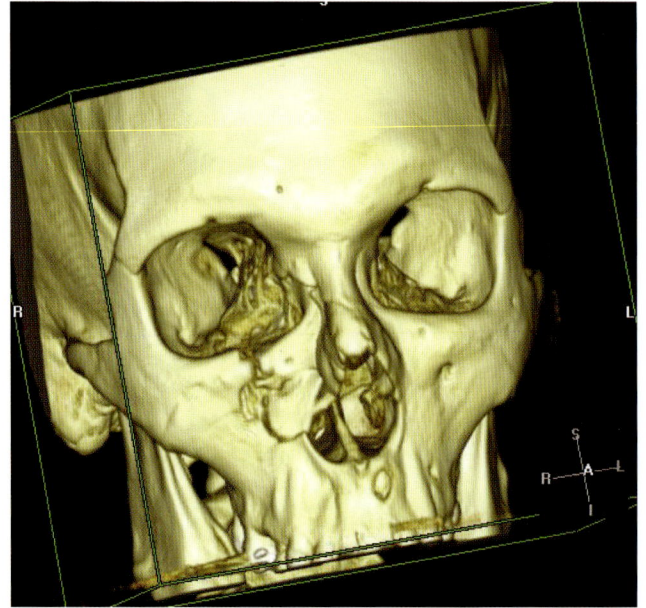

Fig. 13.8 Naso-orbital-ethmoid fracture. The boundaries of the fracture segment that define the central segment to which the medial canthal tendon attaches are demonstrated on the CT scan of this patient

Cheek soft tissues are suspended superolaterally to either correct or prevent tissue ptosis. This complements correction of lower lid distraction by decreasing the downward pull of the cheek soft tissue on the lower lid. Suspension with an appropriate vector, as executed in rhytidectomy surgery, should be performed.[54,61,95] Often superior reduction of the zygoma will restore the position of the lateral canthus.[49,56] Otherwise, lateral canthopexy is performed.[54,56,61]

◆ Naso-orbital-ethmoid Fractures

The naso-orbital-ethmoid (NOE) region represents the anatomic convergence of several subunits of the midface. The importance of injury in this area is heightened by its border with the frontal sinus and anterior skull base.[100] NOE fractures include disruption of the angular process of the maxilla, the medial orbital wall, the medial infraorbital rim, the pyriform aperture and the lateral nasal wall.[101] These fracture lines are the boundaries of what is known as the central segment (**Fig. 13.8**). It contains the medial canthal tendon, and its proper reduction is essential for restitution of the form and function of the tendon. The medial canthal tendon attaches to the lacrimal bone via three extensions of the orbicularis oculi muscle. A horizontal limb attaches to the anterior lacrimal crest, a vertical (superior) limb attaches to the frontal process of the maxilla at its articulation with the frontal bone, and the third (posterior) limb inserts posteriorly to the lacrimal sac on the posterior lacrimal crest.[102,103] NOE fractures result in lateral displacement of the medial orbital wall and the tendon along with it. The normal distance between the medial canthi is 30 mm.[104] Telecanthus is one of the central physical findings and should be quantified. Epicanthal folds and rounding and displacement of the medial commissure inferiorly and anteriorly complete the medial orbital deformity.[53,103,105,106] The nasal bones and septum are often fractured as well, resulting in collapse of the nasal dorsum and a saddle nose deformity.[100,103,105] The nasal length is shortened from the telescoping effect of the nasal bone collapse.[100,103,105] Loss of dorsal nasal height often exaggerates the appearance of telecanthus and exacerbates the development of epicanthal folds.

Complications of NOE fractures include their accompanying orbital and nasal deformity.[105] Stabilization of the medial canthal tendon aims to neutralize the forces that tend to pull the canthus laterally. If the medial canthus is attached to a large, stable bone segment, it can be osteotomized and reduced to correct the deformity.[105] If a more severe disruption of the canthal attachment is present, the tendon itself is wire-fixated and medialized by securing the wire transnasally to the contralateral supra-orbital rim or medial orbit.[101,103,105] The wire is threaded through the remaining lacrimal bone posterior to the lacrimal fossa. It is essential that the tendon be pulled in a superior-posterior direction.[101,102,105] Saddle nose deformity is managed with autogenous or alloplastic grafting materials. Cranial bone grafts and costochondral grafts are most frequently used.[100,101,105] The use of alloplastic materials for dorsal augmentation has shown success, but caution is advised.

Injury to the lacrimal system requiring a secondary bypass procedure may occur in 17–24% of NOE fractures.[106–108] Soft-tissue injury to the medial lower eyelid is another significant cause of obstruction of the nasolacrimal system.[109] Compression of the lacrimal sac or bone fragments of the nasolacrimal duct during surgical manipulation to accomplish reduction can also produce obstruction.[106] Nasolacrimal injuries will result in epiphora and persistent stenosis that may lead to dacryocystitis.[51,106,110] In some instances, the obstruction is temporary, and definitive management should be postponed because some patients will regain function three to six months after the injury.[107,110] In patients with midfacial fractures, the distal portion of the nasolacrimal system is most often injured.[107,108] It is important to recognize more proximal injuries, particularly to the inferior canaliculus, because primary repair over a stent may prevent long-term sequelae.[111] Prophylactic stenting of the nasolacrimal duct is recommended in significant injuries in the area of the lacrimal fossa or the bony canal.[112] Spinelli et al. placed lacrimal stents (Guibor silicone tubes) in all patients with NOE fractures. Of 19 patients, only three developed epiphora, which spontaneously resolved in all.[112] The duration of intubation varied among the group of patients. The Jones I and II tests are used to determine the site of obstruction.[106,112] Dacryocystography is performed by cannulating the lower canaliculus and injecting radiopaque dye, after which an anterior-posterior skull X-ray is taken, which should identify the site of the lesion.[106] Initially, conservative therapy is attempted, consisting of lower eyelid massage and the application of steroid eye drops to the medial fornix.[106] If drainage problems persist, a dacryocystorhinostomy (DCR) can bypass the obstruction by diverting drainage from the lacrimal fossa into the nasal cavity.[106,107] More proximal injuries require additional oculoplastic techniques to reestablish drainage.[106]

◆ Midfacial Fractures

Malocclusion is one of the most significant negative functional sequelae of fractures of the maxilla.[25,113] As discussed in the section on mandible fractures, the same principles of bone healing apply to the maxilla. However, delayed union and nonunion are less frequent complications, as the maxilla is subject to lower functional loads.[7] Facial height and width alteration are commonly seen after malunion, in addition to an anterior open bite malocclusion secondary to posterior-superior rotation of the maxilla.[114] This results when MMF is not established before placement of rigid fixation, along with failure to disimpact an impacted maxilla.[114] It was also more common in the past, when the

use of Adams suspension wires to prevent facial elongation actually resulted in rotation and foreshortening.[115] A simultaneous palatal fracture allows changes in the transverse dimension and a resulting posterior crossbite.[114] Often a midfacial fracture is a component of a panfacial fracture, and malunion of other areas of the facial skeleton may be preventing proper reduction of the midface. A thorough survey of these other areas should be undertaken.

Late malocclusion that results after maxillary fractures is approached in the same way as other dentofacial abnormalities. The evaluation includes maxillofacial CT scans with true coronal images, a lateral cephalogram, and Panorex for assistance with presurgical planning.[25,43,113] Dental models are also obtained and mounted on an articulator to recreate the malocclusion.[25,43,113] Model surgery is performed to simulate the osteotomies that will be performed intraoperatively.[43] The LeFort I osteotomy is the mainstay of corrective surgery.[23] Segmentation of the maxilla may be used to correct transverse deficiency, and asymmetric impaction procedures (posterior>anterior for an anterior open bite) are variations that can be employed to correct more complex malocclusions.[23]

◆ Frontal Sinus

Many classification systems and treatment algorithms exist to guide management of frontal sinus fractures.[116–122] Simply put, treatment seeks to reduce the fracture and restore proper function. In certain injuries, however, attempts at restoration of function potentially lead to life-threatening complications.[117,118,121,123,124] Of all the regions of the facial skeleton discussed thus far, the frontal sinus is the one area in which lack of function is an outcome that the patient can tolerate.[118,121,125,126]

Over all, complication rates after frontal sinus trauma range from 0 to 67%.[116–119,122,124,126] Major complications listed in multiple case reviews are cerebrospinal fluid leak (2–10%[116–118,121]), mucocele or mucopyocele (1–6%[116,117,121]), frontal sinusitis (1–19%[116,118,119,121,124,126]) meningitis (1–4%[116,117,121,123,124]), and other intracranial infections (2%[124,126]). Other complications often considered to be minor are forehead deformity, forehead numbness, and chronic frontal headache in the absence of drainage problems.[118,121,126] The incidence of some complications is difficult to define, because of the delays in presentation and lack of patient follow-up that are sometimes characteristic of frontal sinus fractures.

When complications arise, several central questions should be considered: (1) Has the forehead contour been reestablished? (2) Can the sinus function reliably? (3) Are the dura/intracranial contents separated from the sinus? Most classification schemes divide frontal sinus fractures into three main groupings[118–121,123]: (a) anterior table fractures with or without displacement or comminution, (b) bitabular fractures with significant disruption of the posterior table [these fractures usually involve the frontal sinus outflow tract (the nasofrontal duct) with exposure of dura or brain], and (c) fractures of the frontal sinus outflow tract with an intact (or minimally disrupted) posterior table. The latter fracture pattern is usually seen when an anterior table fracture extends onto the floor of the sinus or when a concomitant NOE fracture is present.[118,120,127]

Complications arising from the first group (group a) include persistent forehead deformity or failure of alloplastic frontal cranioplasty.[118,119,123] Correction involves replacement of missing or displaced bone segments. Autogenous split calvarial bone grafts can be safely harvested and may be contoured to recreate the preinjury forehead contour.[128]

The second group (group b) represents the most severe injuries, for there may be a significant brain injury and concomitant fractures of the skull base. Neurosurgical consultation is usually mandated. Sinus function may need to be sacrificed because of the high risk of intracranial infection. In these instances, cranialization removes the posterior table of the sinus and all sinus mucosa lining the remaining anterior wall. The frontal ducts must be obliterated to seal off and compartmentalize the nasal cavity below.[125] Cranialization itself is not without complications, which include mucocele or mucopyocele, cerebrospinal fluid leak, pneumocephalus, meningitis, or other intracranial infections that can result when a watertight and airtight seal does not exist between the sinus and brain.[117,118] Exploration in the setting of one of these complications must identify and reseal the frontal ducts and ensure that the dural repair is intact.[119,125] Reinforcement of the anterior skull base with a pericranial flap during the initial cranialization may prevent communication between the sinus and intracranial cavities.[123,127]

Nasofrontal duct injury (the third group, c) can result in permanently impaired sinus drainage with the development of frontal sinusitis, mucocele or mucopyocele, or osteomyelitis of the frontal bone.[124] In the setting of a co-existing posterior table fracture that does not require cranialization, these complications carry the more significant potential consequence of intracranial extension. Historically, high rates of these complications and the inability to reestablish duct function bolstered recommendations that sinus function be sacrificed in this setting.[124,126] To accomplish frontal sinus obliteration, the surgeon removed mucosa from the frontal sinus cavity and occluded the nasofrontal duct to prevent the growth of respiratory mucosa from the middle meatus, creating a safe sinus.[122,127,129] Until recently, frontal sinus obliteration using an osteoplastic flap to access the frontal sinus was considered the gold standard treatment option.[116,118,127,130] The success of endoscopic frontal sinus procedures for the treatment of chronic sinus disease, however, has prompted a reexamination of the applicability of frontal sinus obliteration to every injured nasofrontal duct.[129-133]

With these considerations in mind, several reasonable management options may be chosen. First, repair of the anterior table fracture alone is performed. The patient must adhere to a close, regular follow-up with a sinus CT scan, initially at six-month intervals. If a complication develops, surgery is offered to improve sinus drainage via endoscopic techniques, or the sinus is obliterated.[132-134] Reestablishment of nasofrontal duct function has the potential to obviate the need for sinus obliteration, unless patency is not restored. The modified Lothrop or Draf III procedure allows widening of both nasofrontal ducts, with removal of the intersinus septum and a portion of the frontal sinus floor.[129,130] Less extensive endoscopic procedures include simply stenting the duct for several months.[118,119] Har-el and Kennedy support the use of endoscopic sinus surgery for the treatment of mucoceles.[135,136] Mucoceles are mucous-filled cysts that emanate from remnants of respiratory mucosa in the frontal sinus.[137] Impaired sinus drainage allows them to expand into adjacent structures, including the orbit, ethmoid sinus, and brain.[135-137] A mucopyocele is an infected mucocele. Traditionally, mucoceles are treated aggressively with wide exposure and removal of the cyst.[135,136] Cranialization may be necessary if the mucocele has resulted in destruction of the posterior table of the frontal sinus. The goal of endoscopic management is to marsupialize the mucocele and improve sinus drainage by using the extended frontal sinusotomy procedures described above.[135,136]

Success with endoscopic frontal sinus surgery has disproven the notion that frontal sinus function cannot be reestablished by operating on the nasofrontal duct.[118,119,129,130,132,133] Now more than ever, management of frontal sinus fractures includes endoscopic techniques for both observation and treatment. If endoscopic methods are ineffective, traditional frontal sinus obliteration is available as a salvage operation. It should be underscored that complications after frontal sinus trauma can present after a long delay, sometimes many years after the initial injury.[116,119,137] Long-term yearly follow-up of patients is widely advocated to allow the detection of functional sinus problems before a more serious complication develops.[127,137]

◆ Soft-Tissue Trauma

Scar contracture, webbing, notching, hypertrophic or keloidal scars that violate subunits or relaxed skin tension lines, and soft-tissue depression are among the undesired outcomes after soft-tissue trauma healing.[138-142] Associated functional deficits can include ectropion, entropion, epiphora, lagophthalmos, alar stenosis, lip incompetence or oral commissure webbing with drooling, and ear canal stenosis with conductive hearing loss. Scar revision procedures, as well as techniques used in rhinoplasty, cheiloplasty, and oculoplastic surgery, are all employed to improve secondary deformities and are covered in depth in several excellent references.[51,53,140–142]

Lacerating injuries to the parotid gland and lateral cheek warrant special consideration due to the techniques that are required in their management. Tissue that is not viable is debrided, and primary repair is performed with attention to repairing the gland's capsule.[143] Vulnerable structures include Stensen's duct and the facial nerve, and these must be explored carefully if injury is suspected[143–146] (**Fig. 13.9**). Trauma significant enough to lacerate the parotid duct has been reported to have a 40–55% association with injury of adjacent facial nerve branches—most frequently the buccal branch.[143,144] Associated facial nerve injuries mandate immediate exploration of the nerve ends. Debate still exists about the decision to undertake primary repair of parotid duct transection. Primary repair of the duct is recommended

in its course along the masseter muscle.[143,144,146–148] Proximal injuries or intraglandular injuries may not be amenable to repair, and distal injuries (beyond the anterior edge of the masseter) can be successfully managed by reimplantation of the distal stump to reestablish intraoral drainage.[143,145,146,148] Microsurgical techniques are readily adapted to use in the management of acute duct injuries.[145] A stent is placed in the duct for 7–21 days.[143–146]

The complications that accompany parotid duct injuries include sialocele, salivary fistula, and chronic parotitis.[133,144,148] The rarity of parotid duct injuries does not allow the benefit of consulting results from large case studies. One of the three patients reported by Landau and Stewart who had primary duct repair developed a fistula.[144] The three cases reported by Tachmes et al. had no reported complications.[143] Patients whose injuries were initially unrecognized compose the majority of cases that develop impaired duct function after trauma.

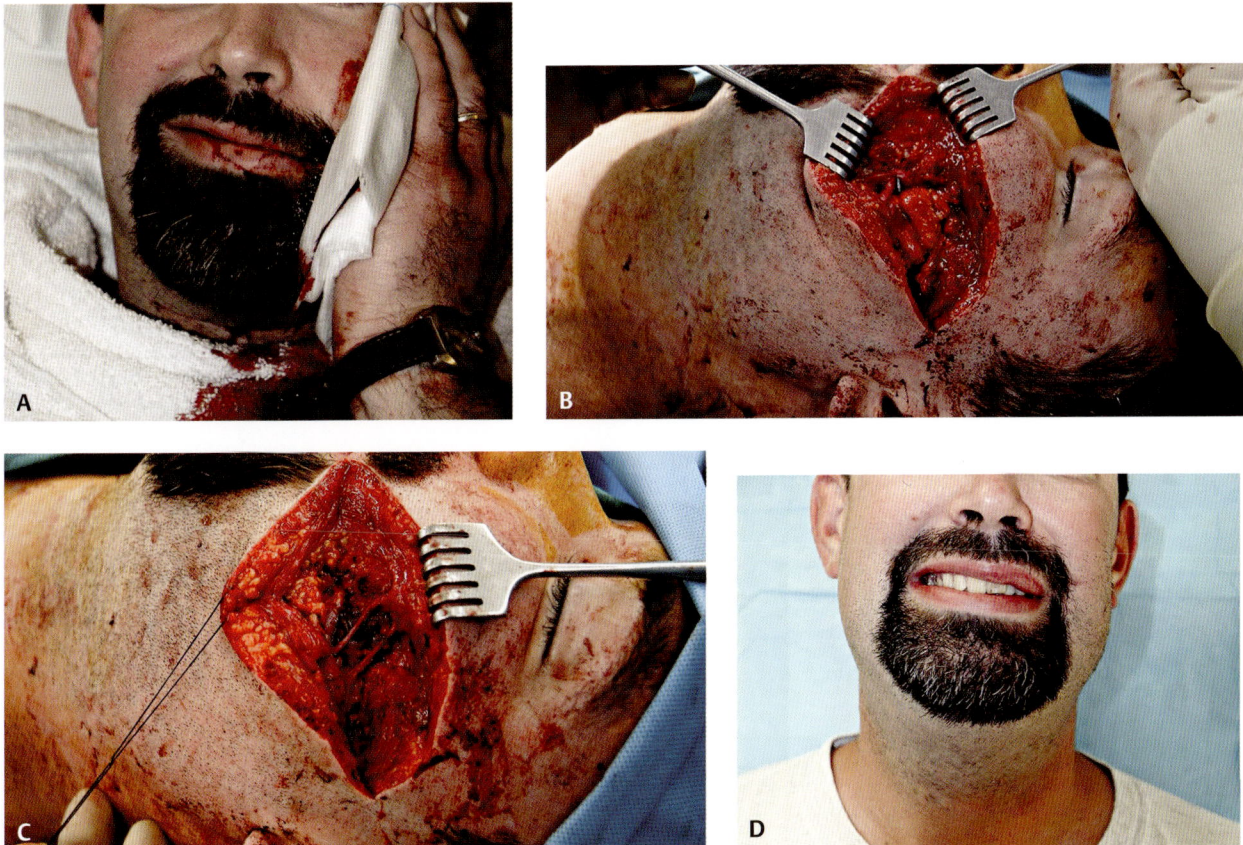

Fig. 13.9 Parotid and facial nerve injury. A 30-year-old patient sustained a penetrating trauma to the left cheek with a laceration of the parotid duct and buccal branches of the facial nerve. **(A)** Preoperatvie photograph showing paralysis of upper lip elevators and flattening of the nasolabial fold. **(B)** Intraoperative photograph shows cannulation of the distal parotid duct via the intraoral opening of Stensen's duct. **(C)** Intraoperative photograph showing repair of Stensen's duct inferiorly (over a polyethelene stent left in place for 10 days) and the two transected buccal branches. **(D)** One year postoperative photograph showing marked improvement in function of lip elevators. Patient regained full resting symmetry as well. The patient initially had impaired salivary flow that was transient.

In a review of posttraumatic fistulae and sialoceles, Landau and Stewart reported that 11 of the 14 patients with penetrating trauma to the cheek did not have this injury addressed within 24 hours of the initial trauma.[144]

A sialogram is perhaps the most sensitive method for determining the site of leakage once a parotid duct complication has developed; however, sialoendoscopy is a newer method that allows direct visualization of Stensen's duct.[144,146,147] Medical management of these complications includes needle aspiration of salivary collections, pressure dressings, anticholinergic drugs, and the substitution of enteral feeding for oral intake until normal salivary flow is reestablished.[144–149] Parekh et al. outlined their successful strategy for medical management.[147] This requires that the patient take nothing by mouth (enteral feeds or total parental nutrition are given) until the fistula or sialocele has resolved. Adjunctive measures were not considered necessary with this regimen.

Intraparotid botulinum toxin A injections are becoming more commonplace after parotid duct injury because of their efficacy and safety. Marchese-Ragona et al. used EMG-guidance for precise injection into the gland and for prevention of inadvertent masticator muscle or facial muscle injection.[150,151] Others use ultrasound guidance, and in some reports simple percutaneous injection is performed.[152,153] Most reports indicate a clinical response within two weeks of the first injection and an effect that lasts at least three months.[150–153] In several cases, only one injection was required, with no recrudescence after several months of follow-up.[150–154]

Patients with sialoceles or salivary fistulae who do not respond to any of these interventions may require ligation of the duct or total parotidectomy.[146,147] A safer surgical alternative has been described,[148] whereby the deep surface of the sialocele or fistula tract is marsupialized into the oral cavity with blunt instruments. The external communication is closed, and the intraoral wound allowed to drain into the mouth.

◆ Conclusion

The adherence to time-tested principles of fracture healing is the foundation of proper management and the key to avoiding complications after trauma to the facial skeleton. This review has also highlighted evolving trends in management that can be applied to the treatment of complications. Access to high-resolution imaging capabilities and image guidance can improve surgical outcomes and decrease the morbidity associated with revision surgery. The use of surgical planning on models of the patient is being extended to areas of the craniofacial skeleton beyond the mandible, where model surgery is commonly performed. Finally, collaboration with other specialists, including ophthalmologists, neurosurgeons, neuroradiologists, and dental specialists, is encouraged to manage these complex cases.

PEARLS OF WISDOM

Comminuted or atrophic mandible fractures should be repaired with load-bearing reconstruction plates and bicortical screws to ensure bony union. Note that atrophic bone does not bear load well, so in such cases load-bearing repair becomes even more critical.

Jaw physiotherapy for treatment of condylar fractures that do not require ORIF should be started early to restore occlusion, especially in pediatric patients, who are at higher risk of developing TMJ ankylosis with long periods of rigid maxillomandibular fixation, which, of course, should be discouraged in both children and adults.

All facial trauma surgeons must be prepared to perform a lateral canthotomy and cantholysis when they suspect the development of a retrobulbar hematoma clinically. Patients can present with a hematoma as a result of the orbital trauma itself or from the repair of an orbital fracture. Given the short time window before irreversible vision loss can develop, clinicians must be able to diagnose this complication quickly, based on history and physical examination. Imaging can result in the loss of valuable time before intervention.

It is important to inform patients with naso-orbital-ethmoid fractures of the possibility of the development of nasolacrimal dysfunction as result of the bony injuries, even after adequate repair. It is reasonable to discuss the appropriateness of prophylactic nasolacrimal intubation with the ophthalmology team and add this to the procedure in the appropriate patient.

In the pediatric population, conservative (nonoperative) therapy of fractures has a more significant role in treatment algorithms than in adults. Especially in the mandible, overly aggressive procedures with extensive periosteal stripping can result in growth disturbances. Bony healing is faster in children, with a narrower therapeutic window for reduction procedures.

In pediatric patients (up to about ages 14–15 years), many surgeons remove fixation implants once bony union has been achieved, for fear of growth disturbance and potential implant migration.

References

1. Alpert B. Management of the complications of mandibular fracture treatment. Oper Tech Plast Reconstr Surg 1998;5(4):325–333
2. Berstein L, McClurg FL. Mandibular fractures: a review of 156 consecutive cases. Laryngoscope 1977;87(6):957–961
3. Fox AJ, Kellman RM. Mandibular angle fractures: two-miniplate fixation and complications. Arch Facial Plast Surg 2003;5(6):464–469
4. James RB, Fredrickson C, Kent JN. Prospective study of mandibular fractures. J Oral Surg 1981;39(4):275–281
5. Nakamura S, Takenoshita Y, Oka M. Complications of miniplate osteosynthesis for mandibular fractures. J Oral Maxillofac Surg 1994;52(3):233–238, discussion 238–239
6. Terris DJ, Lalakea ML, Tuffo KM, Shinn JB. Mandible fracture repair: specific indications for newer techniques. Otolaryngol Head Neck Surg 1994;111(6):751–757

7. Kellman RM. Clinical applications of bone plating systems to facial fractures. In: Papel ID, ed. Facial Plastic and Reconstructive Surgery. New York: Thieme; 2002:720–737

8. Ellis E III, Walker L. Treatment of mandibular angle fractures using two noncompression miniplates. J Oral Maxillofac Surg 1994;52(10):1032–1036, discussion 1036–1037

9. Furr AM, Schweinfurth JM, May WL. Factors associated with long-term complications after repair of mandibular fractures. Laryngoscope 2006;116(3):427–430

10. Haug RH, Schwimmer A. Fibrous union of the mandible: a review of 27 patients. J Oral Maxillofac Surg 1994;52(8): 832–839

11. Mathog RH, Toma V, Clayman L, Wolf S. Nonunion of the mandible: an analysis of contributing factors. J Oral Maxillofac Surg 2000;58(7):746–752, discussion 752–753

12. Prein J, Rahn BA. Scientific and Technical Background. In: Prein J, ed. Manual of Internal Fixation in the Cranio-Facial Skeleton. Berlin: Springer; 1998:1–49

13. Mathog RH. Nonunion of the mandible. Otolaryngol Clin North Am 1983;16(3):533–547

14. Costantino PD, Wolpe M. Facial Plating Systems. In: Papel ID, ed. Facial Plastic and Reconstructive Surgery. New York: Thieme; 2002:769–781

15. Kellman RM, Marentette LJ. Atlas of Craniomaxillofacial Fixation. New York: Raven; 1995

16. Rudderman RH, Mullen RL. Biomechanics of the facial skeleton. Clin Plast Surg 1992;19(1):11–29

17. Levy FE, Smith RW, Odland RM, Marentette LJ. Monocortical miniplate fixation of mandibular angle fractures. Arch Otolaryngol Head Neck Surg 1991;117(2):149–154

18. Schilli W. Mandibular Fractures. In: Prein J, ed. Manual of Internal Fixation in the Cranio-Facial Skeleton. Berlin: Springer; 1998:57–93

19. Kellman RM, Wright DT. Management of posttraumatic osteomyelitis of the mandible. In: Greenberg AM, Prein J, eds. Craniomaxillofacial Reconstructive and Corrective Bone Surgery: Principles of Internal Fixation Using the AO/ASIF Technique. New York: Springer; 2002:433–438

20. Chaushu G, Manor Y, Shoshani Y, Taicher S. Risk factors contributing to symptomatic plate removal in maxillofacial trauma patients. Plast Reconstr Surg 2000;105(2):521–525

21. Barber HD, Bahram R, Woodbury SC, Silverstein KE, Fonseca RJ. Mandibular Fractures. In: Fonseca RJ, Walker RV, Betts NJ, Barber HD, Powers MP, eds. Oral and Maxillofacial Trauma. St. Louis: Elsevier; 2005:479–522

22. Proffit WR, White RP. Combining Surgery and Orthodontics: Who Does What, When? In: Proffit WR, White RP, Sarver DM, eds. Contemporary Treatment of Dentofacial Deformity. St. Louis: Mosby; 2003:245–267

23. Turvey TA, White RP. Maxillary Surgery. In: Proffit WR, White RP, Sarver DM, eds. Contemporary Treatment of Dentofacial Deformity. St. Louis: Mosby; 2003:288–311

24. Blakey GH, White RP. Mandibular Surgery. In: Proffit WR, White RP, Sarver DM, eds. Contemporary Treatment of Dentofacial Deformity. St. Louis: Mosby; 2003

25. Tatum SA. Correction of post-traumatic maxillofacial deformities involving occlusion. Facial Plast Surg Clin North Am 1998;6(4):535–556

26. Nagase DY, Courtemanche DJ, Peters DA. Plate removal in traumatic facial fractures: 13-year practice review. Ann Plast Surg 2005;55(6):608–611

27. Iizuka T, Lindqvist C. Sensory disturbances associated with rigid internal fixation of mandibular fractures. J Oral Maxillofac Surg 1991;49(12):1264–1268

28. Marchena JM, Padwa BL, Kaban LB. Sensory abnormalities associated with mandibular fractures: incidence and natural history. J Oral Maxillofac Surg 1998;56(7):822–825, discussion 825–826

29. Ellis E III, Tharanon W. Facial width problems associated with rigid fixation of mandibular fractures: case reports. J Oral Maxillofac Surg 1992;50(1):87–94

30. Kademani D, Rombach DM, Quinn PD. Trauma to the temporomandibular joint region. In: Fonseca RJ, Walker RV, Betts NJ, Barber HD, Powers MP, eds. Oral and Maxillofacial Trauma. St. Louis: Elsevier; 2005:522–568

31. Kellman RM. Endoscopically assisted repair of subcondylar fractures of the mandible: an evolving technique. Arch Facial Plast Surg 2003;5(3):244–250

32. Ellis E III, Throckmorton G. Facial symmetry after closed and open treatment of fractures of the mandibular condylar process. J Oral Maxillofac Surg 2000;58(7):719–728, discussion 729–730

33. Ellis E III, Simon P, Throckmorton GS. Occlusal results after open or closed treatment of fractures of the mandibular condylar process. J Oral Maxillofac Surg 2000;58(3):260–268

34. Schön R, Fakler O, Gellrich NC, Schmelzeisen R. Five-year experience with the transoral endoscopically assisted treatment of displaced condylar mandible fractures. Plast Reconstr Surg 2005;116(1):44–50

35. Smartt JM Jr, Low DW, Bartlett SP. The pediatric mandible: II. Management of traumatic injury or fracture. Plast Reconstr Surg 2005;116(2):28e–41e

36. Ellis E III, McFadden D, Simon P, Throckmorton G. Surgical complications with open treatment of mandibular condylar process fractures. J Oral Maxillofac Surg 2000;58(9):950–958

37. Raveh J, Vuillemin T, Lädrach K. Open reduction of the dislocated, fractured condylar process: indications and surgical procedures. J Oral Maxillofac Surg 1989;47(2):120–127

38. Stacey DH, Doyle JF, Mount DL, Snyder MC, Gutowski KA. Management of mandible fractures. Plast Reconstr Surg 2006;117(3):48e–60e

39. Zide MF, Kent JN. Indications for open reduction of mandibular condyle fractures. J Oral Maxillofac Surg 1983;41(2): 89–98

40. Worsaae N, Thorn JJ. Surgical versus nonsurgical treatment of unilateral dislocated low subcondylar fractures: a clinical study of 52 cases. J Oral Maxillofac Surg 1994;52(4):353–360, discussion 360–361

41. Rubens BC, Stoelinga PJ, Weaver TJ, Blijdorp PA. Management of malunited mandibular condylar fractures. Int J Oral Maxillofac Surg 1990;19(1):22–25

42. Becking AG, Zijderveld SA, Tuinzing DB. Management of posttraumatic malocclusion caused by condylar process fractures. J Oral Maxillofac Surg 1998;56(12):1370–1374, discussion 1374–1375

43. Proffit WR, Sarver DM. Treatment Planning: Optimizing Benefit to the Patient. In: Proffit WR, White RP, Sarver DM, eds. Contemporary Treatment of Dentofacial Deformity. St. Louis: Mosby; 2003

44. Kaban LB, Perrott DH, Fisher K. A protocol for management of temporomandibular joint ankylosis. J Oral Maxillofac Surg 1990;48(11):1145–1151, discussion 1152

45. Posnick JC, Goldstein JA. Surgical management of temporomandibular joint ankylosis in the pediatric population. Plast Reconstr Surg 1993;91(5):791–798

46. Kaban LB, Perrott DH, Fisher K. A protocol for management of temporomandibular joint ankylosis. (discussion) J Oral Maxillofac Surg 1990;48:1152

47. Lei Z. Auricular cartilage graft interposition after temporomandibular joint ankylosis surgery in children. J Oral Maxillofac Surg 2002;60(9):985–987

48. Dean A, Alamillos F. Mandibular distraction in temporomandibular joint ankylosis. Plast Reconstr Surg 1999;104(7): 2021–2031

49. Byrd HS, Hobar PC. Optimizing the management of secondary zygomatic fracture deformities. Aesthetic and functional considerations. Clin Plast Surg 1992;19(1):259–273

50. Thaller SR, Zarem HA, Kawamoto HK. Surgical correction of late sequelae from facial bone fractures. Am J Surg 1987;154(1):149–153

51. Wolfe SA. Treatment of post-traumatic orbital deformities. Clin Plast Surg 1988;15(2):225–238

52. Dufresne CR, Manson PN, Iliff NT. Early and late complications of orbital fractures. Clin Plast Surg 1988;15(2):239–253

53. Hardesty RA, Coffey JA Jr. Secondary craniomaxillofacial deformities. Current principles of management. Clin Plast Surg 1992;19(1):275–300

54. Kellman RM, Bersani T. Delayed and secondary repair of posttraumatic enophthalmos and orbital deformities. Facial Plast Surg Clin North Am 2002;10(3):311–323

55. Longaker MT, Kawamoto HK Jr. Evolving thoughts on correcting posttraumatic enophthalmos. Plast Reconstr Surg 1998;101(4):899–906

56. Pearl RM. Treatment of enophthalmos. Clin Plast Surg 1992; 19(1):99–111

57. Burnstine MA. Clinical recommendations for repair of isolated orbital floor fractures: an evidence-based analysis. Ophthalmology 2002;109(7):1207–1210, discussion 1210–1211, quiz 1212–1213

58. Catone GA, Morrissette MP, Carlson ER. A retrospective study of untreated orbital blow-out fractures. J Oral Maxillofac Surg 1988;46(12):1033–1038

59. Hawes MJ, Dortzbach RK. Surgery on orbital floor fractures. Influence of time of repair and fracture size. Ophthalmology 1983;90(9):1066–1070

60. Mathog RH, Hillstrom RP, Nesi FA. Surgical correction of enophthalmos and diplopia. A report of 38 cases. Arch Otolaryngol Head Neck Surg 1989;115(2):169–178

61. Yaremchuk MJ. Changing concepts in the management of secondary orbital deformities. Clin Plast Surg 1992;19(1): 113–124

62. Putterman AM, Stevens T, Urist MJ. Nonsurgical management of blow-out fractures of the orbital floor. Am J Ophthalmol 1974;77(2):232–239

63. Ellis E. Fractures of the Zygomatic Complex and Arch. In: Fonseca RJ, Walker RV, Betts NJ, Barber HD, Powers MP, eds. Oral and Maxillofacial Trauma. St. Louis: Elsevier; 2005:569–642

64. Folkestad L, Westin T. Long-term sequelae after surgery for orbital floor fractures. Otolaryngol Head Neck Surg 1999; 120(6):914–921

65. Souyris F, Klersy F, Jammet P, Payrot C. Malar bone fractures and their sequelae. A statistical study of 1.393 cases covering a period of 20 years. J Craniomaxillofac Surg 1989;17(2): 64–68

66. Zingg M, Chowdhury K, Lädrach K, Vuillemin T, Sutter F, Raveh J. Treatment of 813 zygoma-lateral orbital complex fractures. New aspects. Arch Otolaryngol Head Neck Surg 1991;117(6):611–620, discussion 621–622

67. Markowitz BL, Manson PN. Zygomatic complex fractures. In: Manual of Internal Fixation in the Cranio-Facial Skeleton. Berlin: Springer; 1998:133–147

68. Mathog RH, Archer KF, Nesi FA. Posttraumatic enophthalmos and diplopia. Otolaryngol Head Neck Surg 1986;94(1): 69–77

69. Farwell DG, Sires BS, Kriet JD, Stanley RB Jr. Endoscopic repair of orbital blowout fractures: use or misuse of a new approach? Arch Facial Plast Surg 2007;9(6):427–433

70. Klug C, Schicho K, Ploder O, et al. Point-to-point computer-assisted navigation for precise transfer of planned zygoma osteotomies from the stereolithographic model into reality. J Oral Maxillofac Surg 2006;64(3):550–559

71. Ansari MH. Blindness after facial fractures: a 19-year retrospective study. J Oral Maxillofac Surg 2005;63(2):229–237

72. Li KK, Meara JG, Joseph MP. Reversal of blindness after facial fracture repair by prompt optic nerve decompression. J Oral Maxillofac Surg 1997;55(6):648–650

73. MacKinnon CA, David DJ, Cooter RD. Blindness and severe visual impairment in facial fractures: an 11 year review. Br J Plast Surg 2002;55(1):1–7

74. Girotto JA, Gamble WB, Robertson B, et al. Blindness after reduction of facial fractures. Plast Reconstr Surg 1998;102(6): 1821–1834

75. Bater MC, Ramchandani PL, Brennan PA. Post-traumatic eye observations. Br J Oral Maxillofac Surg 2005;43(5): 410–416

76. Popat H, Doyle PT, Davies SJ. Blindness following retrobulbar haemorrhage—it can be prevented. Br J Oral Maxillofac Surg 2007;45(2):163–164

77. Rosdeutscher JD, Stadelmann WK. Diagnosis and treatment of retrobulbar hematoma resulting from blunt periorbital trauma. Ann Plast Surg 1998;41(6):618–622

78. Bailey WK, Kuo PC, Evans LS. Diagnosis and treatment of retrobulbar hemorrhage. J Oral Maxillofac Surg 1993;51(7): 780–782

79. Chang EL, Bernardino CR. Update on orbital trauma. Curr Opin Ophthalmol 2004;15(5):411–415

80. Winterton JV, Patel K, Mizen KD. Review of management options for a retrobulbar hemorrhage. J Oral Maxillofac Surg 2007;65(2):296–299

81. Hayreh SS, Kolder HE, Weingeist TA. Central retinal artery occlusion and retinal tolerance time. Ophthalmology 1980;87(1):75–78

82. Levin LA, Beck RW, Joseph MP, Seiff S, Kraker R, The International Optic Nerve Study Group. The treatment of traumatic optic neuropathy: the International Optic Nerve Trauma Study. Ophthalmology 1999;106(7):1268–1277

83. Steinsapir KD. Treatment of traumatic optic neuropathy with high-dose corticosteroid. J Neuroophthalmol 2006;26(1): 65–67

84. Jungell P, Lindqvist C. Paraesthesia of the infraorbital nerve following fracture of the zygomatic complex. Int J Oral Maxillofac Surg 1987;16(3):363–367

85. Taicher S, Ardekian L, Samet N, Shoshani Y, Kaffe I. Recovery of the infraorbital nerve after zygomatic complex fractures: a preliminary study of different treatment methods. Int J Oral Maxillofac Surg 1993;22(6):339–341

86. Vriens JPM, Moos KF. Morbidity of the infraorbital nerve following orbitozygomatic complex fractures. J Craniomaxillofac Surg 1995;23(6):363–368

87. Ziccardi VB, Zuniga JR. Traumatic injuries of the trigeminal nerve. In: Fonseca RJ, Walker RV, Betts NJ, Barber HD, Powers MP, eds. Oral and Maxillofacial Trauma. St. Louis: Elsevier; 2005:877–914

88. Bodker FS, Cytryn AS, Putterman AM, Marschall MA. Postoperative mydriasis after repair of orbital floor fracture. Am J Ophthalmol 1993;115(3):372–375

89. Stromberg BV, Knibbe M. Anisocoria following reduction of bilateral orbital floor fractures. Ann Plast Surg 1988;21(5):486–488

90. Marmulla R, Niederdellmann H. Surgical planning of computer-assisted repositioning osteotomies. Plast Reconstr Surg 1999;104(4):938–944

91. Westermark A, Zachow S, Eppley BL. Three-dimensional osteotomy planning in maxillofacial surgery including soft tissue prediction. J Craniofac Surg 2005;16(1):100–104

92. Baumann A, Ewers R. Transcaruncular approach for reconstruction of medial orbital wall fracture. Int J Oral Maxillofac Surg 2000;29(4):264–267

93. Frodel JL, Marentette LJ. The coronal approach. Anatomic and technical considerations and morbidity. Arch Otolaryngol Head Neck Surg 1993;119(2):201–207, discussion 140

94. Freihofer PM, Borstlap WA. Reconstruction of the zygomatic area. A comparison between osteotomy and onlay techniques. J Craniomaxillofac Surg 1989;17(6):243–248

95. Hammer B, Prein J. Correction of post-traumatic orbital deformities: operative techniques and review of 26 patients. J Craniomaxillofac Surg 1995;23(2):81–90

96. Costantino PD, Hiltzki DH, Fried CD, et al. Alloplastic Plating Techniques in Orbital Fracture Repair. In: Holck DE, Ng JD, eds. Evaluation and Treatment of Orbital Fractures: A Multidisciplinary Approach. Philadelphia: Elsevier; 2006:261–288

97. Baumann A, Burggasser G, Gauss N, Ewers R. Orbital floor reconstruction with an alloplastic resorbable polydioxanone sheet. Int J Oral Maxillofac Surg 2002;31(4):367–373

98. Freihofer HPM. Effectiveness of secondary post-traumatic periorbital reconstruction. J Craniomaxillofac Surg 1995;23(3):143–150

99. Kushner BJ. Management of diplopia limited to down gaze. Arch Ophthalmol 1995;113(11):1426–1430

100. Gruss JS. Naso-ethmoid-orbital fractures: classification and role of primary bone grafting. Plast Reconstr Surg 1985;75(3):303–317

101. Markowitz BL, Manson PN, Sargent L, et al. Management of the medial canthal tendon in nasoethmoid orbital fractures: the importance of the central fragment in classification and treatment. Plast Reconstr Surg 1991;87(5):843–853

102. Ducic Y. Medial canthal ligament reattachment in skull base surgery and trauma. Laryngoscope 2001;111(4 Pt 1):734–737

103. Sargent LA, Rogers GF. Nasoethmoid orbital fractures: diagnosis and management. J Craniomaxillofac Trauma 1999;5(1):19–27

104. Holt GR, Holt JE. Nasoethmoid complex injuries. Otolaryngol Clin North Am 1985;18(1):87–98

105. Yaremchuck MJ. Evaluation and Management of Chronic Naso-orbito-ethmoid Fractures. In: Holck DEE, Ng JD, eds. Evaluation and Treatment of Orbital Fractures: A Multidisciplinary Approach. Philadelphia: Elsevier; 2006:183–192

106. Osguthorpe JD, Hoang G. Nasolacrimal injuries. Evaluation and management. Otolaryngol Clin North Am 1991;24(1):59–78

107. Gruss JS, Hurwitz JJ, Nik NA, Kassel EE. The pattern and incidence of nasolacrimal injury in naso-orbital-ethmoid fractures: the role of delayed assessment and dacryocystorhinostomy. Br J Plast Surg 1985;38(1):116–121

108. Stranc MF. The pattern of lacrimal injuries in naso-ethmoid fractures. Br J Plast Surg 1970;23(4):339–346

109. Lindsey JT. Lacrimal duct injuries revisited: a retrospective review of six patients. Ann Plast Surg 2000;44(2):167–172

110. Becelli R, Renzi G, Mannino G, Cerulli G, Iannetti G. Posttraumatic obstruction of lacrimal pathways: a retrospective analysis of 58 consecutive naso-orbito-ethmoid fractures. J Craniofac Surg 2004;15(1):29–33

111. Harris GJ, Fuerste FH. Lacrimal intubation in the primary repair of midfacial fractures. Ophthalmology 1987;94(3):242–247

112. Spinelli HM, Shapiro MD, Wei LL, Elahi E, Hirmand H. The role of lacrimal intubation in the management of facial trauma and tumor resection. Plast Reconstr Surg 2005;115(7):1871–1876

113. Staffenberg DA, Kawamoto HK. Revisional surgery for midface fractures:malocclusion and malposition. Oper Tech Plast Reconstr 1998;5(4):302–311

114. Forrest CR, Phillips JH, Prein J. Craniofacial Fractures. In: Prein J, ed. Manual of Internal Fixation in the Cranio-Facial Skeleton. Berlin: Springer; 1998:108–126

115. Ellis E. Advances in Maxillofacial Trauma Surgery. In: Fonseca RJ, Walker RV, Betts NJ, Barber HD, Powers MP, eds. Oral and Maxillofacial Trauma. St. Louis: Elsevier; 2005:329–375

116. Chen KT, Chen CT, Mardini S, Tsay PK, Chen YR. Frontal sinus fractures: a treatment algorithm and assessment of outcomes based on 78 clinical cases. Plast Reconstr Surg 2006;118(2):457–468

117. Duvall AJ III, Porto DP, Lyons D, Boies LR Jr. Frontal sinus fractures. Analysis of treatment results. Arch Otolaryngol Head Neck Surg 1987;113(9):933–935

118. Gossman DG, Archer SM, Arosarena O. Management of frontal sinus fractures: a review of 96 cases. Laryngoscope 2006;116(8):1357–1362

119. Ioannides C, Freihofer HP. Fractures of the frontal sinus: classification and its implications for surgical treatment. Am J Otolaryngol 1999;20(5):273–280

120. Stanley RB Jr, Becker TS. Injuries of the nasofrontal orifices in frontal sinus fractures. Laryngoscope 1987;97(6):728–731

121. Wallis A, Donald PJ. Frontal sinus fractures: a review of 72 cases. Laryngoscope 1988;98(6 Pt 1):593–598

122. Wolfe SA, Johnson P. Frontal sinus injuries: primary care and management of late complications. Plast Reconstr Surg 1988;82(5):781–791

123. Gerbino G, Roccia F, Benech A, Caldarelli C. Analysis of 158 frontal sinus fractures: current surgical management and complications. J Craniomaxillofac Surg 2000;28(3):133–139

124. Larrabee WF Jr, Travis LW, Tabb HG. Frontal sinus fractures—their suppurative complications and surgical management. Laryngoscope 1980;90(11 Pt 1):1810–1813

125. Donald PJ. Frontal sinus ablation by cranialization. Report of 21 cases. Arch Otolaryngol 1982;108(3):142–146

126. Wilson BC, Davidson B, Corey JP, Haydon RC III. Comparison of complications following frontal sinus fractures managed with exploration with or without obliteration over 10 years. Laryngoscope 1988;98(5):516–520

127. Swinson BD, Jerjes W, Thompson G. Current practice in the management of frontal sinus fractures. J Laryngol Otol 2004;118(12):927–932

128. Kellman RM. Safe and dependable harvesting of large outer-table calvarial bone grafts. Arch Otolaryngol Head Neck Surg 1994;120(8):856–860

129. Weber R, Draf W, Kratzsch B, Hosemann W, Schaefer SD. Modern concepts of frontal sinus surgery. Laryngoscope 2001;111(1):137–146

130. Sillers MJ. Frontal sinus obliteration: an operation for the archives or modern armamentarium. Arch Otolaryngol Head Neck Surg 2005;131(6):529–531

131. Mathur KK, Tatum SA, Kellman RM. Carbonated apatite and hydroxyapatite in craniofacial reconstruction. Arch Facial Plast Surg 2003;5(5):379–383

132. Davis WE. Growing obsolescence of the frontal sinus obliteration procedure. Arch Otolaryngol Head Neck Surg 2005;131(6):532–533

133. Lanza DC. Frontal sinus obliteration is rarely indicated. Arch Otolaryngol Head Neck Surg 2005;131(6):531–532

134. Smith TL, Han JK, Loehrl TA, Rhee JS. Endoscopic management of the frontal recess in frontal sinus fractures: a shift in the paradigm? Laryngoscope 2002;112(5):784–790

135. Koudstaal MJ, van der Wal KGH, Bijvoet HWC, Vincent AJPE, Poublon RMI. Post-trauma mucocele formation in the frontal sinus; a rationale of follow-up. Int J Oral Maxillofac Surg 2004;33(8):751–754

136. Har-El G. Endoscopic management of 108 sinus mucoceles. Laryngoscope 2001;111(12):2131–2134

137. Kennedy DW, Josephson JS, Zinreich SJ, Mattox DE, Goldsmith MM. Endoscopic sinus surgery for mucoceles: a viable alternative. Laryngoscope 1989;99(9):885–895

138. Loevner LA, Yousem DM, Lanza DC, Kennedy DW, Goldberg AN. MR evaluation of frontal sinus osteoplastic flaps with autogenous fat grafts. AJNR Am J Neuroradiol 1995;16(8):1721–1726

139. Weber R, Draf W, Keerl R, et al. Magnetic resonance imaging following fat obliteration of the frontal sinus. Neuroradiology 2002;44(1):52–58

140. Powers MP, Beck BW, Holton JB. Management of Soft Tissue Injuries. In: Fonseca RJ, Walker RV, Betts NJ, Barber HD, Powers MP, eds. Oral and Maxillofacial Trauma. St. Louis: Elsevier; 2005:751–819

141. Thomas JR, Frost TW. Scar Revision and Camouflage. In: Baker SR, Swanson NA, eds. Local Flaps in Facial Reconstruction. St. Louis: Mosby; 1995:587–595

142. Tatum SA. Concepts in midface reconstruction. Otolaryngol Clin North Am 1997;30(4):563–592

143. Tachmes L, Woloszyn T, Marini C, et al. Parotid gland and facial nerve trauma: a retrospective review. J Trauma 1990;30(11):1395–1398

144. Landau R, Stewart M. Conservative management of post-traumatic parotid fistulae and sialoceles: a prospective study. Br J Surg 1985;72(1):42–44

145. Lewkowicz AA, Hasson O, Nahlieli O. Traumatic injuries to the parotid gland and duct. J Oral Maxillofac Surg 2002;60(6):676–680

146. Steinberg MJ, Herréra AF. Management of parotid duct injuries. Oral Surg Oral Med Oral Pathol Oral Radiol Endod 2005;99(2):136–141

147. Parekh D, Glezerson G, Stewart M, Esser J, Lawson HH. Post-traumatic parotid fistulae and sialoceles. A prospective study of conservative management in 51 cases. Ann Surg 1989;209(1):105–111

148. Van Sickels JE. Parotid duct injuries. Oral Surg Oral Med Oral Pathol 1981;52(4):364–367

149. Lewis G, Knottenbelt JD. Parotid duct injury: is immediate surgical repair necessary? Injury 1991;22(5):407–409

150. Marchese-Ragona R, Blotta P, Pastore A, Tugnoli V, Eleopra R, De Grandis D. Management of parotid sialocele with botulinum toxin. Laryngoscope 1999;109(8):1344–1346

151. Marchese-Ragona R, De Filippis C, Staffieri A, Restivo DA, Restino DA. Parotid gland fistula: treatment with botulinum toxin. Plast Reconstr Surg 2001;107(3):886–887

152. Ellies M, Gottstein U, Rohrbach-Volland S, Arglebe C, Laskawi R. Reduction of salivary flow with botulinum toxin: extended report on 33 patients with drooling, salivary fistulas, and sialadenitis. Laryngoscope 2004;114(10):1856–1860

153. von Lindern JJ, Niederhagen B, Appel T, Bergé S, Reich RH. New prospects in the treatment of traumatic and postoperative parotid fistulas with type A botulinum toxin. Plast Reconstr Surg 2002;109(7):2443–2445

154. May M. Nerve Repair. In: May M, Schaitkin BM, eds. The Facial Nerve. New York: Thieme; 2000:571–611

14

Complications of Facial Reanimation

Patrick J. Byrne and Christopher R. Cote

Successful management of facial paralysis requires an experienced understanding of its cause, duration, and the prognosis for facial paralysis recovery. Skills in both reconstructive and aesthetic surgery are required to use contemporary techniques to rehabilitate fully the patient with facial paralysis (**Fig. 14.1**). It is helpful during the consultation process for the surgeon to divide the face into upper, middle, and lower thirds. In each facial region, reinnervation procedures as well as static resuspension procedures are available for the patient. Procedures to be considered first assist with periorbital rehabilitation—procedures that improve eyelid closure, eye protection, and brow position. Such periorbital procedures include techniques to load the upper eyelid, reposition the denervated lower eyelid, and reposition the brow. Midfacial procedures are then considered to correct nasal obstruction, provide support for the retracted lower eyelid, reduce oral incompetence, and improve facial symmetry. These goals are accomplished with procedures such as midface lifts, static slings, free

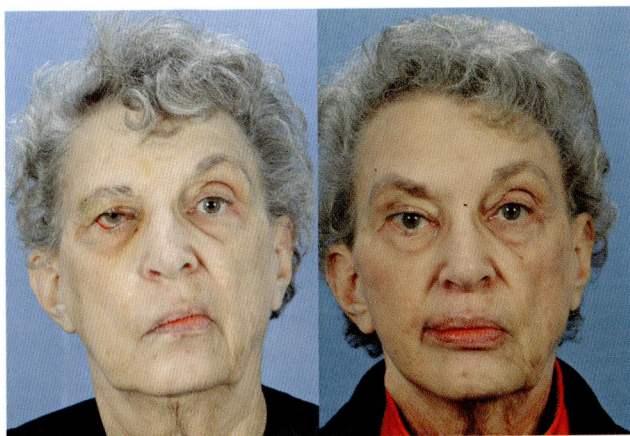

Fig. 14.1 Contemporary management of facial paralysis. This patient was initially treated with gold weight placement, and subsequently underwent endoscopic browlift, lateral canthal suspension with midface lift, and temporalis tendon transfer. (Chan JY, Byrne PJ. Management of facial paralysis in the 21st century. Facial Plast Surg Aug 2011;27(4):346–357.)

muscle transfer, local muscle transfer, and nerve transfers. Lower facial procedures address oral incompetence, speech difficulties, facial asymmetry, and the inability to smile, and they include procedures such as facelift, necklift, and oral commissuroplasty. This chapter will address the prevention and management of complications in facial paralysis rehabilitiation by region. The most common complication is failure to achieve the desired improvement. Other complications, such as hematomas, failure of wound healing, and infection may also occur. The diversity of patient presentations and treatment options makes this topic quite complex. Therefore, each surgeon must understand the advantages and disadvantages of the procedures and balance those with their comfort level and the procedures' application to their individual patients.

◆ Preoperative Prevention Strategies

General Points

Avoidance of complications with facial reanimation begins with the most fundamental aspects of patient care: careful diagnosis and selection of appropriate treatment. It is crucial to engage in thoughtful planning before entering the operating room and beginning a path of treatment that could be inappropriate.

Understanding the causes of facial paralysis and its pathophysiology will guide the surgeon's assessment. Although the differential diagnosis of facial palsy is very extensive, usually a small number of causes account for most cases that present to the surgeon's office. Trauma, acoustic neuroma surgery, parotid neoplasms, and Bell's palsy with incomplete return of function compose the bulk of encountered etiologies.

Treatment planning requires taking an extensive history, performing a physical examination, and possible testing to determine what procedures may be beneficial to the patient. Initial consultations are often detailed, because subsequent decisions are complex. The surgeon should consider several questions to help guide the decision-making process (**Table 14.1**).

Table 14.1

Questions to Aid with Facial Paralysis Surgical Planning
What is the etiology and duration of the paralysis?
What is the prognosis for recovery?
What is the patient's age?
Is the paralysis complete or incomplete?
Are there areas of hyperfunction in addition to areas of paresis?
What troubles the patient most?
How much tissue laxity is present?
How compliant is the patient?
What are the patient's expectations with regard to outcome, recovery period, and the time necessary to assess the success of an intervention?

The answers to these and many other questions will direct the thoughtful surgeon's choices for the timing of any intervention, medical versus surgical management of the eye, static versus dynamic facial suspension, reanimation versus observation for recovery, free tissue transfer versus local muscle transfer versus nerve crossovers, reversible or nonreversible measures, or concomitant contralateral procedures performed to improve symmetry. This analysis can be extensive, and it is required before operating on the patient. More detailed discussion of these considerations is beyond the scope of this text. Nonetheless, this list highlights the importance of the preoperative consultation.

Diagnostic facial nerve testing may be considered before undertaking a surgical procedure. A thorough evaluation and work-up may require imaging studies (CT or MRI) and electrodiagnostic testing. Well-known tests for prognosis include the maximum stimulation test, the nerve excitability test, electromyography (EMG), and electroneuronography (ENOG). Although most cases do not require such testing, it is appropriate in others. This is a topic beyond the scope of this chapter.[1]

Nonsurgical options may be chosen for management of the patient's facial paralysis, depending on the individual's circumstances. A compliant patient, for example, may do well with aggressive medical eye protection. Facial retraining has a role in many cases, and this form of physical therapy may result in improved outcomes, particularly if it is instituted early.

We suggest allotting an appropriate amount of time in the clinic for such a complex discussion with any new facial paralysis patient. We typically allocate more time for this consultation than any other new facial plastic surgery patient visit. Spending one hour on the initial visit is typical. This is the first step toward prevention of untoward outcomes. The patient needs to be educated about multiple issues and must be able to make an informed decision regarding his or her treatment options. A frank acknowledgment of the realistic potential for improvement must be made early. If there has been a complete facial nerve transection, then the chance for a normal outcome does not exist with the current state of medical knowledge. The patient and family need to be made aware of this. The patient and family also need to be engaged in the decision-making process as they consider their options for reanimation.

The Eye

The first priority for facial paralysis management is eye protection. Visual field preservation and correction of eye or brow asymmetry are important but secondary. Procedures to consider include browlifting (direct, coronal, or endoscopic), upper lid loading (gold or platinum weight), and lower lid tightening or elevation (tarsal strip canthoplasty, transorbital canthopexy, spacer grafts, midface lifts). There are several things to look out for to prevent complications. First, perform a careful physical examination. Attention is directed toward the patient's current ability to protect the eye and also to be aware of chronic exposure. A useful mnemonic to help identify patients who are especially at risk for exposure keratitis is BAD: Look for the presence or absence of a Bell phenomenon (B); if it is absent, that represents a risk factor for exposure keratitis due to diminished ability to protect the cornea. An absence of corneal reflex (A for anesthesia) indicates that the patient is also at increased risk for exposure keratitis due to a diminished ability to sense the irritation that would normally accompany an exposed cornea. A patient with preexisting dry eye (D) has poor tear production and is a higher-risk patient. The risk for corneal exposure complications in patients with dry eyes, absent Bell phenomenon, and diminished corneal sensation is very real. The mental status and compliance of the patient are also important. Appropriate eye protection and lubrication requires placement of lubricating ointment, use of artificial tears, moisture chambers, and eyelid taping. The physician must realistically assess the patient's ability to follow a course of treatment and if it is compromised, a more aggressive treatment, such as tarsorrhaphy, may be appropriate in select cases.

A careful preoperative evaluation of the upper eyelid will reduce the chance of ptosis caused by loading techniques. The patient is observed and questioned while trying on several sizes of gold weights. This can be facilitated by securing the weight to the lid with double-sided tape. The goal is to maximize closure while minimizing induced ptosis. Some iatrogenic ptosis is acceptable, but only what remains asymptomatic to the patient.

Likewise, the lower eyelid must be carefully examined. Laxity of a paralyzed eyelid may demonstrate ectropion, lid retraction, lacrimal dysfunction, and insufficient globe coverage. Lower eyelid elevation may be accomplished by a variety of methods. The tarsal strip canthopexy is quite commonly performed. However, certain anatomic findings can affect the outcome. For example, patients with maxillary hypoplasia and the so-called negative vector, with relative proptosis, may be done a disservice if canthopexy is performed (**Fig. 14.2**). Such lower lid tightening may cause the eyelid margin to be pulled under the convexity of the globe, thus worsening lid position and eye protection. Alternative techniques to elevate the lid, such as space grafting and midface lifting, are preferable in such patients.

Midface and Lower Face

The procedures used here include facial nerve grafts, cross face grafts, hypoglossal facial nerve transfers, free muscle transfer, dynamic regional muscle transfer, and static facial slings. Several preoperative considerations are important when the surgeon evaluates a patient for facial reanimation. First, the surgeon must choose a treatment option with a reasonable likelihood of success. Reinnervation techniques of native facial musculature (cross face grafts, hypoglossal nerve (XII)–facial nerve (VII) anastomoses) are unlikely to be successful if they are performed after a prolonged period of denervation. This duration is in most cases approximately one year. Cases of spontaneous reinnervation, as well as successful surgical reanimation, have certainly occurred after delays longer than one year in particular patients; however, this is the exception. The older the patient, the less likely it is that either spontaneous recovery will occur or that reinnervation techniques will be successful.

Patients who have undergone radiation treatments are more likely to require revisions to static facial slings from descent of the initially suspended soft tissues. Implants may be more likely to extrude after radiation therapy (**Fig. 14.3**). These patients also are at greater risk of wound-healing complications in general. Caution is advised in such patients, and they deserve to be appropriately counseled about such risks.

◆ Identification and Management of Intraoperative Complications

Browlifting

Browlift incisions are placed in or along the hairline with careful avoidance of follicle injury to prevent hair loss. This can be done by making incisions parallel to follicles and avoiding electrocautery injury to or suture strangulation of follicles.

The rich vasculature of the brow region makes it especially at risk for the formation of a hematoma after a subcutaneous browlift (direct or indirect browlift) is performed. Particular attention to hemostasis is important. It is so common to see this that we routinely hold compression manually after we perform such a procedure as the patient is emerging from anesthesia and being transported to the recovery room. An immediate postoperative pressure dressing, ice, and elevation may mitigate this complication.

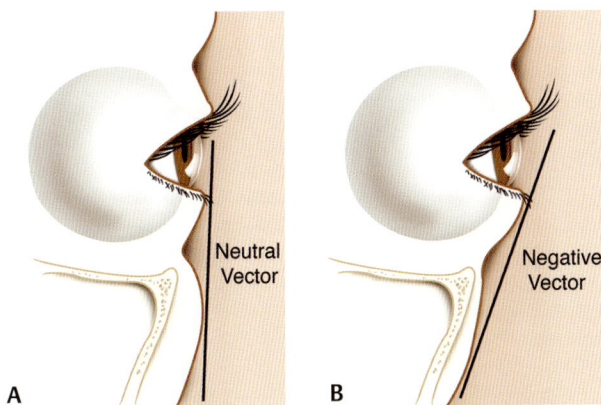

Fig. 14.2 The negative vector. This refers to an anatomical observation **(A)** when the cheek tissue at the level of the orbital rim (OR) is posterior to a vertical line drawn from the lower lid margin (LL). A lid tightening procedure **(B)** could have the undesired result of retraction of the lower lid due to a "sliding" down the globe. (*Illustration by Robert Brown.*)

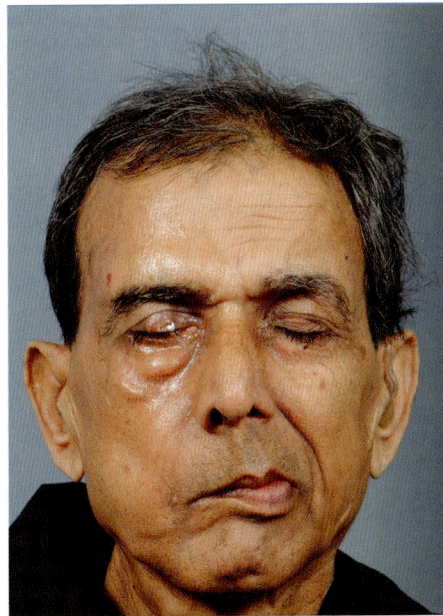

Fig. 14.3 This is an example of upper eyelid gold weight extrusion. Proper placement of the weight deep to the orbicularis oculi muscle and on the tarsus can minimize this problem.

Inadequate or asymmetric brow elevation may occur. The reasons depend upon the technique selected. With direct brow lifts, inadequate elevation is primarily the result of suboptimal fixation of the soft tissue to the periosteum. A skin-only closure will certainly descend with time. We recommend a permanent or long-lasting resorbable suture (such as PDS) to fixate the brow elevation. Place a minimum of three such sutures in each case. Ensure that the suture needle grabs not only the orbicularis muscle near the superior orbital rim but also some deep dermis to obtain a reliable result. Too much dermis will cause long-term dimpling and is best avoided. The endoscopic browlift for facial paralysis requires the same degree of complete bilateral release of the frontal and frontal bar periosteum that a cosmetic endoscopic browlift does. Keep in mind that if an endoscopic approach is preferred, one must perform a bilateral browlift. Attempts to perform a unilateral endoscopic browlift to address paralytic brow ptosis will prove disappointing. Fixation may be performed by any one of a variety of methods.

Upper Lid Loading

Gold or platinum weights can cause ptosis. This is best minimized by a careful preoperative evaluation that includes determining the appropriate size of the weight by taping it to the outer lid prior to surgery with the patient awake. Some manufacturers can provide a sizing kit to make this easier. Intraoperative disruption of the levator mechanism can also cause a significant ptosis once the lid is loaded. To avoid this, make sure that the dissection is in the immediate suborbicular plane. At the same time, extrusion can also occur. This is more likely if the weight is placed too superficially in the immediate subcutaneous plane where the wound may dehisce or skin will thin. Migration, extrusion, and ulceration have been shown to be prevented by suture fixation of the implant securely to the tarsus.

Lower Lid Elevation

Complications will obviously depend on the technique chosen to address the issues of a paralytic lower eyelid. These techniques may include medial or lateral canthoplasty, lateral tarsal strip, wedge excision, and midface lifting. Common considerations include avoiding ectropion and entropion. Trichiasis, which is related to entropion and an inward turning of the eyelashes, is prevented by very careful approximation of the lid and lashes. Many of these procedures involve displacement of the tarsus. Meticulous hemostasis is performed with bipolar electrocautery to minimize the chance of hematoma formation. Over-tightening of the lower lid is best avoided, as this may produce the unintended effect of lowering the lid margin position, especially in the negative vector patient.

Lower Face

Technical points need to be considered when performing any static sling or dynamic muscle transfer. We recommend that when performing a sling, the surgeon choose native material, such as fascia lata, or donor grafts of human acellular dermis and engineered porcine dermis, both which have competing resorption and rates of strength.[2,3] Expanded polytetrafluoroethylene (ePTFE) should be avoided, because extrusion has been found with these implants.[4,5] Reports have been variable regarding long-term success. The sling or muscle must be aggressively secured. Over-correction is recommended. We use a combination of nonresorbable polypropylene sutures and resorbable polyglactin secured to the deep tissues and redundantly to the suspension sling or muscle.

Nerve repair includes many possible outcomes, depending on the methods used. Primary repair is preferred over interposition grafting and crossover grafts when possible. Nerve grafts need to be carefully placed to optimize fascicular size match rather than external diameter match. Magnification is essential for this. A tension-free closure is always important.

◆ Diagnosis and Management of Perioperative and Postoperative Complications

Brow

Hematoma formation can be seen in the early postoperative period and even up to ten days afterward. Early recognition is crucial to avoid infection and tissue injury. When hematoma formation is encountered, immediate evacuation is warranted. On the other hand, serous accumulation may be seen, and observation may be appropriate for it. An immediate postoperative pressure dressing, ice, and elevation may mitigate this complication. The need for additional intervention will depend on the amount of fluid accumulation; small fluid collections may be observed, larger ones aspirated via a needle (followed by a compression dressing), and the largest ones openly drained. A similar hematoma management strategy may be considered in other areas of the face and neck, though a retrobulbar hematoma needs the most acute attention.

Alopecia at incisions may be observed and can often be temporary. Observation for at least three to six months is prudent in case there may be some recovery of hair growth at that time. Patients may be candidates for microfollicular hair transplants should alopecia persist.

Inadequate or asymmetric elevation of the brow is not uncommon. Secure over-fixation intraoperatively is imperative, because descent due to gravity is significant as a result of lack of muscle tone. It is crucial that the method of fixation include anchoring to periostium or bone. Some fixation methods may better facilitate a revision. For example, the Endotine device (MicroAire, Charlottesville, VA) allows some revision in the early postoperative period in the clinic setting.

Eyelids

Upper Eyelid Procedures

Certain problems related to improper weight position and size may be observed. Inadequate lid descent occurs when there was improper or no preoperative assessment of the weight size. Ptosis may be the result of too heavy an eyelid weight or injury to the levator mechanism of the upper eyelid. If weight placement is too high on the lid (not just above the lashes), the patient may even experience lagophthalmos when lying supine.[6]

When load-bearing procedures are used, upper lid weight migration can be related to surgical technique. We recommend a horizontal incision at the supratarsal crease or immediately above the lash line rather than a smaller incision for creating a tight pocket. This will allow careful supratarsal placement with at least three anchoring sutures of 6–0 polyprolylene and positioning deep to the orbicularis muscle. Wound dehiscense and upper lid weight extrusion can occur when the incision is placed at the level of the weight position instead of above or below the weight. When these complications occur, the weight will need to be removed and the wound treated for infection if necessary. The patient can be reassessed for any continued need for the weight. If eye closure is adequate without it, you may choose not to replace the weight. If the patient still needs and wants a weight, then it may be wrapped in temporalis fascia or even processed human pericardium and secured to the tarsus in a suborbicular plane—points emphasized by many experienced surgeons in the literature.[6–10]

Lower Eyelid Procedures

In the paralyzed face, lower eyelid procedures are usually selected to address the paralytic ectropion or lid retraction. Elderly patients with involutional ectropion may be at higher risk. Such dysfunction may affect eye cosmesis, eye protection, and the lacrimal drainage system. Postoperative follow-up should include careful attention to the position of the eyelid, so that early intervention can begin.

Postoperative ectropion may be temporary from swelling, but it also could be due to an early cicatricial ectropion. Choices for early intervention may include eyelid taping suspension, a suspension Frost suture, and tarsorrhaphy. Additional intermediate intervention could include a steroid injection to soften scar formation. Careful attention during an examination should note whether ectropion involves the entire lid or occurs medially or laterally. This will direct the surgeon as to how to address the problem surgically. Later options may include revision canthopexy, anterior or posterior spacer grafting, and midface lifting.

Conversely, the patient may present postoperatively with trichiasis and entropion caused by posterior lamellar scarring from transconjunctival approaches or lid malposition during canthopexy. Focal areas may be addressed with removal of hair follicles. Temporary epilation is not likely to work long term, and some alternative methods may include permanent hair removal or wedge excision. Nonetheless, these approaches are not anatomic, and addressing the underlying cause may be a better option. Posterior lamellar lid spacer grafts can be used to address cicatrix, while revision of canthopexy can also be considered.

Lid retraction is manifested as increased scleral show and may be accompanied by ectropion or entropion. Treatment is similar to the options listed above.

Finally, hematoma formation may occur due to inadequate hemostasis. Careful attention to this in the early postoperative period may prevent a rare but devastating complication—blindness. More commonly, a preseptal hematoma would be encountered since most procedures involve the anterior lamella. Management of this would include a thorough ocular exam and wound evacuation. When significant orbital work has been performed, there is an increased concern for this risk, and we recommend overnight observation with visual field checks. Bleeding within the orbit may be manifested as severe eye pain, loss of visual acuity, proptosis, afferent papillary defect, ophthalmoplegia, and increased intraocular pressure. Immediate consultation with an ophthalmologist is strongly encouraged if a hematoma is suspected. Computerized tomography can confirm a diagnosis, though only if it is necessary, since any delay of treatment can be catastrophic. Intervention with lateral canthotomy and cantholysis should result in improvement in pain, vision, and intraocular pressure.[11]

Corneal exposure keratitis is a complication that deserves special emphasis, because this is a potentially catastrophic complication related to facial paralysis and inadequate eye protection. The immediate postoperative period should include all medical measures for protection of the eye while the patient is healing and being followed for the outcome of the eyelid procedures. These measures include frequent lubrication of the eye using artificial tears, use of nighttime moisture chambers, or more aggressive temporary measures, such as tarsorrhaphy and lid suspensions. Taping or eye patches are not advisable. Consider cooperation with an ophthalmologist who can perform corneal exams if there is any question of compromised protection. Patient compliance can be an important factor during this decision-making process. If the patient fails to achieve the desired protection, modification of the medical regimen or more aggressive procedures should be considered.

Midface and Lower Face

Hematoma formation after a standard facelift has been reported in the range of 1 to 10%, so patients undergoing more complex elevations will fall into that risk category as well. Recognition of postoperative asymmetrical swelling, bruising, and pain will prompt early evacuation. Inattention to this can contribute to skin necrosis and sloughing. In those cases, the patient may need wound debridement and revision of scarring as indicated.

Salivary leaks or sialoceles can occur when there is an injury to the parotid gland and its associated structures. For instance, facial suspension may be performed in the setting of parotidectomy, and a sialocele can be an early or subacute complication that may require needle aspiration and pressure dressing. The patient can be followed on a regular basis, with needle aspirations repeated as needed. This may be done multiple times and may take weeks for resolution. For recalcitrant cases, open drainage or even parotidectomy may be considered. In addition, parotid duct injury should be anticipated when dissection occurs in the deep planes of the face, such as during a temporalis tendon transfer. Immediate repair or diversion at a later point can be considered.

Sling or muscle transfer dehiscence with descent of oral commissure may be an early or late result. This may be a result of inadequate anchoring of the suture or excessive tension, resorption of the sling from inflammation, infection, or foreign body rejection. See our comments above on how to avoid this intraoperatively. When this is encountered in the postoperative period, revision suspension is often recommended. Be sure that the patient is counseled on this possibility. Postoperative radiation after a sling increases the risk for dehiscense, and for these patients in particular it can be more difficult to achieve the desired results when their slings are revised.

Lack of cross face graft reinnervation is a possibility in all cases, and the patient and surgeon must be prepared to wait for successful results. Age, radiation history, and reoperation can all affect the outcome, and the patient must be counseled on the need to wait for a reasonable outcome. End-to-end anastomosis confers the best facial function, followed by cable nerve graft interposition and then classic facial-hypoglossal transposition. Some reports have observed a delay of up to two years before even partial function is observed. Success in this area is usually determined by a House-Brackmann score of III or IV and is never better than this. This can be achieved in approximately 61–85% of cases for primary closure, 56% for cable graft interposition, and 25–79% for crossover grafts.[12–15]

Donor site morbidity is a consideration when crossover grafts are used. For example, the classic VII-XII crossover procedure involves a complete transection of the hypoglossal nerve. Transection of the 12th cranial nerve can cause speech and swallowing dysfunction in the tongue, although this is the exception rather than the rule. Such problems have been reported in up to 45% of patients.[16,17] Full transection should not be done in a patient with a preexisting contralateral 12th nerve injury, because such a patient may become an oral cripple if the opposite side is transected. We have found that performing 12-7 crossovers with only a partial transection of the hypoglossal nerve is safe and effective. The use of partial transection and a jump graft is an attempt to reduce morbidity. With this, the hypoglossal nerve is only partially transected and a cable graft is interposed to the distal facial nerve. Similar complications can occur, but less commonly. Some authors report no incidence of this in small series.

Recurrent asymmetry is expected in the paralyzed face. The denervated side of the face ages more rapidly than the normal side. This is secondary to advanced muscle atrophy, volume loss, and continued effects of gravity. Proper counseling preoperatively is important, and patients may benefit from multiple procedures over their lifetimes.

Oral commissure incompetence can be exacerbated by static suspension procedures of the midface by creating an oral gap from elevation of the upper lip. Loss of tone in the lower lip also contributes to problems with drooling, air leakage, and discoordination when chewing. These problems may be alleviated by several dynamic procedures, including the mobilization of the anterior belly of the digastric or simple lip wedge excision with commissuroplasty (**Fig. 14.4**). When per-

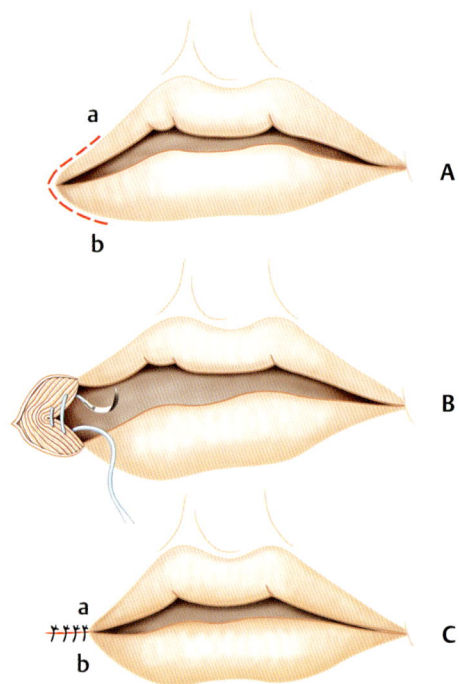

Fig. 14.4 Commissuroplasty. One option for addressing lower lip laxity is to incise along the vermilion border of the oral commissure **(A)**, separate the vermilion mucosa **(B)**, and then reapproximate skin and muscle **(C)**, effectively narrowing the oral aperture. (*Illustration by Robert Brown.*)

forming a wedge excision of the lower lip, the surgeon should remove a full-thickness v-shaped wedge on the paralyzed side with meticulous three-layer closure of mucosa, orbicularis muscle and skin, with careful attention to the vermillion border.

◆ Conclusion

The overarching goal in the treatment of patients with facial paralysis is a safe restoration of form and function. Complications seen in facial paralysis surgery are as myriad as the treatments offered and can range from a lack of achieving the desired outcome (e.g., no improvement) to an aggravation or even worsening of the patient's condition (e.g., worsened corneal exposure or increased asymmetry). Improper selection of treatment can be the first step to failure. Undoubtedly, all surgeons will have their individual comfort levels with the various treatment options, and the success of any given procedure may vary in each surgeon's hands, but with early identification and aggressive management of complications, the surgical results will be optimized. A thorough understanding of facial nerve pathophysiology, a detailed assessment of the patient's condition, meticulous surgical technique, and experience with both good and bad outcomes are all vital to treat the sequelae of facial paralysis successfully.

PEARLS OF WISDOM

Spend a generous amount of time with the patient in the preoperative period for surgical planning and counseling so as to select the most appropriate treatment.

Remember B.A.D. to identify patients at risk for exposure keratitis: absence of Bell's phenomenon, absence of corneal reflex, and dry eyes.

Beware of negative vector lower eyelids.

Master your lid loading technique. Complications should be minimal.

Regarding nerve repairs and grafts, prepare the patient for a long wait and realization that normal function return will not occur.

Classic XII-VII crossover grafts have better alternatives, such as the XII-VII interposition jump graft. Hemiglossal dysfunction can be problematic.

Careful follow-up, education and re-education of the patient will maximize their satisfaction.

References

1. Crumley RL, Armstrong WB, Byrne PJ. Rehabilitation of Facial Paralysis, Chapter 35 of Cummings Otolaryngology: Head & Neck Surgery, 4th ed. Philadelphia: Mosby; 2005

2. Rose EH. Autogenous fascia lata grafts: clinical applications in reanimation of the totally or partially paralyzed face. Plast Reconstr Surg 2005;116(1):20–32, discussion 33–35

3. Vural E, McLaughlin N, Hogue WR, Suva LJ. Comparison of biomechanical properties of alloderm and enduragen as static facial sling biomaterials. Laryngoscope 2006;116(3): 394–396

4. Constantinides M, Galli SK, Miller PJ. Complications of static facial suspensions with expanded polytetrafluoroethylene (ePTFE). Laryngoscope 2001;111(12):2114–2121

5. Yousif NJ, Matloub M D And H, Summers AN. The midface sling: a new technique to rejuvenate the midface. Plast Reconstr Surg 2002;110(6):1541–1553, discussion 1554–1557

6. Baylis HI, Goldberg RA, Wilson MC. Complications of Surgery of the Upper Eyelid. In: Putterman AM, ed. Cosmetic Oculoplastic Surgery: Eyelid, Forehead, and Facial Techniques, 3rd ed. Philadelphia: WB Saunders Co; 1998

7. Harrisberg BP, Singh RP, Croxson GR, Taylor RF, McCluskey PJ. Long-term outcome of gold eyelid weights in patients with facial nerve palsy. Otol Neurotol 2001;22(3):397–400

8. Misra A, Grover R, Withey S, Grobbelaar AO, Harrison DH. Reducing postoperative morbidity after the insertion of gold weights to treat lagophthalmos. Ann Plast Surg 2000;45(6): 623–628

9. Thomas DA, Khalifa YM. Temporalis fascia in the management of gold eyelid weight extrusion. Ophthal Plast Reconstr Surg 2005;21(2):153–155

10. Foster JA, Perry JD, Cahill KV, Holck DE, Kugler L. Processed human pericardium barrier for gold weight implantation. Ophthal Plast Reconstr Surg 2004;20(2):107–109

11. Baylis HI, Goldberg RA, Groth MJ. Complications of Surgery of the Lower Eyelid. In: Putterman AM, ed. Cosmetic Oculoplastic Surgery: Eyelid, Forehead, and Facial Techniques, 3rd ed. Philadelphia: WB Saunders Co; 1998

12. Malik TH, Kelly G, Ahmed A, Saeed SR, Ramsden RT. A comparison of surgical techniques used in dynamic reanimation of the paralyzed face. Otol Neurotol 2005;26(2):284–291

13. Saeed SR, Ramsden RT. Rehabilitation of the paralysed face: results of facial nerve surgery. J Laryngol Otol 1996;110(10): 922–925

14. Samii M, Matthies C. Management of 1000 vestibular schwannomas (acoustic neuromas): the facial nerve—preservation and restitution of function. Neurosurgery 1997;40(4): 684–694, discussion 694–695

15. Ryzenman JM, Pensak ML, Tew JM Jr. Facial paralysis and surgical rehabilitation: a quality of life analysis in a cohort of 1,595 patients after acoustic neuroma surgery. Otol Neurotol 2005;26(3):516–521, discussion 521

16. May M, Sobol SM, Mester SJ. Hypoglossal-facial nerve interpositional-jump graft for facial reanimation without tongue atrophy. Otolaryngol Head Neck Surg 1991;104(6): 818–825

17. Hammerschlag PE. Facial reanimation with jump interpositional graft hypoglossal facial anastomosis and hypoglossal facial anastomosis: evolution in management of facial paralysis. Laryngoscope 1999;109(2 Pt 2, Suppl 90):1–23

15

Surgical Correction of Congenital Anomalies and Associated Complications

Sherard Austin Tatum III and Sven-Olrik Streubel

Surgical correction of anomalies associated with congenital malformation is both rewarding and challenging. Few areas in facial plastic surgery display such myriad presentations that require careful analysis and exact surgical planning. Many of the procedures are complex and dangerous, requiring highly specialized training and experience, so it is not surprising that surgery for congenital anomalies is associated with complications. This chapter discusses many of these complications and their management. As with all untoward results, prevention is the best practice, and attention to detail and early acknowledgment of complications are paramount to their management.

◆ Complications of the Surgical Treatment of Craniosynostosis

Congenital craniofacial surgery refers to the correction of congenital or developmental defects, such as those resulting from premature fusion of cranial sutures or branchial arch abnormalities. The surgical treatment of craniosynostosis began in the latter half of the nineteenth century. Many of the techniques developed then are still used today in modified form. As might be imagined, any surgery involving the cutting and moving of craniofacial bones has significant risks. These include death, eye or brain damage, hemorrhage, infection, anesthesia problems, need for revision surgery, and others. Mitigating factors include patient age and size, severity of the deformity and the subsequent complexity of surgery, and comorbidities.

Reported mortality rates range from zero to 3%, and morbidity rates range from 1 to 40%, with the lowest rates associated with the simplest surgeries (strip craniectomy or synostectomy) on the least significant deformities.[1–4] The incidence of neurologic deficits after strip craniectomies was less than 1%. In the Shillito and Matson series, the frequency of reoperation secondary to resynostosis was 13.3% after correction of single sutures and 38% after repair of multiple sutures.[1] Complication rates increase

with the complexity of the surgical procedure. As more bone is exposed, there is an increased occurrence of blood loss, infection rate, risk of subgaleal collections, air embolism, dural tears associated with cerebrospinal fluid (CSF) leak, and direct injury to the brain or eye.

Preventing Airway Complications

The prevalence of obstructive sleep apnea syndrome in children with syndromic craniofacial synostosis has been reported to be as high as 40%.[5,6] Airway management remains a constant and significant problem in craniofacial dysostosis. Children with craniofacial dysostoses often have airway problems related to distortion of the oropharynx by the cranial base. Midface retrusion and acute skull base angles bring the soft palate against the posterior pharyngeal wall, leading to breathing problems and sleep apnea. Small nasal airways contribute to the problem as well. In addition, laryngotracheal anomalies may be associated with craniofacial problems. Signs associated with increased respiratory difficulties include swallowing or gagging problems, increased reflexes and spasticity, and sleep apnea (often described by the parent as a worsening in the child's snoring). Preoperative endoscopic evaluation is essential. In some cases, a tracheostomy must be established before surgery. Of children with syndromes involving bony deformities of the face and skull, 20% unambiguously required tracheostomy in a study of 251 patients by Sculerati et al.[7] Tracheostomy also reduces the risk of postoperative problems, such as airway edema, aspiration pneumonia, or pneumocephalus after monobloc advancement. In some cases, Chiari malformations must be decompressed to reduce brainstem dysfunction.

Complications Related to Timing of Surgery

The main issues regarding timing of surgery are skull thickness and malleability, patient size and blood volume, brain growth potential, and intracranial constraint. In the first year of life, the human brain grows from roughly 335 g to 925 g, almost tripling in mass. Fused sutures may restrict the skull growth required to accommodate this brain growth. Before 1965, surgical correction was undertaken later rather than earlier (i.e., after an age of 1 year) because of anesthesia and blood volume issues. During the 1970s and into the 1980s, arguments were advanced for surgery from one to six months of age to leverage the growth potential and reduce elevated ICP. Scheduling surgery at four to nine months of age allows for relative safety due to patient size, takes advantage of rapid brain growth to support and enhance the correction, and provides for malleable skull bone that is thick enough to hold fixation materials without being too thick and stiff to allow easy remodeling. The osteogenic dural stimulus in the infant (age less than 12 months) allows for filling in of bony gaps after repositioning, so bony defects are rare at this age. If ICP is elevated, then an early operation is necessary to prevent brain damage.

Blood Loss, Air Embolism, and Pneumocephalus

Excessive blood loss is still the most worrisome complication.[8] This problem results from constant slow ooze throughout cases requiring ten hours or more as well as from acute bleeding from vascular injury. Dissection over dural sinuses, particularly more posteriorly, risks massive hemorrhage from dural sinus injury, especially in the region of the torcular herophili (**Fig. 15.1A,B**). Knowledge of the locations of these vessels relative to the skull surface anatomy is critical. Sagittal sinus liga-

tion to control hemorrhage can result in serious neurologic injury or death if it is done posterior to the anterior one-third of the sinus. Most deaths and serious neurologic sequelae associated with craniosynostosis surgery reflect an inability to maintain adequate blood volume perioperatively. Hypovolemia also increases the risk of air embolism. Blood should be available from the beginning of the procedure, and the patient's hematocrit should be monitored routinely throughout the procedure. To reduce blood loss, some centers maintain systemic hypotension (a mean blood pressure of 50 mm Hg) during the operation. Epinephrine is injected into the skin before the incision is made. Hemostasis at the incision site is achieved with Raney clips or with cauterizing instruments, such as the Shaw scalpel or the Colorado needle. Topical agents like thrombin and collagen reduce blood loss as well. Systemic aminocaproic acid also reduces blood loss in select cases. Many centers now routinely arrange for donation of pedigree blood from the family before surgery.

Pneumocephalus is expected after such dissections, but tension pneumocephalus is a life-threatening emergency and must be managed with decompression. Subdural and epidural fluid collections are likewise expected, but hematomas exerting a mass effect should also be decompressed. Brain contusion or hemorrhage may occur as a result of excessive retraction, and it will be visible on postoperative computed tomography (CT) imaging. The contusions and hemorrhage generally are self-limiting and resolve, but neurologic sequelae may result. The best way to manage complications is to avoid them with gentle retraction on the dura. The tempo-

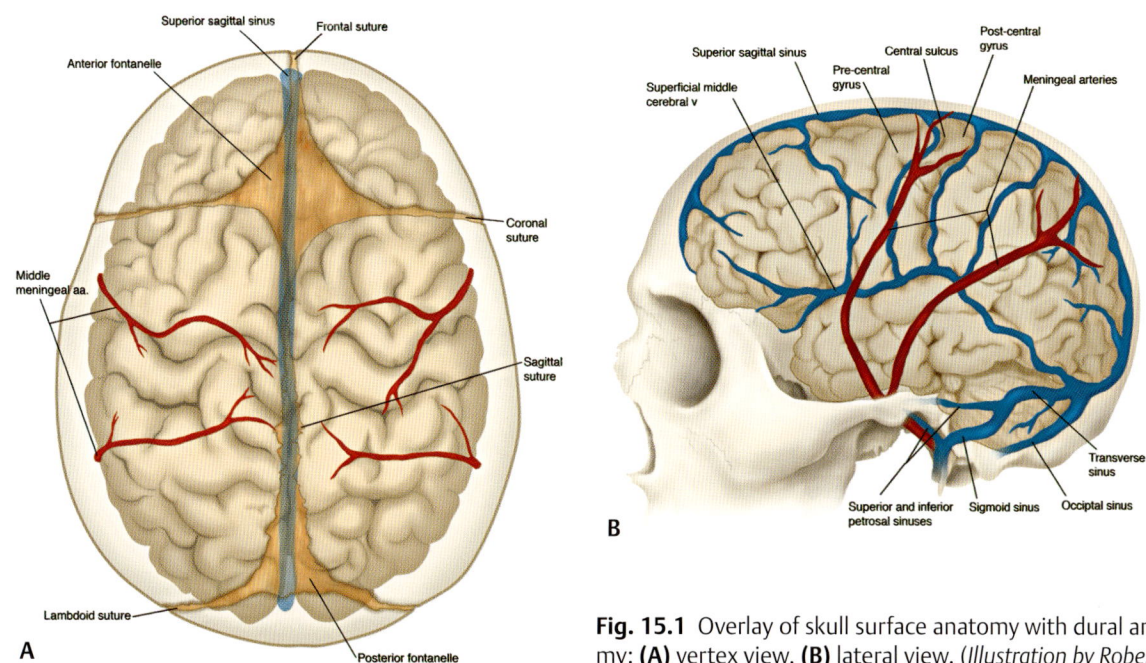

Fig. 15.1 Overlay of skull surface anatomy with dural and brain anatomy: **(A)** vertex view, **(B)** lateral view. (*Illustration by Robert Brown.*)

ral branch of the facial nerve can be damaged sharply during scalp elevation or injured by cautery or traction. Again, avoidance is the best management. Widening of the scalp scar (**Fig. 15.2A,B**) can result from excessive tension on the closure or damage to the adjacent hair follicles. Careful tissue handling and wound closure generally avoid these problems. In particularly long cases, strangulating scalp clips or sutures should be used with caution.

Hydrocephalus and Intracranial Pressure

Hydrocephalus and increased intracranial pressure, although not synonymous, are closely related. They may exist together or separately. Findings include neurologic dysfunction, irritability, and visual disturbance. Complete neurologic, ophthalmologic, and CT radiographic examinations are necessary if these conditions are suspected. Hydrocephalus is uncommon in children with isolated single-suture synostosis but becomes more frequent in multisuture synostosis and in cases involving the skull base (i.e., craniofacial dysostosis such as Crouzon and Apert syndromes). Various series have reported hydrocephalus in less than 50% of cases.[1,9,10] Renier et al. performed intraoperative ICP monitoring on an extensive series of patients and found that the risk of increased ICP in children with Kleeblattschädel or multiple suture

closures can be as high as 95%. Many patients present with surgical emergencies because of increased ICP.[11] The decision of when to place a ventriculoperitoneal (VP) shunt for cerebrospinal fluid (CSF) diversion can be complex. If the child has symptoms and signs of elevated ICP caused by hydrocephalus, then a VP shunt is placed first. If the child is asymptomatic, it is best to wait until after the craniofacial reconstruction to reduce the risk of infection from a VP shunt in the field of surgery. Elevated ICP often causes severe erosion of the skull bone (**Fig. 15.3**). These erosions are seen as scalloping of the inner table of the calvarium on plain films or full-thickness defects on CT scanning (**Fig. 15.4**). The dura can erode through the bone, making it technically difficult to elevate the pericranium from the dura.

Complications Due to Altered Anatomy

Children with craniofacial dysostoses have skull base anomalies, the most common of which is the Chiari malformation, and associated distortions of the foramen magnum.[12] Consequently, a thorough preoperative evaluation with magnetic resonance imaging (MRI) or CT is essential to evaluate the brain stem and cervicomedullary junction. Appropriate preoperative evaluation prevents postoperative quadriplegia from spinal cord or brain stem compression caused by inappropriate surgical positioning during craniofacial reconstruction (i.e., cervical hyperextension). Children with metopic synostosis commonly have a maldeveloped, foreshortened anterior fossa. A frontal lobe pseudoherniation often occurs, moving the lobes downward to a position between the orbits. In coronal synostosis, the temporal lobe tends to be located very anterior in the lateral orbital wall. These abnormalities increase the risk of dura and brain injury requiring careful brain retraction

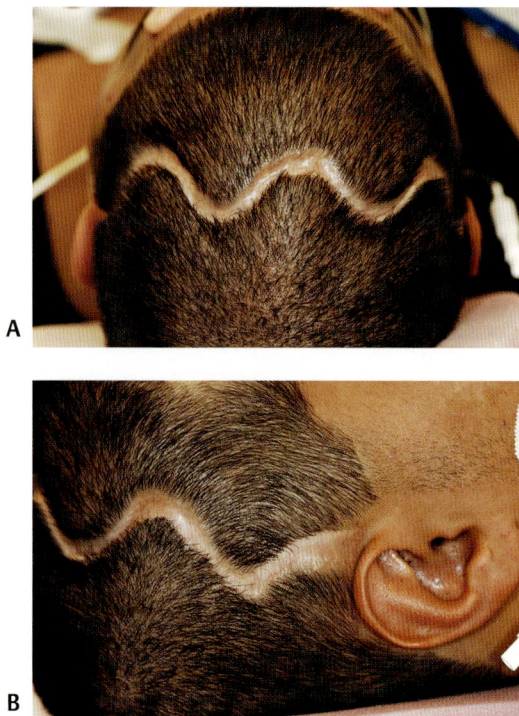

A

B

Fig. 15.2 Widened scalp scar: **(A)** top view, **(B)** lateral view.

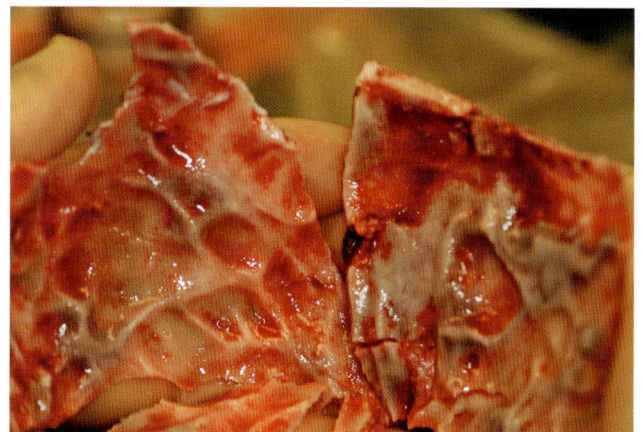

Fig. 15.3 Intraoperative view showing inner table calvarial scalloping.

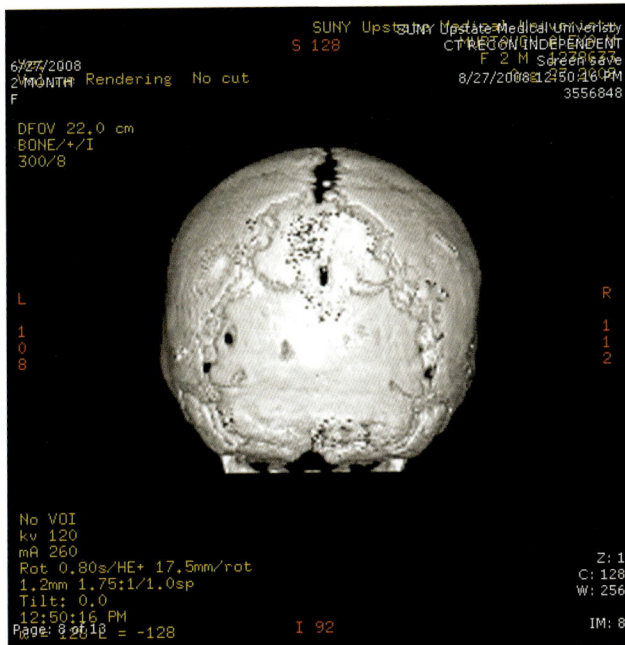

Fig. 15.4 3D CT showing calvarial defects.

(**Fig. 15.5**). Preoperative computed tomography (CT) or magnetic resonance imaging (MRI) helps to discover such problems, allowing modification of the surgical approach as necessary to avoid these injuries.

Infection

Most operative series for craniosynostosis have been associated with an infection rate of 3 to 5%.[13,14] The duration of the operation is directly related to the relative risk of infection, with shorter operations (e.g., strip craniectomies) carrying a 3% risk of infection. Longer operations may lead to increases in rates of infection of up to 8%. A key factor in infection is the age of the child and the developmental status of the sinuses. If the frontal sinus communicates with the epidural space, the rate of infection increases greatly, especially when advancement procedures leave a dead space. In most cases, such operations are performed before pneumatization of the sinuses occurs at 3 years of age. Monobloc procedures have the highest risk, because they cause connection between the nasal and cranial cavities. Pericranial flaps and tissue sealants are used to reduce the risks. Osseodistraction rather than acute advancement is also associated with lower risks. Surgical prophylaxis should target the typical offenders, mainly *Streptococcus* and *Staphylococcus*. Copious irrigation to remove bone debris and blood aids in the prevention of infections. Infection poses the risk of losing the osteotomized bone.

Cerebrospinal Fluid Leak

Dural tears with subsequent cerebrospinal fluid (CSF) leak occur most commonly at the bony sutures where the dura is tightly attached in children under the age of one year. Also, the skull erosion associated with elevated ICP leads to direct pericranium to dura contact that increases the risk of tears. These tears increase the incidence of postoperative CSF leakage and the risk of meningitis. Therefore, meticulous attention must be paid to closing such tears when leaks are present. If the dura is torn, a watertight repair must be performed. At the completion of the operation, it is advisable to check with a Valsalva maneuver for persistent CSF leakage. After surgery, large subgaleal collections can occasionally result from CSF pooling. Such collections rarely require treatment, because they usually resolve spontaneously. If a leak persists, a lumbar spinal drain can be placed for five to seven days; the pressure reduction of CSF is usually effective in correcting a CSF leak. Thereafter, the surgical site must be reexplored and the CSF leak site repaired.

Problems with Foreign Materials

In the past, metallic wires and miniplates have led to extrusion through the skin or worse, migration into the brain. Most craniofacial surgeons now use resorbable miniplates or suture material (**Fig. 15.6**). Various commercial products are currently in use, primarily composed of polyglycolic acid (PGA), poly-L-lactic acid (PLLA), and PGA-PLLA copolymers. Miniplates provide additional structural support, particularly when advancement and transposition techniques are performed. The reported complications of resorbable plating systems include pronounced fibrous encapsulation and visibility,[15] palpability,[16,17] sterile sinus formation,[18]

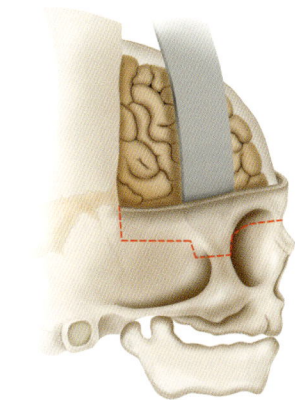

Fig. 15.5 Brain protection during bandeau osteotomies. (*Illustration by Robert Brown.*)

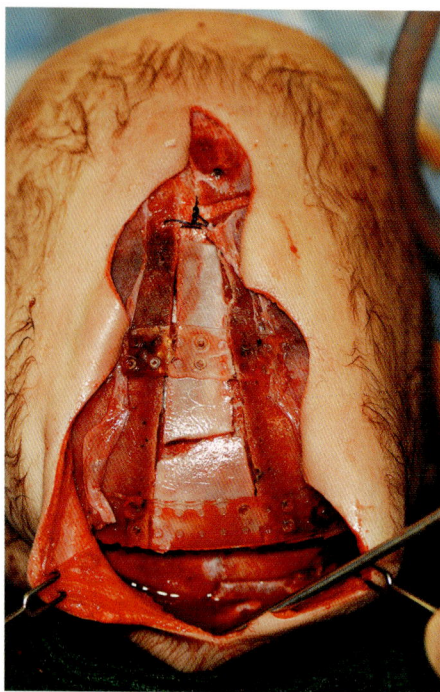

Fig. 15.6 Resorbable plates used for cranial fixation.

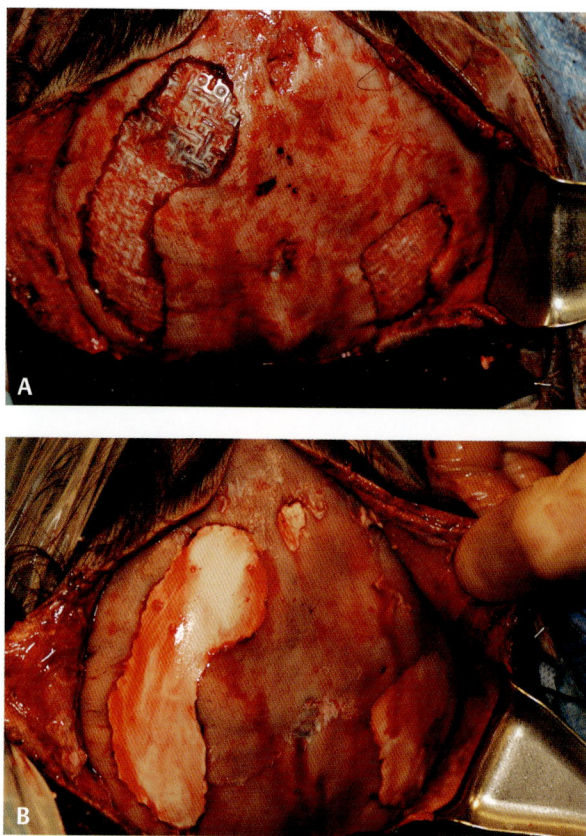

Fig. 15.7 **(A)** Dural pulsation–shielding resorbable plates in preparation for cranioplasty. **(B)** Calcium phosphate cement cranioplasty.

and bone osteolysis.[19] In 1,883 pediatric patients repaired with resorbable plates, Eppley et al. found that significant infectious complications occurred in 0.2%, device instability (primarily resulting from postoperative trauma) was noted in 0.3%, and self-limiting local foreign body reactions were seen in 0.7% of the treated patients.[20] The overall reoperation rate attributable to identifiable device-related problems was 0.3%. Improved stability was gained by using the longest plate geometries and configurations possible and by bone grafting any significant gaps across plated areas that were structurally important. Mackool et al.[21] reported four cases in which a PLLA system—MacroPore (Cytori Therapeutics, San Diego, CA), a copolymer of 70:30 Poly (L-lactide-co-d,L-lactide)—resulted in long-term palpability and visibility, with underlying bone resorption and a significant foreign body giant cell reaction.

Calcium phosphate cements (CPC) are often used as bone graft substitutes for skull defects. Verret et al.[22] reported their experience with CPC in craniofacial reconstruction in 102 patients (**Fig. 15.7A,B**). Twenty-four of the reconstructions were related to trauma and 78 arose secondary to neoplasm. Eleven implants required removal; six were related to placement within the frontal sinus or in contact with the frontal sinus. The remaining five were from other parts of the craniofacial skeleton. Dujovny et al.[23] and Mathur et al.[24] discussed the incomplete setting of CPC, partial resorption of paste, and subsequent volume loss in the presence of a water-based

medium such as blood. Implant migration and microfragmentation related to dural pulsations have also been reported from postoperative CT scans. Avoidance of sinus contact and shielding from dural pulsations reduce these problems.[25]

Skull Irregularities and Defects

Persistent calvarial contour irregularities and defects are a potential problem in all craniofacial reconstructions. Temporal hollowing is a common problem in frontal advancement cases that can be avoided by advancing the body of the muscle forward and reattaching it to the lateral orbital rim. All cut bone edges have the potential to be palpable and even visible, particularly with the thinness of the young scalp. When extensive advancements are performed, sufficient bone for reconstruction of the calvarium may be lacking. In children under 1 year old, most bone defects less than 2.5 cm in size close with time. However, after age 1 the ability of the patient to close bone defects decreases significantly. If a persistent bone defect is encountered, it is reasonable to wait until the child is 3 years old before attempting to repair it. By the time the child is 3, the diploe has formed, and split-thickness bone grafts can be harvested and used to fill in the defects.[26] Defects have also been repaired with distant bone grafts and a myriad of bone graft substitutes, such as the previously mentioned CPC (**Fig. 15.7A,B**). Visible contour irregularities may require burring to improve appearance.

Postoperative Head Injury or Deformity

The frequency of postoperative head trauma tends to be age-related, being highest in children who have reached the crawling and toddler stages. Protective headgear is recommended at this stage if significant defects persist. In addition, helmets may be used postoperatively to re-shape the head further, or they may be used in lieu of surgery for nonsynostotic plagiocephaly cases. Potential health risks associated with the use of helmets include excessive skin breakdown and infection, inappropriate mechanical restriction leading to altered or impaired head growth and development, asphyxiation, and head and neck trauma as well as ocular trauma.[27] The parents should be instructed on how to position their child in cases of plagiocephaly or advancement repair so that the child's sleep position does not add to the forces for skeletal relapse. Techniques for positioning the child with rolled towels should be demonstrated. During the day, parents should be encouraged to keep the child in a walker-type stroller fitted with a circumferential rail that prevents the child from receiving an impact with hard objects. About 6–12 weeks of healing are required to achieve good structural support for the repositioned bone and brain protection. During this critical period, the child must be watched closely. Daycare may be a risk in this period. After 3–6 months, the bone is well fibrosed, and only a hard impact can disrupt the bone units.

Ocular Complications

The visual system is often significantly involved in craniosynostosis.[28] Impaired vision may be an inherent feature of the pathologic process or occur as a secondary complication. In particular, optic disc edema, optic atrophy, and progressive optic nerve dysfunction may accompany increased intracranial pressure without evidence of hydrocephalus and with open fontanels. Uncorrected refractive error (particularly anisometropia), strabismus, ptosis, and corneal exposure problems are an invitation to the development of amblyopia.[29] If not reversed, this condition can lead to permanent visual disability. Proptosis and corneal exposure problems are a third potentially treatable cause of functional blindness. Prompt involvement of an ophthalmologist in the care of children with craniosynostosis is essential. Proptosis resulting in corneal exposure should be urgently managed with tarsorrhaphy. Tarsorrhaphy is also useful intraoperatively to protect the corneas. Papilledema and disc pallor both signal threatened vision and require urgent action. In a review of 141 patients with craniosynostotic syndromes of Apert, Crouzon, Pfeiffer and Saethre–Chotzen, Khan et al.[30] demonstrated a poor visual outcome with an acuity of 6/12 Snellen or worse in the better eye in 39.8% of cases, while 64.6% of cases had this level of vision or worse in either eye. Tay et al.[31] assessed the prevalence and causes of visual impairment in 71 patients with craniosynostotic syndromes of Apert, Crouzon, Pfeiffer, Saethre–Chotzen and CFND and confirmed Hertle's findings.[28] Causes of visual impairment were amblyopia (16.7%), ametropia (25%), optic atrophy (16.7%), exposure keratopathy (4.2%), and infantile nystagmus syndrome (4.2%). Overall, 6.3% of the patients had amblyopia that was attributable to a combination of factors: exotropia (two cases), astigmatism (two cases), and anisometropic hypermetropia (one case). 6.3% patients were found to have optic atrophy. Tay et al. found complete resolution of papilledema in all six patients with it following decompressive surgery.

Orbital repositioning may result in extraocular muscle dysfunction. In most instances, it resolves spontaneously within six months. Persistent problems may require strabismus surgery for correction. Pulsatile ophthalmopathy results from transmitted dural pulsations after fronto-orbital advancements without orbital roof reconstruction. In patients older than 9–12 months, the orbital roofs must have bone grafts. Diamond et al.[32] reported the ocular and adnexal complications of unilateral orbital advancement for plagiocephaly. Ptosis was observed postoperatively in 29% of patients, and strabismus and amblyopia in 18% of the patients. For eye protection during craniofacial corrective surgery, tarsorrhaphy can be performed before surgical draping to protect the cornea. Otherwise, the eyes must be taped securely to avoid corneal injury. During surgery, retraction or pressure on the orbits can cause changes in the patient's pulse rate and blood pressure. Accordingly, during orbital dissection the anesthesiologist should be alerted to monitor the vital signs with particular care, so that the surgical team can immediately be informed of oculocardiac stimulation. Fortunately, the reported number of complications involving the orbits that result in loss of vision is less than 1%.

◆ Distraction Osteogenesis

Distraction osteogenesis is becoming the treatment of choice for the surgical correction of many skeletal deficiencies because of its promise of new bone formation without donor sites, slow movements allowing for soft-tissue accommodation, and suitability for growing patients. Although initially there had been great emphasis on a several day postoperative latency period and a limited distraction rate of 1 mm per day, distraction is now often started on the first postoperative day after distracter insertion and at an increased rate of 2 mm per day without either fibrous union or premature consolidation. Mandibular distraction is less invasive than traditional methods of mandibular reconstruction with bone grafts and has a significantly reduced morbidity rate. It may also be done in infancy to avoid or shorten time with a tracheotomy in cases of micrognathia. Anterior cranial and maxillary distraction share the above benefits plus the lack of a large anterior cranial fossa defect with monobloc distraction compared with traditional advancement. In addition, larger movements are easier with distraction than with traditional techniques. Pitfalls include improper device and osteotomy placement, device failure, poor compliance with device activation, pin track scars, and difficulties with device removal after alteration of the anatomy. Complications can range from infection of the pin track to total failure of the procedure.

Complications of osseodistraction can be divided into placement, osteotomy, and removal complications and distraction process complications. Surgical complications include those found with traditional osteotomies: infection, hematoma, brain or ocular injury, facial or mandibular nerve injury, damage to tooth buds, scars from visible incisions, and incorrect osteotomy or device placement (**Fig. 15.8**). Tooth bud injury can lead to eruption failure or odontogenic cyst formation.[10,33–35] Careful planning and execution are the best ways to avoid these problems.

Distraction process complications occur during activation of the device or in the latency phase. Device failure includes breakage of the distracter, screw or pin loosening, and device binding. Condylar displacement has also been reported.[35,36] Distraction can cause pin migration through the soft tissues and pin tracks in the skin (**Fig. 15.9**). Compliance problems with BID or TID activation with a small tool that must be turned the cor-

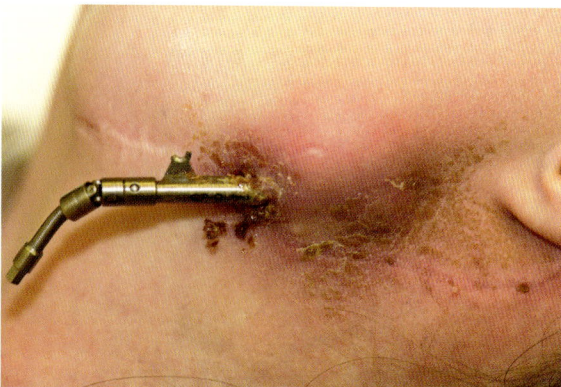

Fig. 15.9 External distracter pins extruded through the chin.

rect way can lead to premature consolidation of the regenerate formation or lack of regenerate formation after what appears to be successful distraction. Lack of compliance with activity level restrictions can lead to device dislodgement. Other causes of failure to form regenerate are patient factors such as local vascular compromise and bone metabolism disorders.

◆ Cleft Lip and Palate

The location of the cleft lip and palate anomaly leads to possible impairments of breathing, eating, hearing, speech, dental relationships, craniofacial growth, and facial appearance, along with possible psychosocial impairment. There is a lack of data on outcomes to direct cleft care. Several factors contribute to this problem. The time lapse between treatment intervention and final growth result is significant. There are no standardized national treatment protocols. Most surgeons follow a protocol that places primary cleft lip repair and tip rhinoplasty between three and six months of age. Millard and Tennison techniques tend to be the ones most commonly used. That is followed by palatoplasty at six to twelve months, usually with some variation of a Langenbeck, Veaux-Wardill-Kilmer, or Furlow technique. Secondary speech surgery, if needed, is performed between the ages of three and seven years. At the age of seven to eleven years, alveolar bone grafting is frequently necessary. Some patients require orthognathic surgery, and in selected cases distraction osteogenesis is performed. Between the ages of 12 and 18 years, secondary rhinoplasties are indicated in most patients.

Cleft Lip Repair

Initial problems with bleeding, infection, or dehiscence are rare. Occasionally, significant respiratory distress may be noted from nasal obstruction, particularly in the

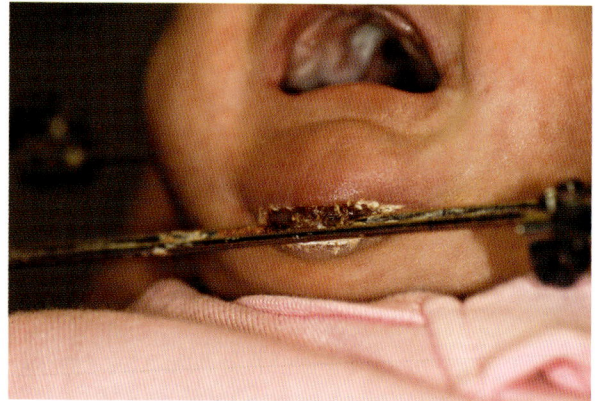

Fig. 15.8 Infected extruding fractured distracter.

repair of bilateral clefts. The problem responds acutely to insertion of nasal stents. Twenty-three hour postoperative observation is recommended for patients younger than four months of age. Avoidance of lip trauma in the first seven to ten days postoperatively with gentle feeding techniques and handling helps ensure good healing with minimal scars.

Cleft lip repair generally involves recruiting tissue flanking the cleft to fill the cleft-related defects. Complications generally result in the need for a revision. Revisions can be divided into small touch-up procedures for minor deficiencies and total lip repair revisions for major problems. Careful analysis of the residual deformity leads to the choice of the appropriate approach. Residual deficiencies can be thought of as tissue deficiency problems, tissue distortion problems, or some combination of both. As is typical, the best management is proper initial technique to avoid residual problems. However, even the best hands still have revisions.

Notching of the lip margin (whistle deformity) is a frequently encountered secondary deformity in cleft lip patients (**Fig. 15.10**). It represents some degree of vertical deficiency in the lip skin, vermilion, muscle, or mucosa. Central mucosal deficiency may be minimized at the time of the initial unilateral lip repair by back-cutting the mucosa in the gingivobuccal sulcus along the medial lip element, where the deficiency is most common, and advancing from lateral to medial and inferiorly. The resulting mucosal defect in the sulcus quickly heals secondarily.

There is a natural vermilion deficiency in clefts (worse in bilateral clefts) as the wet line fuses with the white roll at the cleft margin. This is best managed during primary repair with vermilion flaps from the lateral segments being brought into the philtral tubercle. Vermilion deficiency can occur under the lip scar(s) or centrally as a philtral tubercle deficiency. Minor de-

ficiencies may be addressed with dermal fat grafts or V–Y mucosal advancement, but mucosa outside of the wet line can lead to chapping and color mismatch. More significant deficiency is due to vertical skin or muscle deficiency, and depending on degree, it requires a scar revision or total lip revision. Severe bilateral cleft lip vermilion deficiencies can be corrected with a lower lip vermilion flap.

Cleft-side high peaking of Cupid's bow or vertical skin deficiency without lip notching is commonly seen early after the Millard rotation advancement repair due to scar contracture.[37] This usually resolves with gentle massage and scar maturation. If the problem persists beyond one year postoperatively, then it should be surgically corrected. In cases in which the lip is short by up to 2 mm, a diamond-shaped excision of the scar and reclosure can add adequate length. When the whole lip is short due to scar contracture, total excision of the scar eliminates contracture and allows for normal alignment. If additional lengthening is needed, Z-plasties, rotation-advancement, or triangular flap techniques can be used just in the skin. Greater vertical deficiency or a shortage of subcutaneous tissue and muscle necessitates complete revision. If the orbicularis muscle is dehiscent, it should be released from its abnormal insertions and approximated. The most severe defects may require an Abbe flap. Less commonly, excess in the vertical dimension results in a long upper lip. Reduction is achieved with an excision of the skin and muscle just below the nasal ala and sill.

Misalignment without significant tissue deficit can be corrected by readjustment of available local tissue. The degree of misalignment again dictates whether there will be a minor procedure or complete revision. The most obvious abnormalities include misalignment of the white roll and the wet line. Popular techniques include scar excision and reclosure with proper alignment, a small asymmetric Z–plasty, V–Y advancement, and serial excision to move structures with minimal secondary distortion. Severe misalignment may involve a complete revision of the lip with mobilization and formal realignment of the muscle and surface structures.

Horizontal abnormalities can result from deficiency or excess. A deficiency in the distance from the low point of Cupid's bow to the cleft-side peak is produced by improper marking in the initial repair. The deficiency is very difficult to repair and is best avoided. In the bilateral cleft lip, asymmetry can be addressed by moving the scar on the wider side of the philtrum closer to the midline. Inadequate undermining and recruitment of tissue from lateral to medial can lead to excess tension, hypertrophic scarring, keloids, subcutaneous tissue dehiscence, or a tight lip. Infection or reaction to suture material can also cause unfavorable scars. This complication can be improved with a normal straight scar excision or with the wave line method of Pfeifer. Dermabrasion may help in mild cases. It is important to

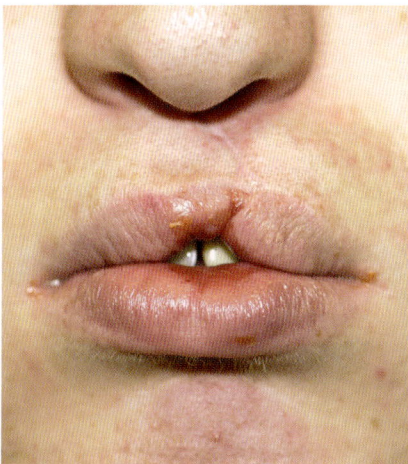

Fig. 15.10 Whistle deformity.

ensure proper alignment of the orbicularis muscle fibers and minimal tension. A tight, thin upper lip can often be corrected by total revision with wide recruitment of lateral tissue, but an Abbe flap or Bruns lip-lengthening technique may be necessary. An overly wide philtrum occurs mostly in a bilateral cleft lip and is created when the philtrum is designed too widely at the initial lip repair (greater than 4–5 mm). Any excess philtrum and muscle or connective tissue should be excised and the lip scars medialized.

Unilateral Cleft Lip Nasal Deformity

It is generally the residual associated nasal deformity that stigmatizes affected children rather than the repaired cleft lip. The anomalous anatomy of the cleft lip nose was clearly defined in the 1950s by Huffman and Lierle[38] (**Fig. 15.11**). If the cleft lip is repaired without correction of the malpositioned alar cartilage, the nostril rim droops on the side of the cleft, the lower border of the alar cartilage pushes up an oblique ridge within the vestibule, and the nostril flares.

Primary (i.e., synchronous with cleft lip repair) correction of nasal alar deformity has become commonplace during the past 25 years and has reduced the severity of the residual deformity. Primary treatment consists of correcting the caudal rotation of the alar cartilage at the time of lip repair. The alar cartilage, with the attached vestibular lining, is lifted to lengthen the nose on the side of the cleft. The arch swings forward and establishes the vault of the vestibule before closure of the nostril floor. McComb and Coghlan[37] published an 18-year follow-up of ten consecutive patients who underwent primary correction of their cleft lip nasal deformity to elevate the displaced alar cartilage at the time of cleft

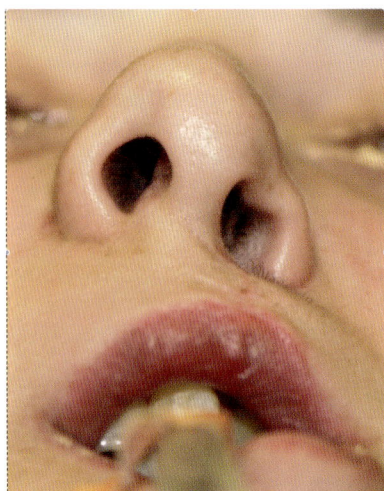

Fig. 15.11 Cleft lip nasal deformity.

lip repair. The results support the observation that nasal growth on the cleft side of the nose is unaffected by early primary nasal surgery and that the vertical lengthening of the nose by the alar lift technique is preserved into adult life. Ariyan and Krizek[39] recommended suture fixation of the cleft-sided lower lateral cartilage to the non-cleft upper lateral cartilage, while Dingman and Natvig[40] felt suture fixation to the cleft-sided upper lateral cartilage was superior. Black et al.[41] described box suture fixation to correct the cleft lateral crus. Many advocate postoperative nostril stenting to maintain nostril shape.

Nasal airway obstruction may be caused by irregularity of nasal floor on the cleft side, inferior turbinate hypertrophy into the cleft, a deviated nasal septum common to nearly all unilateral cleft lip-palates and many bilateral clefts, and decreased nostril and nasal cavity size. A 25% diminution of the nasal airway using pressure flow studies was documented by Warren.[42] Severe obstruction may necessitate early corrective nasal surgery (intermediate septorhinoplasty). Caudal septal deflection is corrected with minimal dissection and very conservative septoplasty. The septum is repositioned to the midline and secured to the nasal spine with a suture. Most posterior deviation requires limited septal spur resection. Inferior turbinate reduction and nasal valve surgery may also be required.

Other secondary cleft nose deformities include a widened or constricted nostril, hooding in the soft triangle, inadequate correction of the lower lateral cartilage, and flaring of the alar base. A mildly stenotic nostril can be addressed early through dilation with nasal silicone stents. Moderate or severe stenosis requires vestibular surgery, possibly with grafting. The soft-tissue triangle hooding can be addressed during the primary rhinoplasty. Later it can be directly excised, resulting in an external scar. Alternatively, once the new high point of the cleft-side dome has been established during secondary rhinoplasty, careful closure of the marginal incision under the dome will pull the soft triangle up. Defatting the cleft-side lateral alar lobule may also help with nostril narrowing. A wide nostril can be corrected with a sill excision or V-Y advancement of the alar base. Lower lateral cartilage and tip correction can be performed with standard open septorhinoplasty techniques. A turned-out alar base can be improved by a perialar Z-plasty. Tip asymmetries and dorsal deviations are correctable with standard open rhinoplasty techniques. Inferior turbinate reduction and nasal valve surgery may also be required.

Bilateral Cleft Lip Nasal Deformity

The classic bilateral cleft lip nasal deformity is characterized by a poorly projecting bulbous bifid tip, splayed alar cartilages, short columella, flared alar rims, and a wide alar base (**Fig. 15.12**). The nostril rims are oriented transversely instead of at the usual 45° angle to the fa-

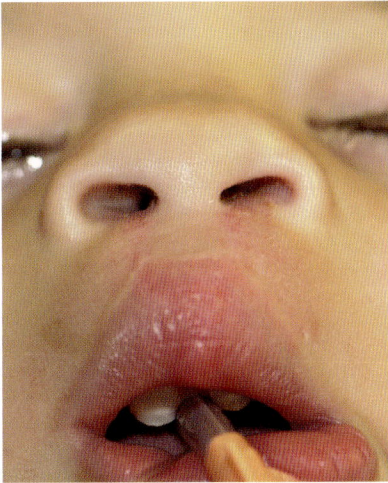

Fig. 15.12 Bilateral nasal deformity.

cial plane. The nose generally forms an obtuse nasolabial angle.[43] Columellar shortening and poor nasal tip projection require V-to-Y advancement of tissue from the upper lip.

Simple techniques include the use of suture fixation of the lower lateral cartilage to adjacent nasal structures after extensive dissection and mobilization. McComb[44] described suture fixation of the lower lateral cartilage to the nasion and nasal bridge. To maintain the outcome, others like Cenzi and Guarda[45] have advocated nostril splints to oppose the contractile forces during healing. Unfortunately, these suturing methods have tended to result in an inadequate correction of the bilateral cleft lip nasal deformities, with a high incidence of recurrence.

Structural grafts also help to correct the bilateral cleft lip nasal deformity. Barsky[46] advocated the use of nasal tip grafts of autologous cartilage to improve tip projection. Columellar struts are commonly employed. Some authors[47,48] have advocated multiple cartilage and bone grafts to provide structural support and improve the projection of the nose.

Columellar lengthening typically requires a combination of skin lengthening and structural support with cartilage grafting and suture techniques. To gain maximum tip projection, the surgeon must often augment both the internal structures and the skin envelope. Cartilage composite grafts support the nasal rim and prevent alar retraction. Raspall et al.[49] used a columellar strut and a small V-Y advancement from the nasal sill to lengthen the columella and minimize columellar and philtral incisions. Others have used advanced vestibular flaps, philtral scars or banked fork flaps from the prolabium into the columella, skin or composite grafting, or narrowing of the nasal tip with central excision of tip skin. Lateral crural flaps have similarly been advanced toward the tip.[50–52] The lip, sill, and grafting techniques lengthen the

columella at the expense of creating a scarred, abnormally wide columella. Inadequate and incomplete correction, noticeable external scars, an unnatural columellar appearance, inadequate alar support with resultant vestibular narrowing, external nasal valve collapse, and alar base asymmetry have all been problems associated with these techniques. Alar asymmetry and notching, as well as persistent deformities in the lower lateral cartilages, may also be seen.[53–56] Other procedures involve the use of external nasal tip and columellar incisions to lengthen the columella from the tip down rather than from the lip and sill up. This approach achieves both columellar lengthening and tip narrowing[57,58] with the cost of external incisions and subsequent midline columellar and tip scars. However, this type of approach is gaining popularity. Placing an alar base cinch suture improves the ratio of the nasal length to the alar base width and creates a more aesthetically pleasing and balanced nasal contour. Defatting the tip and placing interdomal sutures improves the bulbous nasal tip and gives it a more narrowed and refined shape.

Palatoplasty

The multidimensionality of cleft outcomes includes the effects of the anomaly and its repair on respiration, nutrition, speech, hearing, appearance, dental occlusion, craniofacial growth and psychosocial function. Modification of surgical techniques or timing to optimize one of these variables may induce untoward consequences in another; for example, it has been shown that delayed closure of the hard palate, recommended to minimize maxillary growth disturbances because of palatoplasty, increases speech impairment.[59] The best outcomes are achieved with an interdisciplinary, coordinated, and uniform approach to treatment.

Modern palatoplasty techniques have focused on reducing postoperative velopharyngeal insufficiency. However, negative growth effects remain a concern as well as fistula rates. Palatal lengthening, improved muscle function, and reduction of anteroposterior scar contraction have been goals. The Veau-Wardill-Kilner pushback operation is aimed at palatal lengthening by posterior palatal tissue mobilization. In the hope of improving speech results, the palatal musculature was reoriented. This operation, popularized by Kriens[60] as intravelar veloplasty, has been adopted by many cleft surgeons during the past three to four decades. However, neither anatomical reports nor historical comparative data have established the efficacy of intravelar veloplasty. The only prospective study in the literature does not show a statistically significant difference that would warrant its routine application.[61]

More recently, palatal lengthening and levator repositioning have been combined in the Furlow double-opposing Z-plasty repair.[62] Retrospective studies of the Furlow palatoplasty by Spauwen et al.,[63] Yu et al.,[64] and

Sie et al.[65] have demonstrated complete resolution or substantial improvement of velopharyngeal insufficiency postoperatively. However, Spauwen et al.[63] found no significant differences between the Furlow palatoplasty and von Langenbeck palatoplasty techniques in respect to articulatory skills, language comprehension, and language production as well as hearing.

Concerning the use of a vomer flap, the literature is contradictory about whether it interferes with maxillary growth. Friede et al.[66] presented data that seem to indicate disturbance of maxillary growth when a vomer flap was used to close the hard palate in infancy. Others use a vomer flap to close the hard palate at the time of lip repair and have not found significant growth alteration. The Oslo Cleft Palate group believes that the vomer flap allows early closure of the cleft alveolus, thereby decreasing the frequency of alveolar nasal fistulas without producing significant maxillary growth attenuation.[67]

Oronasal Fistulas

A palatal fistula may occur anywhere along the site of the original cleft as a complication of palatoplasty (**Fig. 15.13**). The reported incidence of fistulization varies widely, ranging from zero to 34% of all patients with repaired clefts.[68,69] Multiple etiologic factors have been suggested for the formation of oronasal fistulas, including wound breakdown secondary to closure site tension,[70] infection,[71-73] postoperative flap trauma,[74] hematoma,[75] and hypoxemia.[76] Care should be taken to avoid pedicle damage during flap elevation. If a flap appears ischemic, it should be explored for tension on the pedicle. Tension may be reduced by notching the pedicle out of the back of the hard palate, dissecting a few millimeters of the pedicle off of the flap, circumferential dissection of the periosteum around the pedicle, and hamulus fracture or tensor transposition. A palatal fistula may result in audible nasal air escape during speech, hypernasality, increased nasal resonance, nasal regurgitation during

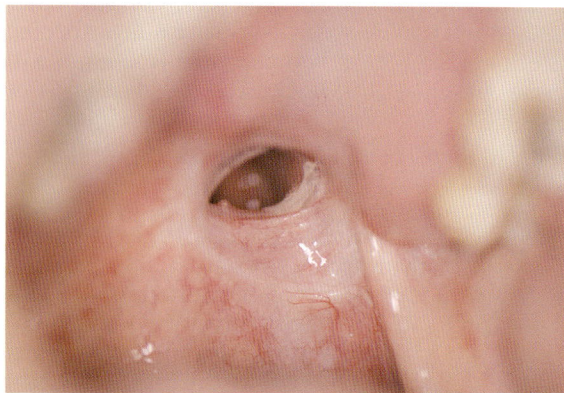

Fig. 15.13 Oronasal fistula.

drinking and eating, difficulties with oral hygiene, and production of socially undesirable sounds. A symptomatic fistula may cause deterioration in speech quality and intelligibility. Many opinions have been expressed in the surgical literature concerning which fistulas are likely to be symptomatic.[68,69] The most common variables discussed are the size and location of the fistula. Larger fistulas may be associated with more significant hypernasality and nasal emission, but the size of a fistula alone does not correlate with the change in speech symptoms when a fistula is temporarily obturated or repaired. This finding is supported by data from Henningsson and Isberg[77] that indicated that improvement in speech is not caused solely by the reduction of air flow through the fistula. Using videofluoroscopy, they demonstrated that the occlusion of a fistula could cause concomitant improvement in velopharyngeal valving.

Prior palatal surgery inevitably results in formation of scarred tissue that often makes successful wound healing after oronasal fistula repair problematic. Consequently, the likelihood of recurrent fistula formation after an attempted repair is quite high, with reported rates ranging from 9 to 65%.[68,69,78-82] Several options for fistula repair have been reported, including paring of fistula margins with reclosure, local turnover flaps,[83] tongue flaps,[74,83] buccal fat pad grafting,[75,84] pedicled flaps from adjacent oral tissue,[83] free flaps,[84-91] distraction osteogenesis,[92] tissue expansion,[93,94] and free cartilage grafts.[95-97] The multitude of techniques is testament to the fact that no particular procedure reliably yields satisfactory results. Furthermore, these options can require cumbersome, lengthy procedures and may result in significant donor-site morbidity, even as they still carry high rates of recurrence. More recently, Clark et al.[98] and Kirschner et al.[99] have successfully used acellular dermis as an interposition graft in the repair of cleft palate fistulae.[100]

Velopharyngeal Dysfunction

Approximately 20% of children who undergo cleft palate repair develop speech production disorders, most commonly velopharyngeal dysfunction, that require additional intervention.[101] This percentage seems independent of the type of palatoplasty. Velopharyngeal dysfunction is diagnosed clinically by a constellation of symptoms that include abnormal nasal resonance (hypernasality), misarticulation, escape of air through the nose (nasal emissions), and aberrant facial movements (grimacing). Trost-Cardamone[102] has proposed a taxonomy for velopharyngeal disorders that is based on causative factors. Velopharyngeal dysfunction may result from anatomic, myoneural, and behavioral disorders or from a combination of these disorders. Although it is now possible to separate various etiologies of velopharyngeal dysfunction by using instrumental evaluations, contemporary treatments for velopharyngeal dysfunction were developed irrespective of its etiology. The efforts of an international working group to standardize fluoroscopic and endoscopic velopharyngeal functional evaluations[103] may permit development of differential treatments based on differential diagnosis.

Partial obstruction of the velopharyngeal port is the unifying feature of most surgical treatments for velopharyngeal dysfunction. Two classes of operations are currently used to manage velopharyngeal dysfunction: (1) lengthening and reorienting the muscles of the palate by retropositioning of the velum (V-Y pushback; intravelar veloplasty; double-opposing Z-plasty) and (2) reducing the size of the opening between the nasal and oral pharynges. Velopharyngeal port reduction can be accomplished by central obstruction (pharyngeal flap), posterolateral narrowing (sphincter pharyngoplasty),[104-106] or posterior pharyngeal wall augmentation.[107-109] Although outcome reports for each of these interventions have been published[107-109] that document variable success rates and associated morbidity, comparative data are unavailable. All these procedures are capable of producing iatrogenic postoperative airway obstruction. They should be used very cautiously in patients who are at risk for airway complications because of cardiopulmonary or neurologic conditions or in patients who already have airway concerns.

Failure of the pharyngeal flap or sphincter pharyngoplasty operations results from inadequate obstruction (persistent hypernasality) or too much obstruction (mouth breathing, rhinorrhea, increase in ear and sinus infections, and sleep apnea). Tailoring the intervention to the patient's needs based on visualization studies (fluoroscopy and endoscopy) is thought to be one of the best ways to achieve appropriate obstruction. Attempts have been made to define the reasons for morbidity and failure after sphincter pharyngoplasty. Riski et al.[110] documented the necessity for proper anatomic placement of the myomucosal flaps that comprised the neosphincter and the improvement in velopharyngeal function after attention to anatomic placement during a six-year experience. Witt et al.[107-109] identified the risk of identifiable syndromes, microretrognathia, or perinatal respiratory and feeding difficulties for development of post-sphincter airway problems and Chegar et al.[111] described pharyngeal flap modifications that resulted in reduced risk of obstruction from wide pharyngeal flaps. Persistent airway obstruction may necessitate port dilation, revision surgery, or even removal of the obstructing tissue with the likely attendant reduction in the speech result. Various palatal prosthetic lifts or obturators may be used as reversible methods of velopharyngeal management. A comparison of speech outcomes using prosthetic versus surgical management showed no difference for patients who complied with the prostheses.[112] However, because nearly 30% of patients referred for prostheses did not comply, surgery was more efficacious overall. Recognized infection is uncommon, but it might contribute to post-operative dehiscence. Certainly there is at least a theoretical concern for mediastinal or vertebral spread after these procedures, but it is rare, even though the posterior oropharyngeal donor site in pharyngeal flap surgery is typically left open to heal by secondary intention.[113]

Alveolar Bone Grafting

Patients with clefts through the maxillary alveolus have osseous discontinuity of the alveolus and maxillary basal bone. Succedaneous teeth cannot erupt through the bone defect and may be unstable when flanking the bony cleft even if soft-tissue closure of the alveolar gap has been achieved. Any patient born with a complete cleft should be considered for alveolar grafting. The benefits and goals of this procedure are well recognized and include the stabilization of the maxillary arch, elimination of oronasal fistulae, creation of bony support for subsequent tooth eruption, and reconstruction of the hypoplastic pyriform aperture and soft-tissue nasal base support. Losquadro and Tatum[114] more recently described their results for gingivoperiosteoplasty at the time of cleft palate repair as a method to reduce or eliminate alveolar bone grafting.

Based on its timing, alveolar bone grafting is classified into primary (before palate repair or in children younger than two years of age) and secondary bone grafting (at any time thereafter). The main concerns with bone grafting are its effect on maxillary growth and the height and width of the neo-alveolar ridge. Early techniques of primary bone grafting were characterized by extensive hard palatal dissection around and across the vomerine-premaxillary suture and led to long-term midfacial growth disturbance. With more recent modifications, there are no differences in facial growth between operated and unoperated patients.[115,116]

Although the need for secondary augmentation of the primarily grafted alveolus is reported to be low,[117] delayed secondary grafting of the cleft alveolus with iliac cancellous bone has gained widespread acceptance because of the predictable production of viable bone with adequate cross-sectional width for tooth eruption, orthodontic tooth movement, or endosteal implant placement. This procedure typically provides greater than 80% root coverage of incisors and cuspids adjacent to the cleft.[118] When teeth are present and erupt into the grafted alveolus, often with the aid of surgical exposure and orthodontic assistance, alveolar bone height is retained. When teeth are not present to erupt through the graft within six months, partial resorption of the graft occurs, even when it is overfilled intraoperatively.[119] However, total secondary graft failures are uncommon. Poor tissue quality is the most common reason for compromised results.[119] Other complications include tooth injury or loss, along with recurrent fistulization. Complications at the iliac donor site include bleeding, infection, bowel or hip joint damage, cutaneous nerve damage, inguinal ligament separation, scarring, chronic hip pain, gait disturbance and contour defect. Other donor sites have included the skull, mandible, ribs, and tibia.

◆ Microtia Repair

Malformations of the external ear occur in newborn infants with a frequency of less than 1%. The majority of those are minor, such as preauricular skin tags. The incidence of isolated microtia is 1:10,000,[120] occurring more often in right ears and in males.[121] Whites and blacks appear to have a lower incidence of microtia than Hispanics and Asians.[122] The cause of microtia is thought to be multifactorial, and most cases are sporadic, with fewer than 15% having a positive family history. If associated with a syndrome (e.g., Treacher-Collins, Goldenhar, etc.) the incidence is higher. Microtia is unilateral in 70% of cases, and the commonest associations are facial abnormalities and hearing loss. There is no universally accepted classification system for microtia. One widely adopted system, originally described by Weerda and simplified by Aguilar, assigns a grade from I to III based on the severity of the deformity.[121]

Auricular Reconstruction with Costal Cartilage

In 1971, Tanzer[123] described his four-stage reconstruction that consisted of (1) lobule transposition, (2) cartilage framework carving and placement, (3) elevation of the ear with postauricular skin grafting, and (4) tragus construction with conchal excavation. In 1992, Brent[124,125] published his own experience with 600 cases over 20 years, with a median follow-up of five years. He describes his four-stage technique that consisted of (1) framework placement, (2) lobule transposition, (3) tragus construction and conchal excavation, and (4) elevation of the ear framework. With experience, sequencing the stages of reconstruction is flexible depending on the degree of deformity and the surgeon's preference. With regard to timing, there is usually sufficient rib cartilage by the age of six years, and the auricle has reached 95% of its adult size.[126] Reconstruction can often begin at an earlier age if an alloplastic framework is being used, because there is no need to harvest a large quantity of rib cartilage.[124,125,127,128] An alternative to reconstruction is the use of a prosthetic ear. Despite the introduction of osseointegrated prostheses, most patients prefer a rib graft repair.[129] Because the placement of osseointegrated implants requires the removal of skin and soft tissue in the area of the repair, future autogenous rib reconstruction is precluded. However, rib reconstruction does not prevent later prosthesis placement.

Complications associated with autogenous rib cartilage graft harvest include a chest scar, a visible anterior chest wall deformity, pneumothorax, and postoperative pain. Ohara et al.[130] evaluated donor site morbidity in 18 patients who underwent microtia repair. He observed chest deformities in 64% of children under the age of ten years and 20% in older children. The surgical incision should be placed in the medial inframammary fold, especially in female patients. Leaving the deep perichondrium down during cartilage removal reduces the risk of pneumothorax. The anesthesiologist should perform a Valsalva maneuver at the time of closing to check for an air leak. Small pleural tears can be repaired over a suction catheter that can be removed after airtight wound closure. Tube thoracostomy is rarely required. Costal cartilage harvest is associated with significant pain. It is helpful to place a small-diameter infusion catheter in the wound bed at the time of graft harvest for instillation of anesthetic solution.

Complications also occur at the ear reconstruction site. Thinning of the skin flap is desirable to enhance visible cartilage contours. However, too much thinning or pressure dressings may compromise the skin envelope.[124,125] Exposure of the carved cartilage framework secondary to skin flap necrosis may necessitate complete removal of the framework. Small areas of skin loss (less than 1 cm) can be treated with topical and systemic antibiotic therapy as well as limited debridement, but this usually leads to a contour defect (**Fig. 15.14**). Infection occurs in less than 0.5% of cases. Hematoma formation has been reported in 0.3% of patients.[131] The use of stainless steel wire instead of sutures to coapt the cartilage elements of the framework has been associated with a higher incidence of construct notching and wire extrusion.[132] Long-term complications include extrusion of suture material or necrotic cartilage, resorption of cartilage, and poor anatomic detail (**Fig. 15.15**). Careful attention to detail and conservative tissue handling improve results.

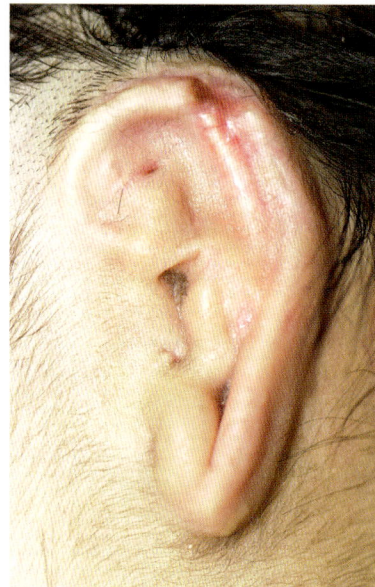

Fig. 15.14 Neohelix defect from cartilage exposure.

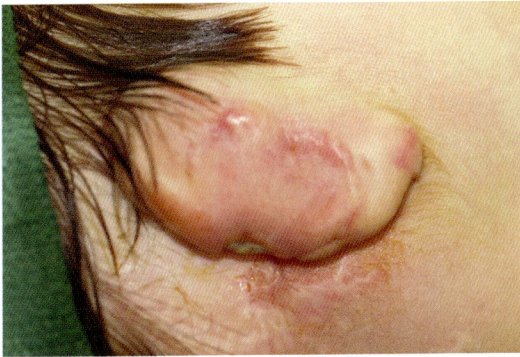

Fig. 15.15 Poor auricular definition and exposed cartilage.

Alloplastic Framework Reconstruction

By using an alloplastic framework, reconstruction may begin at an earlier age because the size of the child's rib cartilage is not an issue. Cronin and Ohmori described excellent initial aesthetic results from the use of a silicone framework, but long-term follow-up revealed an unacceptably high failure rate from implant exposure.[126] Exposure and subsequent failure may occur many years after implantation, even with minor trauma. The use of silicone for ear reconstruction has thus been abandoned. More recently, reconstruction with a porous polyethylene (MEDPORE, Porex Surgical, Inc., Newnan, GA) framework has been advocated with increasing enthusiasm. Porous polyethylene causes minimal tissue reaction, and its porosity allows ingrowth of soft tissue, thereby providing greater stability. The use of a temporoparietal fascia flap that completely surrounds the porous polyethylene implant has significantly reduced its initial failure rate,[124,125] although long-term results are lacking[127,128] and a lifelong risk of exposure remains.

Prosthetic Reconstruction

Prosthetic reconstruction usually requires only one operative procedure after removal of the congenitally malformed auricular remnants. Depending on the thickness of the temporal bone, the implant can be attached to a bone-anchored abutment or (if there is insufficient bone thickness) to an implant-carrying plate system. Complications of placement include meningitis, dural penetration, hemorrhage, and brain injury. Meticulous hygiene around the transcutaneous abutments is necessary to avoid infection of the implant site. Implant integration failure and rejection remain persistent risks. Psychological difficulties might arise from the social impact of the dislodgement of an auricular prosthesis, in a classroom setting for instance. Replacement of the prosthetic ear is required every two to five years.

Otoplasty

Otoplasty typically refers to surgery to correct an overly prominent auricle, generally from some combination of conchal excess and antihelical fold deficiency. The approach is usually a postauricular incision or excision, with cartilage weakening or cutting and suturing. Early complications after otoplasty include hematoma formation and infection. The incidence of postoperative hematoma after otoplasty is low. Bleeding results from local factors, such as an improper dissection plane or inadequate hemostasis, and from systemic factors such as hypertension or undiagnosed coagulopathy. Excessive pain should prompt exploration of the wound to rule out a hematoma. If a blood clot is found and removed, the incision is loosely closed over a passive drain, followed by replacement of a conforming dressing or possibly even sutured dental rolls, along with treatment by a broad-spectrum antibiotic. If the hematoma is left untreated, wound infection, perichondritis, chondritis and postoperative cauliflower deformity may result. The risk of infection is reduced by strict observance of sterile technique, perioperative parenteral and topical antibiotic administration, and postoperative application of antibiotic ointment to the suture line.

Patients may be dissatisfied with the result of the otoplasty; for example, over-correction may put the ear too flat against the head, or overly aggressive cartilage weakening techniques may lead to an unnatural operated look with sharp contours. Over-resection of the central postauricular skin can lead to a telephone ear deformity, in which the ear is close to the head in its middle portion but projects at the upper and lower poles (**Fig. 15.16**).

Hypertrophic scarring, hypesthesia, and suture-related complications such as granuloma formation or suture exposure are also potential problems. Suture-related complications such as localized skin inflammation, stitch abscess formation, or foreign-body granulomas are easily dealt with by removal of the offending suture when the wound has matured. Extrusion of sutures is more prevalent with scaphoconchal Mustarde sutures than with conchomastoid Furnas sutures. If they are placed too far away from the antihelical fold, these sutures may then bowstring across the gap, even becoming exposed and causing both an aesthetic and functional deformity, particularly for patients who wear eyeglasses. Over-excision of postauricular skin may result in tense skin closure and poor suture coverage. Finally, improper conchomastoid suture placement may be responsible for anterior displacement of the conchal cartilage, leading to external auditory canal narrowing.

Relapse or loss of correction is one of the more common postoperative complications encountered, with reported rates ranging from 6.5 to 12%.[133,134] It is frequently observed with postoperative trauma and cartilage-sparing techniques. Improper type, location, or quantity of sutures may result in excessive tension and

Fusiform Skin Excision   Telephone Ear Deformity

Dumbell Skin Excision   No Deformity

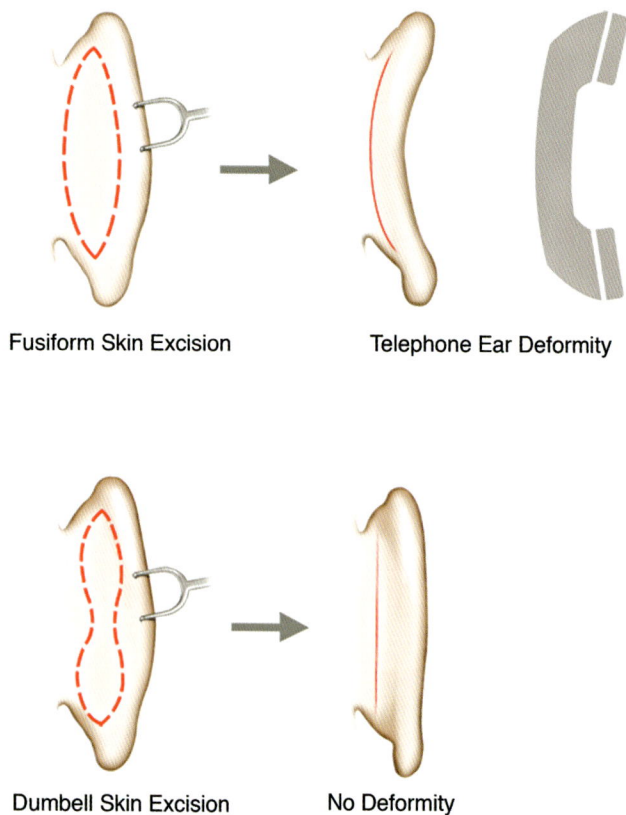

Fig. 15.16 Telephone deformity of the auricle. (*Illustration by Robert Brown.*)

pull-through of sutures. Other causes of insufficient long-term correction include insufficient conchal set-back or inadequate weakening of particularly inflexible cartilage. The patient should be made aware of the consequences of external trauma in the postoperative healing phase. The untoward effects of external trauma may be lessened by careful placement of sutures with attainment of adequate purchase on the anterior perichondrium to avert suture pull-through and by placement of conchotemporal tension-relieving sutures to help reinforce the correction. Hypertrophic scarring or keloid formation occurs most commonly in susceptible individuals of African, Asian, or Scandinavian descent. Younger patients are also more vulnerable, especially in the setting of postauricular incisions. Preventive modalities include avoidance of excessive wound-closing tension and minimization of tissue trauma or infection. Management may include steroid injections and scar revision. Persistent paresthesias or sensory deficits after otoplasty are rare. Although injury to the greater auricular nerve may give rise to these symptoms initially, they usually resolve spontaneously over several months. A more likely symptom relates to cold temperature insensitivity and increased risk of frostbite after otoplasty.

◆ Conclusion

Surgery for the correction of congenital anomalies is both rewarding and challenging. There is a myriad of presentations, each requiring careful analysis and planning. Many of the procedures are complex and dangerous, requiring specialized training and experience. As has been stated, prevention is the best way to manage complications. Attention to detail and early acknowledgment are paramount to complication management. Thorough preoperative counseling will help to maintain the patient's confidence during the trying times of postoperative complications.

PEARLS OF WISDOM

Remain constantly aware of hemostasis and volume replacement throughout infantile craniofacial surgery. Although these procedures have become routine, they are still very dangerous.

Pay close attention to the security of the endotracheal tube during craniofacial cases. It is best to avoid reintubation after the calvarium has been removed.

In distraction osteogenesis, the regenerate is as only as big as the cross-section of the original osteotomy. Choose a large area of bone stock to make the osteotomy.

Avoid absorbable skin sutures on primary cleft lip repairs. They can leave marks on delicate infant skin.

Tension is the enemy of palate repair. Learn multiple maneuvers to reduce tension.

Remember that pharyngeal flaps are intended to partially obstruct the nasopharynx. Additional obstruction at the oropharyngeal level can occur if the flap is too low or the donor-site healing narrows the pharynx.

In alveolar bone grafting, it is critical to expose the entire margins of the bony cleft from the alveolar ridge to the floor of the nose and lateral pyriform crest.

Consider waiting to start microtia correction until the child is over eight years old. The larger cartilages are easier to work with.

Avoid cartilage cutting techniques until you have become very comfortable with otoplasty. They are much harder to use to achieve a natural appearance.

References

1. Shillito J Jr, Matson DD. Craniosynostosis: a review of 519 surgical patients. Pediatrics 1968;41(4):829–853
2. Harrop CW, Avery BS, Marks SM, Putnam GD. Craniosynostosis in babies: complications and management of 40 cases. Br J Oral Maxillofac Surg 1996;34(2):158–161
3. Kadri H, Mawla AA. Incidences of craniosynostosis in Syria. J Craniofac Surg 2004;15(4):703–704

4. Nonaka Y, Oi S, Miyawaki T, Shinoda A, Kurihara K. Indication for and surgical outcomes of the distraction method in various types of craniosynostosis. Advantages, disadvantages, and current concepts for surgical strategy in the treatment of craniosynostosis. Childs Nerv Syst 2004;20(10):702–709

5. Kakitsuba N, Sadaoka T, Motoyama S, et al. Sleep apnea and sleep-related breathing disorders in patients with craniofacial synostosis. Acta Otolaryngol Suppl 1994;517:6–10

6. Järund M, Lauritzen C. Craniofacial dysostosis: airway obstruction and craniofacial surgery. Scand J Plast Reconstr Surg Hand Surg 1996;30(4):275–279

7. Sculerati N, Gottlieb MD, Zimbler MS, Chibbaro PD, McCarthy JG. Airway management in children with major craniofacial anomalies. Laryngoscope 1998;108(12):1806–1812

8. Goodrich JT. Craniofacial surgery: complications and their prevention. Semin Pediatr Neurol 2004;11(4):288–300

9. Fishman MA, Hogan GR, Dodge PR. The concurrence of hydrocephalus and craniosynostosis. J Neurosurg 1971;34(5):621–629

10. Golabi M, Edwards MS, Ousterhout DK. Craniosynostosis and hydrocephalus. Neurosurgery 1987;21(1):63–67

11. Renier D, Sainte-Rose C, Marchac D, Hirsch JF. Intracranial pressure in craniostenosis. J Neurosurg 1982;57(3):370–377

12. Thompson DN, Jones BM, Harkness W, Gonsalez S, Hayward RD. Consequences of cranial vault expansion surgery for craniosynostosis. Pediatr Neurosurg 1997;26(6):296–303

13. Fialkov JA, Holy C, Forrest CR, Phillips JH, Antonyshyn OM. Postoperative infections in craniofacial reconstructive procedures. J Craniofac Surg 2001;12(4):362–368

14. Fearon JA, Yu J, Bartlett SP, Munro IR, Chir B, Whitaker L. Infections in craniofacial surgery: a combined report of 567 procedures from two centers. Plast Reconstr Surg 1997;100(4):862–868

15. Bergsma JE, de Bruijn WC, Rozema FR, Bos RR, Boering G. Late degradation tissue response to poly(L-lactide) bone plates and screws. Biomaterials 1995;16(1):25–31

16. Eppley BL, Sadove AM, Havlik RJ. Resorbable plate fixation in pediatric craniofacial surgery. Plast Reconstr Surg 1997;100(1):1–7, discussion 8–13

17. Tharanon W, Sinn DP, Hobar PC, Sklar FH, Salomon J. Surgical outcomes using bioabsorbable plating systems in pediatric craniofacial surgery. J Craniofac Surg 1998;9(5):441–444, discussion 445–447

18. Imola MJ, Hamlar DD, Shao W, Chowdhury K, Tatum S. Resorbable plate fixation in pediatric craniofacial surgery: long-term outcome. Arch Facial Plast Surg 2001;3(2):79–90

19. Böstman OM. Osteolytic changes accompanying degradation of absorbable fracture fixation implants. J Bone Joint Surg Br 1991;73(4):679–682

20. Eppley BL, Morales L, Wood R, et al. Resorbable PLLA-PGA plate and screw fixation in pediatric craniofacial surgery: clinical experience in 1883 patients. Plast Reconstr Surg 2004;114(4):850–856, discussion 857

21. Mackool R, Yim J, McCarthy JG. Delayed degradation in a resorbable plating system. J Craniofac Surg 2006;17(1):194–197, discussion 197–198

22. Verret DJ, Ducic Y, Oxford L, Smith J. Hydroxyapatite cement in craniofacial reconstruction. Otolaryngol Head Neck Surg 2005;133(6):897–899

23. Dujovny M, Aviles A, Anger C. An innovative approach for cranioplasty using hydroxyapatite cement. Surg Neurol 1997;48(3):294–297

24. Mathur KK, Tatum SA, Kellman RM. Carbonated apatite and hydroxyapatite in craniofacial reconstruction. Arch Facial Plast Surg 2003;5(5):379–383

25. Dupoirieux L, Gard C. Hydroxyapatite cement for calvarial reconstruction. Oral Surg Oral Med Oral Pathol Oral Radiol Endod 2000;89(2):140–142

26. Psillakis JM, Grotting JC, Casanova R, Cavalcante D, Vasconez LO. Vascularized outer-table calvarial bone flaps. Plast Reconstr Surg 1986;78(3):309–317

27. Littlefield TR. Food and Drug Administration regulation of orthotic cranioplasty. Cleft Palate Craniofac J 2001;38(4):337–340

28. Hertle RW, Quinn GE, Minguini N, Katowitz JA. Visual loss in patients with craniofacial synostosis. J Pediatr Ophthalmol Strabismus 1991;28(6):344–349

29. Gray TL, Casey T, Selva D, Anderson PJ, David DJ. Ophthalmic sequelae of Crouzon syndrome. Ophthalmology 2005;112(6):1129–1134

30. Khan SH, Nischal KK, Dean F, Hayward RD, Walker J. Visual outcomes and amblyogenic risk factors in craniosynostotic syndromes: a review of 141 cases. Br J Ophthalmol 2003;87(8):999–1003

31. Tay T, Martin F, Rowe N, et al. Prevalence and causes of visual impairment in craniosynostotic syndromes. Clin Experiment Ophthalmol 2006;34(5):434–440

32. Diamond GR, Katowitz JA, Whitaker LA, Bersani TA, Bartlett SP, Welsh MG. Ocular and adnexal complications of unilateral orbital advancement for plagiocephaly. Arch Ophthalmol 1987;105(3):381–385

33. Hurmerinta K, Hukki J. Vector control in lower jaw distraction osteogenesis using an extra-oral multidirectional device. J Craniomaxillofac Surg 2001;29(5):263–270

34. Hollier LH, Kim JH, Grayson B, McCarthy JG. Mandibular growth after distraction in patients under 48 months of age. Plast Reconstr Surg 1999;103(5):1361–1370

35. Karaharju-Suvanto T, Peltonen J, Laitinen O, Kahri A. The effect of gradual distraction of the mandible on the sheep temporomandibular joint. Int J Oral Maxillofac Surg 1996;25(2):152–156

36. Carls FR, Sailer HF. Seven years clinical experience with mandibular distraction in children. J Craniomaxillofac Surg 1998;26(4):197–208

37. McComb HK, Coghlan BA. Primary repair of the unilateral cleft lip nose: completion of a longitudinal study. Cleft Palate Craniofac J 1996;33(1):23–30, discussion 30–31

38. Huffman WC, Lierle DM. Studies on the pathologic anatomy of the unilateral harelip nose. Plast Reconstr Surg (1946) 1949;4(3):225–234

39. Ariyan S, Krizek TJ. A simplified technique for correction of the cleft lip nasal deformity. Ann Plast Surg 1978;1(6):568–574

40. Dingman RO, Natvig P. The infracartilaginous incision for rhinoplasty. Plast Reconstr Surg 1982;69(1):134–135

41. Black PW, Hartrampf CR Jr, Beegle P. Cleft lip type nasal deformity: definitive repair. Ann Plast Surg 1984;12(2):128–138

42. Warren DW. A quantitative technique for assessing nasal airway impairment. Am J Orthod 1984;86(4):306–314

43. Ozaki W, Chaffoo RA, Vu KC, Markowitz BL. Comprehensive rhinoplasty technique to correct the bilateral cleft lip nasal deformity using conchal composite grafts. J Craniomaxillofac Surg 2006;34(3):150–155

44. McComb H. Primary repair of the bilateral cleft lip nose. Br J Plast Surg 1975;28(4):262–267

45. Cenzi R, Guarda L. A dynamic nostril splint in the surgery of the nasal tip: technical innovation. J Craniomaxillofac Surg 1996;24(2):88–91

46. Barsky AJ. Principles and Practice of Plastic Surgery. Baltimore: Williams and Wilkins; 2007:159–198

47. Ortiz Monasterio F, Ruas EJ. Cleft lip rhinoplasty: the role of bone and cartilage grafts. Clin Plast Surg 1989;16(1): 177–186

48. Omori M, Takato T, Eguchi T, Mori Y, Tomizuka K. Secondary correction of the wide nasal root in bilateral nasal deformity associated with cleft lip in five Oriental patients. Scand J Plast Reconstr Surg Hand Surg 2003;37(4):216–219

49. Raspall G, González-Lagunas J. Management of the nasal tip by open rhinoplasty. J Craniomaxillofac Surg 1996;24(3): 145–150

50. Gilles HD, Kilner TP. Hare-lip: operation for correction of secondary deformities. Lancet 1932;223:1369–1375

51. Gillies HD, Millard DR. The Principles and Art of Plastic Surgery. Boston: Little, Brown & Co; 2007

52. McIndoe A, Rees TD. Synchronous repair of secondary deformities in cleft lip and nose. Plast Reconstr Surg 1959; 24:150–161

53. Millard DR Jr. Earlier correction of the unilateral cleft lip nose. Plast Reconstr Surg 1982;70(1):64–73

54. Rees TD, Guy CL, Converse JM. Repair of the cleft lip-nose: addendum to the synchronous technique with full-thickness skin grafting of the nasal vestibule. Plast Reconstr Surg 1966;37(1):47–50

55. Vissarionov VA. Correction of the nasal tip deformity following repair of unilateral clefts of the upper lip. Plast Reconstr Surg 1989;83(2):341–347

56. Kirschbaum JD, Kirschbaum CA. The chondromucosal sleeve for the secondary correction of the unilateral cleft lip nasal deformity. Ann Plast Surg 1992;29(5):402–407

57. Cho BC, Lee JH, Cohen M, Baik BS. Surgical correction of unilateral cleft lip nasal deformity. J Craniofac Surg 1998;9(1): 20–29

58. Mulliken JB. Repair of bilateral complete cleft lip and nasal deformity—state of the art. Cleft Palate Craniofac J 2000; 37(4):342–347

59. Bardach J, Morris HL, Olin WH. Late results of primary veloplasty: the Marburg Project. Plast Reconstr Surg 1984; 73(2):207–218

60. Kriens OB. An anatomical approach to veloplasty. Plast Reconstr Surg 1969;43(1):29–41

61. Marsh JL, Grames LM, Holtman B. Intravelar veloplasty: a prospective study. Cleft Palate J 1989;26(1):46–50

62. Furlow LT Jr. Cleft palate repair by double opposing Z-plasty. Plast Reconstr Surg 1986;78(6):724–738

63. Spauwen PH, Goorhuis-Brouwer SM, Schutte HK. Cleft palate repair: Furlow versus von Langenbeck. J Craniomaxillofac Surg 1992;20(1):18–20

64. Yu CC, Chen PK, Chen YR. Comparison of speech results after Furlow palatoplasty and von Langenbeck palatoplasty in incomplete cleft of the secondary palate. Chang Gung Med J 2001;24(10):628–632

65. Sie KC, Tampakopoulou DA, Sorom J, Gruss JS, Eblen LE. Results with Furlow palatoplasty in management of velopharyngeal insufficiency. Plast Reconstr Surg 2001;108(1):17–25, discussion 26–29

66. Friede H, Enocson L, Lilja J. Features of maxillary arch and nasal cavity in infancy and their influence on deciduous occlusion in unilateral cleft lip and palate. Scand J Plast Reconstr Surg Hand Surg 1988;22(1):69–75

67. Semb G. A study of facial growth in patients with unilateral cleft lip and palate treated by the Oslo CLP Team. Cleft Palate Craniofac J 1991;28(1):1–21, discussion 46–48

68. Cohen SR, Kalinowski J, LaRossa D, Randall P. Cleft palate fistulas: a multivariate statistical analysis of prevalence, etiology, and surgical management. Plast Reconstr Surg 1991;87(6):1041–1047

69. Abyholm FE, Borchgrevink HH, Eskeland G. Palatal fistulae following cleft palate surgery. Scand J Plast Reconstr Surg 1979;13(2):295–300

70. Campbell DA. Fistulae in the hard palate following cleft palate surgery. Br J Plast Surg 1962;15:377–384

71. Jolleys A, Savage JP. Healing defects in cleft palate surgery: The role of infection. Br J Plast Surg 1962;16:134

72. McClelland RMA, Patterson TJS. The influence of penicillin on the complication rate after repair of clefts of the lip and palate. Br J Plast Surg 1962;16:144

73. Musgrave RH, Bremner JC. Complications of cleft palate surgery. Plast Reconstr Surg Transplant Bull 1960;26: 180–189

74. Posnick JC, Getz SB Jr. Surgical closure of end-stage palatal fistulas using anteriorly-based dorsal tongue flaps. J Oral Maxillofac Surg 1987;45(11):907–912

75. Honnebier MB, Johnson DS, Parsa AA, Dorian A, Parsa FD. Closure of palatal fistula with a local mucoperiosteal flap lined with buccal mucosal graft. Cleft Palate Craniofac J 2000;37(2):127–129

76. Wood FM. Hypoxia: another issue to consider when timing cleft repair. Ann Plast Surg 1994;32(1):15–18, discussion 19–20

77. Isberg A, Henningsson G. Influence of palatal fistulas on velopharyngeal movements: a cineradiographic study. Plast Reconstr Surg 1987;79(4):525–530

78. Schultz RC. Management and timing of cleft palate fistula repair. Plast Reconstr Surg 1986;78(6):739–747

79. Amaratunga NA. Occurrence of oronasal fistulas in operated cleft palate patients. J Oral Maxillofac Surg 1988;46(10): 834–838

80. Rintala AE. Surgical closure of palatal fistulae: follow-up of 84 personally treated cases. Scand J Plast Reconstr Surg 1980;14(3):235–238

81. Emory RE Jr, Clay RP, Bite U, Jackson IT. Fistula formation and repair after palatal closure: an institutional perspective. Plast Reconstr Surg 1997;99(6):1535–1538

82. Muzaffar AR, Byrd HS, Rohrich RJ, et al. Incidence of cleft palate fistula: an institutional experience with two-stage palatal repair. Plast Reconstr Surg 2001;108(6):1515–1518

83. Bardach J, Salyer K. Surgical Techniques in Cleft Lip and Palate. Chicago: Year Books; 1987

84. Coghlan K, O'Regan B, Carter J. Tongue flap repair of oro-nasal fistulae in cleft palate patients. A review of 20 patients. J Craniomaxillofac Surg 1989;17(6):255–259

85. Egyedi P. Utilization of the buccal fat pad for closure of oro-antral and/or oro-nasal communications. J Maxillofac Surg 1977;5(4):241–244

86. Batchelor AG, Palmer JH. A novel method of closing a palatal fistula: the free fascial flap. Br J Plast Surg 1990;43(3): 359–361

87. Chen HC, Ganos DL, Coessens BC, Kyutoku S, Noordhoff MS. Free forearm flap for closure of difficult oronasal fistulas in cleft palate patients. Plast Reconstr Surg 1992;90(5):757–762

88. Corrêa Chem R, Franciosi LF. Dorsalis pedis free flap to close extensive palate fistulae. Microsurgery 1983;4(1):35–39

89. Inoue T, Harashina T, Asanami S, Fujino T. Reconstruction of the hard palate using free iliac bone covered with a jejunal flap. Br J Plast Surg 1988;41(2):143–146

90. MacLeod AM, Morrison WA, McCann JJ, Thistlethwaite S, Vanderkolk CA, Ryan AD. The free radial forearm flap with and without bone for closure of large palatal fistulae. Br J Plast Surg 1987;40(4):391–395

91. Soutar DS, Scheker LR, Tanner NS, McGregor IA. The radial forearm flap: a versatile method for intra-oral reconstruction. Br J Plast Surg 1983;36(1):1–8

92. Taub PJ, Bradley JP, Kawamoto HK. Closure of an oronasal fistula in an irradiated palate by tissue and bone distraction osteogenesis. J Craniofac Surg 2001;12(5):495–499, discussion 500

93. De Mey A, Malevez C, Lejour M. Treatment of palatal fistula by expansion. Br J Plast Surg 1990;43(3):362–364

94. Van Damme PA, Freihofer HP. Palatal mucoperiosteal expansion as an adjunct to palatal fistula repair: case report and review of the literature. Cleft Palate Craniofac J 1996;33(3):255–257

95. Matsuo K, Kiyono M, Hirose T. A simple technique for closure of a palatal fistula using a conchal cartilage graft. Plast Reconstr Surg 1991;88(2):334–337

96. Ohsumi N, Onizuka T, Ito Y. Use of a free conchal cartilage graft for closure of a palatal fistula: an experimental study and clinical application. Plast Reconstr Surg 1993;91(3): 433–440

97. Mohanna PN, Kangesu L, Sommerlad BC. The use of conchal-cartilage grafts in the closure of recurrent palatal fistulae. Br J Plast Surg 2001;54(3):274

98. Clark JM, Saffold SH, Israel JM. Decellularized dermal grafting in cleft palate repair. Arch Facial Plast Surg 2003;5(1):40–44, discussion 45

99. Kirschner RE, Cabiling DS, Slemp AE, Siddiqi F, LaRossa DD, Losee JE. Repair of oronasal fistulae with acellular dermal matrices. Plast Reconstr Surg 2006;118(6):1431–1440

100. Losee JE, Smith DM, Afifi AM, et al. A successful algorithm for limiting postoperative fistulae following palatal procedures in the patient with orofacial clefting. Plast Reconstr Surg 2008;122(2):544–554

101. Witt PD, D'Antonio LL. Velopharyngeal insufficiency and secondary palatal management. A new look at an old problem. Clin Plast Surg 1993;20(4):707–721

102. Trost-Cardamone JE. Coming to terms with VPI: a response to Loney and Bloem. Cleft Palate J 1989;26(1):68–70

103. Golding-Kushner KJ, Argamaso RV, Cotton RT, et al. Standardization for the reporting of nasopharyngoscopy and multiview videofluoroscopy: a report from an International Working Group. Cleft Palate J 1990;27(4):337–347, discussion 347–348

104. Hynes W. Pharyngoplasty by muscle transplantation. Br J Plast Surg 1950;3(2):128–135

105. Wilk A, Champy M. [Repair of soft palate deficiencies in adults by Orticochea's method (author's transl)]. Rev Stomatol Chir Maxillofac 1981;82(1):22–27

106. Jackson IT. Sphincter pharyngoplasty. Clin Plast Surg 1985; 12(4):711–717

107. Witt PD, D'Antonio LL, Zimmerman GJ, Marsh JL. Sphincter pharyngoplasty: a preoperative and postoperative analysis of perceptual speech characteristics and endoscopic studies of velopharyngeal function. Plast Reconstr Surg 1994;93(6):1154–1168

108. Witt PD, Marsh JL, Muntz HR, Marty-Grames L, Watchmaker GP. Acute obstructive sleep apnea as a complication of sphincter pharyngoplasty. Cleft Palate Craniofac J 1996;33(3): 183–189

109. Witt PD, O'Daniel TG, Marsh JL, Grames LM, Muntz HR, Pilgram TK. Surgical management of velopharyngeal dysfunction: outcome analysis of autogenous posterior pharyngeal wall augmentation. Plast Reconstr Surg 1997;99(5):1287–1296, discussion 1297–1300

110. Riski JE, Serafin D, Riefkohl R, Georgiade GS, Georgiade NG. A rationale for modifying the site of insertion of the Orticochea pharyngoplasty. Plast Reconstr Surg 1984;73(6): 882–894

111. Chegar BE, Shprintzen RJ, Curtis MS, Tatum SA. Pharyngeal flap and obstructive apnea: maximizing speech outcome while limiting complications. Arch Facial Plast Surg 2007;9(4):252–259

112. Marsh JL, Wray RC. Speech prosthesis versus pharyngeal flap: a randomized evaluation of the management of velopharyngeal incompetency. Plast Reconstr Surg 1980;65(5): 592–594

113. Tucker AL, Hubbard JG. Retropharyngeal infection with disc space involvement and osteomyelitis, following a pharyngeal flap operation. Case report. Plast Reconstr Surg 1974;53(4):477–478

114. Losquadro WD, Tatum SA. Direct gingivoperiosteoplasty with palatoplasty. Facial Plast Surg 2007;23(2):140–145

115. Rosenstein S, Dado DV, Kernahan D, Griffith BH, Grasseschi M. The case for early bone grafting in cleft lip and palate: a second report. Plast Reconstr Surg 1991;87(4):644–654, discussion 655–656

116. Rosenstein S, Kernahan D, Dado D, Grasseschi M, Griffith BH. Orthognathic surgery in cleft patients treated by early bone grafting. Plast Reconstr Surg 1991;87(5):835–892, discussion 840–842

117. Eppley BL. Alveolar cleft bone grafting (Part I): Primary bone grafting. J Oral Maxillofac Surg 1996;54(1):74–82

118. Long RE Jr, Paterno M, Vinson B. Effect of cuspid positioning in the cleft at the time of secondary alveolar bone grafting on eventual graft success. Cleft Palate Craniofac J 1996;33(3):225–230

119. Cohen M, Polley JW, Figueroa AA. Secondary (intermediate) alveolar bone grafting. Clin Plast Surg 1993;20(4): 691–705

120. Shaw GM, Carmichael SL, Kaidarova Z, Harris JA. Epidemiologic characteristics of anotia and microtia in California, 1989–1997. Birth Defects Res A Clin Mol Teratol 2004;70(7):472–475

121. Aguilar EF III. Auricular reconstruction of congenital microtia (grade III). Laryngoscope 1996; 106(12 Pt 2, Suppl 82): 1–26

122. Forrester MB, Merz RD. Impact of excluding cases with known chromosomal abnormalities on the prevalence of structural birth defects, Hawaii, 1986–1999. Am J Med Genet A 2004;128A(4):383–388

123. Tanzer RC. Total reconstruction of the auricle. The evolution of a plan of treatment. Plast Reconstr Surg 1971;47(6):523–533

124. Brent B. Auricular repair with autogenous rib cartilage grafts: two decades of experience with 600 cases. Plast Reconstr Surg 1992;90(3):319–374

125. Brent B. Microtia repair with rib cartilage grafts: a review of personal experience with 1000 cases. Clin Plast Surg 2002;29(2):257–271, vii

126. Beahm EK, Walton RL. Auricular reconstruction for microtia: part I. Anatomy, embryology, and clinical evaluation. Plast Reconstr Surg 2002;109(7):2473–2482, quiz 2482

127. Romo T III, Fozo MS, Sclafani AP. Microtia reconstruction using a porous polyethylene framework. Facial Plast Surg 2000;16(1):15–22

128. Reinisch J. Microtia reconstruction using a polyethylene implant: An eight-year surgical experience. 2007. Presented at the 78th Annual Meeting of the American Association of Plastic Surgeons, Colorado Springs, CO.

129. Botma M, Aymat A, Gault D, Albert DM. Rib graft reconstruction versus osseointegrated prosthesis for microtia: a significant change in patient preference. Clin Otolaryngol Allied Sci 2001;26(4):274–277

130. Ohara K, Nakamura K, Ohta E. Chest wall deformities and thoracic scoliosis after costal cartilage graft harvesting. Plast Reconstr Surg 1997;99(4):1030–1036

131. Walton RL, Beahm EK. Auricular reconstruction for microtia: Part II. Surgical techniques. Plast Reconstr Surg 2002;110(1):234–249, quiz 250–251, 387

132. Nagata S. Microtia: Auricular Reconstruction. In: Vanderkolk CA, ed. Plastic Surgery: Indications, Operations, and Outcomes. St. Louis: Mosby; 2007:1023–1056

133. Adamson PA, McGraw BL, Tropper GJ. Otoplasty: critical review of clinical results. Laryngoscope 1991;101(8):883–888

134. Goode RL, Proffitt SD, Rafaty FM. Complications of otoplasty. Arch Otolaryngol 1970;91(4):352–355

16

Complications in Orthognathic Surgery

Travis T. Tollefson, Shepherd G. Pryor V, and Nicholas W. Rotas

Orthognathic surgery is widely used to correct congenital and acquired dentofacial discrepancies. The principles of orthognathic surgery were developed for treatment of facial disharmony and dental malocclusion; however, the techniques are also useful for consideration of maxillofacial tumor resection and as therapy for obstructive sleep apnea syndrome. Orthognathic surgical procedures can produce a high degree of satisfaction for the patient and surgeon, but they remain challenging in both presurgical planning and surgical execution. The benefits of orthognathic surgery include better masticator function, reduced facial pain, and improved facial aesthetics. However, numerous complications have been reported that can be attributed to improper surgical planning, technical errors, or poor wound healing. These can be loosely categorized as (1) vascular or nerve injuries, (2) temporomandibular joint dysfunction, (3) bone or soft-tissue infections, (4) periodontal disease, (5) change in airway (obstructive sleep apnea) or swallowing function, and (6) psychological problems.

The bulk of this chapter is organized according to the complications seen in specific procedures. By reviewing the potential pitfalls that may be encountered in each procedure, this chapter should provide insight to those who perform orthognathic surgery, including head and neck surgeons, oral and maxillofacial surgeons, and facial plastic surgeons.

◆ Common Complications Associated with Orthognathic Surgery

Complications commonly associated with the spectrum of orthognathic surgical procedures are listed in **Table 16.1**. Of these, special attention will be given to infection and relapse as universal complications associated with all procedures.

Infection

Infection after orthognathic surgery may be acute or chronic, local or general. Endogenous bacteria, most likely a mixture of anaerobic and aerobic bacteria, cause most postoperative infections. Factors contributing to this in orthognathic surgery populations may be the usage of steroids, the duration of the surgical procedure, the patient's age, interference with the blood supply to the bony segments, dehydration of the wounds, the presence of foreign bodies or sequestrum, hospitalization in large wards, nutrition, hematoma, and smoking. The surgeon's experience, a good aseptic technique, and gentle tissue handling are also relevant factors.[1]

In the classical wound classification, normal orthognathic surgery wounds fall into the Class II category (clean contaminated wound). An infection rate of 10% to 15% can be expected without use of antibiotics, in comparison to Class III wounds, with an expected infection rate of 20% to 30%. In a clean wound (Class I), the probability of infection is approximately 2%.[1] Studies dealing with infection after mandibular osteotomies report infection rates ranging from 0% to 18%.[2] In maxillary osteotomies, infection rates lower than 6% are mostly reported,[3] but

Table 16.1

Orthognathic Surgery Complications
• Infection
• Hardware exposure
• Unanticipated fractures
• Devitalization of teeth
• Malunion and/or nonunion
• Malocclusion
• Injury to teeth
• Gingival recession and/or periodontal complications
• Respiratory decompensation
• Bleeding
• Relapse

in the study of Zijderveld et al. (1999),[4] a 52.6% infection rate was found in a placebo medication group with bimaxillary surgery.

There is some controversy concerning the need for prophylactic antibiotics,[4] and many different practices exist. The operator must assess dosage, timing, duration of therapy, and side effects when considering the use of antibiotic prophylaxis. Peterson (1990)[5] has outlined the following principles for the rational use of antibiotic prophylaxis in orthognathic surgery: (1) The surgical procedure should involve a significant risk for infection; increased risk is seen with both bone grafts and wound class II (10–15%). (2) Proper antibiotics should be selected. (3) Serum concentrations of the antibiotic should be appropriately high. (4) The chosen antibiotic must be administered in a correct time sequence. (5) The shortest effective antibiotic exposure should be used.

Relapse

Relapse is an unpredictable risk of orthognathic surgery. Many studies reporting relapse have limitations of sample size or the duration of follow-up, involve different surgical techniques being applied in the same sample, or suffer from limitations in the application of cephalometric measurements. Relapse may be dental, skeletal, or both.

In general, mandibular advancement appears to be stable if rigid internal fixation is used[6–8] and if anterior facial height is maintained or increased.[9] Several factors may affect relapse in mandibular advancements: the surgeon's skills; proximal segment control, including condylar positioning and prevention of proximal segment rotation; prevention of counterclockwise rotation of the distal segment in cases with a high mandibular plane angle; the degree of mandibular advancement; and the stretching of the perimandibular tissues, including skin, connective tissues, muscles and periosteum.[10] Mandibular setback is not always stable, and the inclination of the ramus at surgery appears to have an important influence on stability.[9]

The stability of maxillary osteotomies is affected by the magnitude of the anterior movement and the magnitude of the inferior repositioning of the maxilla, the adequacy of mobilization of the downfractured maxilla at surgery, the extent of bone contact in the newly established position of the maxilla, and the type of fixation.[11] On the other hand, Louis et al. (1993)[12] did not find any correlation between relapse and the magnitude of maxillary advancement. The most stable maxillary procedure is superior repositioning, and forward movement is also reasonably stable. Inferior repositioning is the least stable, especially if it causes downward rotation of the mandible and stretching of the elevator muscles of the jaw. Proffit et al. reported that the least stable orthognathic procedure is transverse expansion of the maxilla.[9]

◆ Complications of Mandibular Surgery

Bilateral Sagittal-Split Osteotomy

The most common procedure to correct mandibular deformities is the bilateral sagittal-split osteotomy (BSSO), which is useful for both mandibular setback or advancement (**Fig. 16.1**). The most commonly reported complications for BSSO are listed in **Table 16.2**.

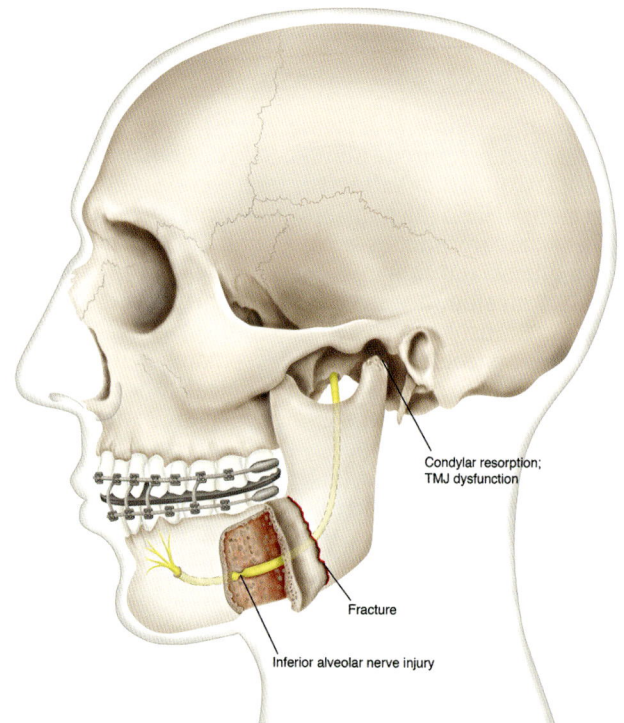

Fig. 16.1 Illustration of the potential complications that can occur with the bilateral sagittal-split osteotomy procedure. (*Illustration by Robert Brown*.)

Table 16.2

Bilateral Sagittal-Split Osteotomy (BSSO) Complications
• Unanticipated fracture or unfavorable split
• Nerve injury
• Bleeding (inferior alveolar artery, masseteric artery)
• Proximal segment malpositioning
• Temporomandibular joint dysfunction
• Condylar resorption
• Avascular necrosis
• Interfragmentary incompatibilities
• Distal segment interference with large setbacks.

Unanticipated Fracture or Unfavorable Splits

Fractures of the osteotomized segments in BSSO (i.e., bad splits) have been reported to occur in 3 to 23% of cases.[13-15] Proper corticotomy technique is the first line of prevention. Many modifications (Hunsuck,[16,17] Epker,[18] Wolford[19]) of the initial procedure by Dal Pont[20] have lessened the chance of unfavorable splits. Of great importance is the position of the burr or saw blade during the medial ramus cut that must be angled parallel to the mandibular occlusal plane. Likewise, adequate but minimal visualization of the lateral ramus allows for appropriate positioning of the medial cut and avoids risking a horizontal ramus fracture. Removal of a small amount of the internal oblique ridge with a large burr in the area of the proposed medial ramal cut may enhance visualization.[21] The vertical lateral corticotomy of the mandibular body should penetrate only the cortex. The corticotomy that connects the medial and lateral corticotomies should be as lateral as possible while still remaining inside the lateral cortex. The inferior border osteotomy must be cut through both cortices to enhance a favorable split. The only time one would not want to cut through both cortices is when an inferior border saw is used.[22]

Some surgeons remove mandibular third molars during the BSSO,[23,24] but most authors routinely recommend this at least six months before BSSO surgery. This allows time for bone healing and helps ensure a favorable split. Often the third molars are not in the center of the buccal and lingual plates, thus increasing the chance of an unfavorable split if they are removed at the time of a BSSO.

Steps to prevent an unfavorable split include careful use of a bibeveled chisel to complete the split after the medial and lateral osteotomies. Another technique uses a Smith spreader to enhance separation of the segments. While inspecting the bone separation, the surgeon adjusts the chisel position to help prevent unfavorable fractures or injury to the inferior alveolar nerve. While the surgeon separates the bone segments, the nerve is carefully released from the proximal segment. A proper split is ensured when the proximal and distal segments have independent movement. A finger on the medial aspect can ensure the proximal (condylar) segment is not moving while minimally moving the distal (tooth-bearing) segment. This technique prevents transmission of heavy prying forces to the proximal and distal segments.

If an unfavorable split occurs, it is most important for the surgeon to decide whether to proceed with the planned procedure or to return the fragments to their native location and abort the surgery. If the surgery is not aborted, the key feature of treatment on an unfavorable fracture is rigid plating. The initial management is to ensure that the osteotomy is completed and that separation of the condylar segment from the distal (tooth-bearing) segment has occurred. The free fractured pieces are fixed to the repositioned mandible with miniplates, making sure the condyle is seated. This can be challenging even in the hands of an experienced surgeon. Depending on the stability of the segments, one may choose to monitor the postoperative occlusion without intermaxillary fixation (MMF) or elect to place the patient in MMF for eight weeks. Counterclockwise rotation of the proximal segment is the most common indicator that healing is delayed and that migration of the fragments has occurred. Periodic radiographs (Panorex) will monitor the condylar and ramal position and bone healing. A second surgery to create osteotomies and bone graft may be warranted if nonunion or malunion is identified.

Nerve Injury

Nerve injuries in orthognathic surgery can be caused by indirect trauma (e.g., from compression by surgical edema), direct trauma with surgical instruments, or stretching during manipulation of the osteotomized bone segments.[14] The most common sensory nerve injury with BSSO occurs to the inferior alveolar nerve (IAN) as it courses through the mandibular canal. The risk of injury to the IAN is a significant disadvantage of the sagittal-split osteotomy. The incidence of transection is reportedly 2–3.5%.[24] A long-term neurological deficit reportedly occurs to some degree in 10–30% of patients, although not all are symptomatic.[25] When a sagittal-split osteotomy is combined with genioplasty, nearly 70% of patients have some degree of neurosensory deficit after one year.[26,27] Patients must accept this tradeoff between benefits and risks before undergoing mandibular surgery. Several factors have been identified that may predispose a patient to IAN injury, including age, the magnitude of mandibular movement, position of the inferior alveolar nerve, concomitant genioplasty, the surgeon's skills, and the degree of manipulation of the IAN.[14,28,29] Even with careful manipulation of the IAN, persistent sensation disturbances are possible.[30-32] The most dependable way to prevent this complication is a controlled osteotomy under direct vision. The inferior alveolar nerve is particularly vulnerable at the anterior aspect of the split, but it may be damaged anywhere from the pterygomandibular space to the vertical osteotomy site. Errant and aggressive drilling, sawing, or chiseling can damage the nerve at any point along its course.

When the IAN has been injured or transected during a procedure, an immediate attempt should be made to assess and repair the damage. Options include apposition of the nerve segments or primary neurorrhaphy, but proximal and distal nerve segments may need to be released from the bone as far as the mental foramen to provide a tension-free closure. There is no reported correlation between operator-observed partial injury and postoperative neurosensory changes.[33] Therefore, extensive dissection must be weighed carefully, and conservative management may be the best choice.

Some patients may complain of postoperative dysthesia in the distribution of the inferior alveolar nerve. This is difficult to diagnose and manage, and often observation is employed. If symptoms are relieved by injecting a nerve block, it may indicate that a nerve decompression could be helpful. Preoperative discussion with the patient must emphasize that nerve decompression may not, however, relieve these symptoms.

Lingual nerve sensory deficits occur less frequently than IAN sensory disturbances. The initial postoperative incidence has been reported between 1% and 19%;[34,35] however, lingual nerve sensory deficits tend to resolve over time. Tissue retraction along the medial mandible and bony fixation methods are the proposed mechanisms of injury.

Facial nerve paralysis is a devastating outcome of BSSO. De Vriese et al. reported a low incidence (0.26%) of facial nerve injuries in a series of 1747 BSSO cases.[36] Steps to prevent this complication include careful subperiosteal elevation and chisel orientation. Facial nerve injury is more common in mandibular set-back procedures done for prognathism.[37] Damage to the marginal mandibular branch of the facial nerve is a well-known complication of extraoral approaches to the mandibular ramus or angle, but these approaches in orthognathic surgery are rare. The presumed traumatic mechanisms have included compression caused by retractors placed behind the posterior ramus, fracture of the styloid process, and direct pressure as a result of distal segment setback. The prognosis is better if there is incomplete loss of function, and worse if the loss of function is immediate and complete.[38]

If facial nerve injury is suspected, the surgeon should provide ample time for the effects of local anesthesia to dissipate. If facial paralysis evolves gradually over a period of days, it may be assumed that a complete return of function will occur over time. If, however, complete paralysis is encountered early, standard facial nerve studies are warranted (e.g., nerve excitability testing or electroneuronography. Evoked electromyography (EMG) is an additional test that can help predict return of function.[39] Nerve exploration with reanastomosis and possible sural nerve grafting may be considered. Protection of the eye with lubrication, moisture chambers, or eyelid taping should be emphasized to prevent corneal exposure and keratopathy.

Bleeding

Uncontrolled hemorrhage may result from either a mechanical disruption of the blood vessels or a congenital or acquired coagulopathy.[40] The most common cause of hemorrhage in orthognathic surgery is a lack of surgical hemostasis.[41] Factors contributing to immediate or secondary hemorrhage may include variations in anatomy (bone or vascular), aggressive dissection, tearing of the periosteum during dissection, and hypotensive intraoperative anesthesia with postoperative hypertension. A more rapid recovery by the patient has been reported when major bleeding is avoided.[42] Prevention of bleeding begins with the patient history. Reports of prior bleeding experiences or a family history suggestive of coagulopathy warrant preoperative coagulation studies.

The most likely sources of bleeding include the inferior alveolar and the masseteric arteries. The inferior alveolar artery courses with the IAN through the mandibular canal and is contained within the pterygomandibular space. Bleeding from this vessel should be treated by pressure, packing, thrombin spray, and possibly even ligation or cautery once the IAN has been identified and retracted. The masseteric artery is not commonly encountered during a controlled dissection.

The facial artery and retromandibular vein are placed at risk if the lateral mandibular periosteum is violated. Proper dissection for a BSSO should require very little lateral mandibular ramal dissection. Transcervical exposure may be necessary to control hemorrhage if packing, direct control with bipolar cautery, or thrombogenic agents are unsuccessful. A pressure dressing may be warranted if immediate postoperative swelling and hemorrhage are seen. If any signs of airway compromise or of rapid expansion of the oral cavity or neck occur, an immediate return to the operating room is warranted for exploration and evacuation of a hematoma.

Temporomandibular Joint (TMJ) Dysfunction

Temporomandibular joint (TMJ) dysfunction must be carefully assessed and discussed preoperatively. Although some patients have improvement of symptoms after orthognathic surgery, others may develop symptoms. Fibrous ankylosis or joint hypomobility following orthognathic surgery has been proposed to be caused by several factors: immobilization of the TMJ by MMF,[43] iatrogenic posterior displacement of the condyle, intra-articular hematoma,[44] or excessive stripping of the periosteum and muscle attachments in the ascending ramus, which can result in myofibrotic tissue formation.[45] Multiple pharmacologic therapies (e.g., doxycycline, vitamin C) have been suggested to help stabilize the joint and may be helpful.

Condylar Resorption

The importance of the preoperative assessment of TMJ health with a detailed history, centric-mounted models, and radiographic exams (lateral cephalogram, baseline tomographs, and Panorex) must be emphasized (**Fig. 16.2**). The final outcome of the surgery may be altered if the condyles are not seated during the modeling. Several risk factors for condylar resorption after orthognathic surgery have been proposed. Preoperative morphological or functional factors include radiological signs of osteoarthrosis, TMJ dysfunction, a posteriorly inclined

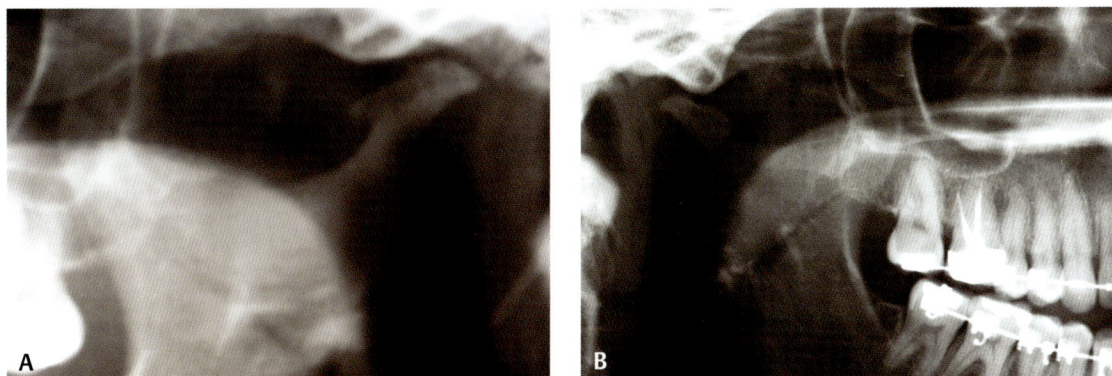

Fig. 16.2 (A) Radiograph of the left mandibular condyle depicting severe condylar resorption prior to orthognathic surgery. **(B)** Radiograph of same patient showing the resorption of the right condyle.

condyle, a high mandibular plane angle, and a low posterior-to-anterior facial height ratio.[46–51] Contributing surgical factors include major mandibular advancement, counterclockwise rotation of the mandibular proximal fragment, rigid internal fixation with incorrect placement of condylar head, or avascular necrosis of the condyle.[46,48,49,51,53–55] Young females (15–30 years) have a higher risk for condylar resorption than males and older females.[47,48,50,51,56] The incidence of postoperative condylar resorption has been reported to vary from 1% to 31%. This wide range probably reflects the great variation in the study populations.[46,49,57,59] Rigid fixation is the most successful way to avoid osteotomy slippage and condylar resorption. Postoperative recommendations are varied and are not standardized. It may be unwise to reoperate on a patient with condylar resorption, as further revision osteotomies may compound the problem. Mandibular splinting may provide relief from myofascial pain if it is present. If the patients fit a high-risk profile as outlined above, often preoperative splinting by the their orthodontist may help prevent further condylar resorption.

Proximal Segment Malposition

Prevention of an undesirable proximal mandibular segment rotation or position begins with careful preoperative planning. Intraoperatively, the inferior border of the proximal and distal mandibular segments should be used as a landmark for correct vertical positioning. Introduction of a rotational component makes alignment more difficult. The inferior border of the distal or proximal segment may lie in a different plane if the mandibular segments are rotated clockwise or counterclockwise. Rigid fixation will help to prevent motion and migration of the planned advancement or setback.[59] Fixation of the proximal segment may also be achieved with either an inferior border wire or a combined superior border wire and MMF.[60]

Postoperatively, a physical exam and determination of the patient's comfort with occlusion are paramount to diagnosing malpositioning. Even when there is an anomaly on a Panorex radiograph, if the patient has no occlusal complaints, observation may be warranted. A more serious problem occurs when shifting of the proximal segment becomes evident. There may be shifting of the mandibular midline or an open bite deformity present that indicates malposition of one or both condyles. This may occur at any time following surgery; however, if it is noted in the first three weeks, it may be reasonable to place the patient in MMF again to allow for additional wound healing and fracture line security. Delayed malalignment often necessitates surgical intervention with osteotomies and bone grafting.

Intraoral Vertical Ramus Osteotomy

Intraoral vertical ramus osteotomy (IVRO) may be used for mandibular setbacks. The operation can be performed more quickly and with less morbidity than BSSO, but it offers less control of the proximal segment and often results in condylar sag, with resultant open bite deformity. IVRO is indicated in cases that require vertical changes between the proximal and distal segments and involve a mandibular setback on at least one side. Hemifacial hyperplasia is one example. The most common complications of IVRO are listed in **Table 16.3**.

Condylar Sag

Condylar sag is the lack of proper seating of the condylar head in the glenoid fossa. One method that some surgeons use to avoid condylar sag is to overcompensate in the presurgical workup by providing a posterior open

Table 16.3

Intraoral Vertical Ramus Osteotomy (IVRO) Complications
• Condylar sag
• Bleeding
• Nerve Injury
• Inappropriate osteotomy
• Anterior open bite

bite in the planned postoperative occlusion. During MMF, the posterior space can be built up slightly with an occlusal wafer. If it is removed before complete healing, closure of the open bite may rotate the osteotomy site. On the other hand, if the splint is removed following complete healing, the condyles are seated using light guiding elastics instead of heavy elastics that may place excessive stress on the condylar head.

Bleeding

The most likely source of excessive bleeding during IVRO is the masseteric artery as it passes through the sigmoid notch of the ramus.[61] During retraction, it is easy to place this vessel on stretch, making it difficult to identify. Every attempt should be made to ligate the vessel directly. As with BSSO, in IVRO the surgeon must carefully avoid the facial artery and retromandibular vein.

Nerve Injury

Sensory nerve injury in IVRO is less likely than in BSSO[62]; however, careful placement of the vertical osteotomy is essential to avoid inadvertent injury to the inferior alveolar nerve as it enters at the mandibular lingula. The osteotomy is completed behind the mandibular foramen from the sigmoid notch to the posterior border of the mandible. The IAN may be injured if the proximal segment slips medial to the distal segment. The vast majority of postoperative dysthesias will resolve over 12–18 months' time. Although it has been reported, facial nerve injury is exceedingly rare in this procedure.[63,64]

Inappropriate Osteotomy

Subcondylar osteotomy has been reported as a complication of the IVRO procedure.[15,65] A poorly placed posterior osteotomy may cause severe proximal segment rotation. Proper exposure and direct visualization of the planned cuts should prevent this complication. One pearl is to identify the antilingula on the buccal (lateral) surface of the mandible for orientation of the lingula.

Open Bite

Open bite deformity (**Fig. 16.3**) is relatively common with IVRO compared with BSSO.[66,67] The surgeon has the least control over the proximal segments with the IVRO technique. The condyle may be seated properly at surgery but sag inferiorly away from the glenoid fossa during healing. This results in a gap above the condyle and inferior to the glenoid fossa. Once MMF is released, the masticator muscles reseat the condyle, and an open bite can occur. Although condylar resorption is a proposed theory, the circumferential condylar blood supply (in contrast to the femoral head blood supply) may make this unlikely.[68] Condylar resorption also tends to occur months or even years postoperatively, making it less likely that such a mechanism may induce an immediate open bite deformity.

Body and Symphysis Osteotomy

Osteotomies performed in the body and symphysis usually pass between teeth and place the inferior alveolar nerve at risk when posterior to the mental foramen. If they are anterior to the foramen, then the surgeon needs to be cognizant of the added rotational forces placed upon the mandible by the muscles of mastication. Complications for these procedures are listed in **Table 16.4**.

Malpositioning

Malpositioning is the most common complication associated with osteotomies of the tooth-bearing section of the mandible.[69] Careful model surgery may enhance the outcome in the preoperative setting. Intraoperatively, rigid fixation and good splint alignment are recommended. Most importantly, after fixation of the segments, the planned occlusion should be verified as

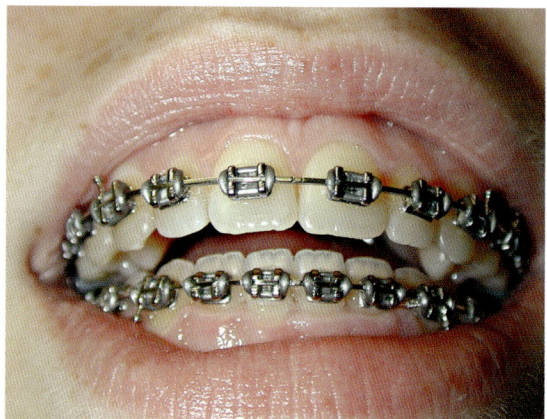

Fig. 16.3 Photograph of patient's occlusion with orthodontic devices in place illustrating an open-bite deformity.

Table 16.4

Body and Symphysis Osteotomy Complications

- Malpositioning of segments
- Nonunion of segments
- Periodontal defects possibly causing loss of teeth adjacent to the osteotomy
- Devitalization of teeth, possibly necessitating endodontic treatment
- Nerve injury
- Loss of entire bony segment due to devitalization and poor blood supply

outlined on the preoperative workup. If the postoperative occlusion is incorrect, then an early return to the operating room or consultation with the patient's orthodontist may be helpful.

Periodontal Defects and Devitalized Teeth

Careful surgical technique and planning of soft-tissue and bony work are essential. The dental papilla should be well preserved intraoperatively. Avoidance of apical tooth roots by staying at least 5 mm above or below the apices of the teeth (depending on the jaw being operated on) limits pulp injury. Osteotomies between teeth require at least 3 mm of space, which can be enhanced with preoperative orthodontic care and planning.[70] Endodontic treatment may be necessary. Periodontal and tooth damage may be encountered, especially in segmental osteotomies. Most problems are caused by errors in surgical technique, which reinforces the need for preoperative planning. The design of the soft-tissue incisions is critical, as vertical incisions in the area of osteotomy will predictably create periodontal problems. Trauma to the lingual mucoperiosteum is a risk. Excessive heat generated by the saw or drill must be countered by copious irrigation and careful protection of the soft tissues from injury. Poor oral hygiene plays some role in periodontal problems. It should be reemphasized that these problems may be minimized if an interdental space is created preoperatively by orthodontic means.[71]

Genioplasty

Genioplasty is a challenging and versatile technique that is useful in isolated cases of horizontal or vertical mandibular discrepancies, as well as in combination with other orthognathic procedures (**Fig. 16.4**). The complications most often associated with genioplasty are list-

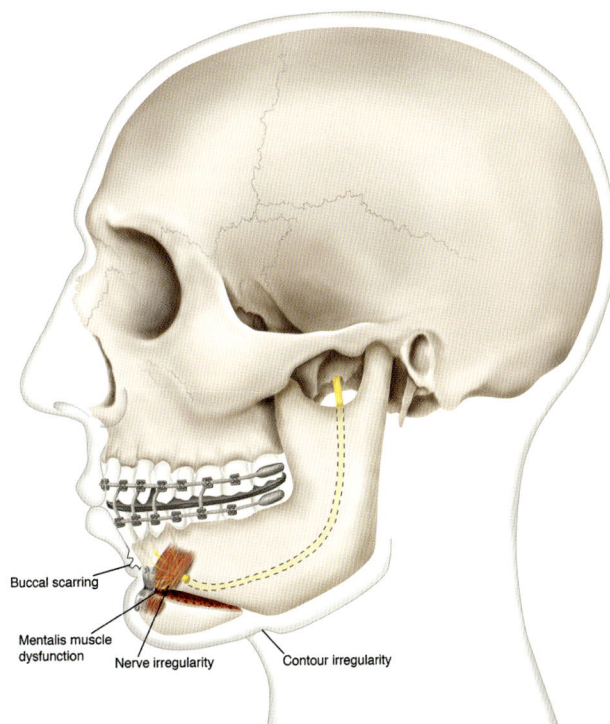

Fig. 16.4 Illustration of the potential complications that can occur with the sliding osseous genioplasty procedure. (*Illustration by Robert Brown.*)

ed in **Table 16.5**. Careful dissection of the mental nerve, reinsertion of the mentalis muscle fibers (with two-layer closure), stepped soft-tissue incision (soft-tissue incision at one level and muscle dissection at a lower level in the chin), and careful subperiosteal dissection plane will limit these complications.

Nerve Injury

Neuropraxia often occurs after genioplasty. This complication may be avoided with meticulous technique and careful surgical planning of the osteotomy sites. Dissec-

Table 16.5

Genioplasty Complications

- Nerve injury (mental nerve)[104]
- Inferior mandibular border contour irregularity and unaesthetic contours[105]
- Chin ptosis and deepening of the labiomental sulcus[106]
- Gingival recession
- Mandibular sulcus scarring

tion of the mental nerves will allow for ease of access and retraction and may help prevent errant injury during bony osteotomy. Careful dissection of the mental nerve, reinsertion of the mentalis muscle fibers with a two-layer closure, stepped soft-tissue incision (soft-tissue incision superiorly and muscle dissection more inferiorly), and meticulous subperiosteal dissection will limit these complications.

Chin Ptosis and Aesthetic Concerns

Ptosis of chin soft tissues may be prevented by minimizing subperiosteal stripping off the mandible and reapproximating the mentalis muscles. To prevent descent, the mentalis may be resuspended to the anterior superior edge of the distal chin, and a pressure dressing may be applied. Botulinum toxin may be used to treat temporary asymmetric mentalis deformities and hyperactivity.[72] Long-term dysfunction of the mentalis should be addressed with resuspension procedures, which have been reported to include drilling holes in the proximal mandible for use in securing the mentalis.[73]

The most common aesthetic concern following genioplasty is characterized by indentations on each side of the genioplasty at the posterior extent of the inferior border cut (keyhole-shaped mandible). Extending the inferior osteotomy posteriorly may prevent this complication; however, this maneuver may place the mental nerve at greater risk. These irregularities may also be improved with a secondary contouring procedure.

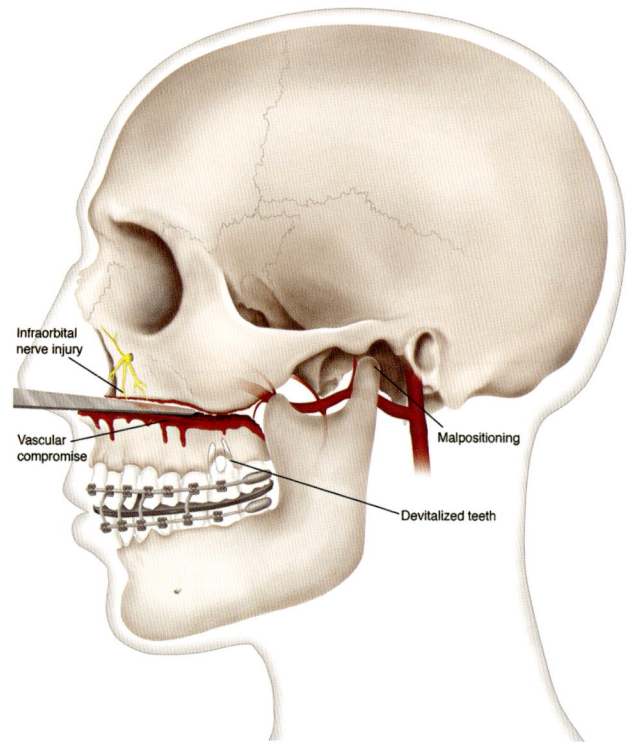

Fig. 16.5 LeFort 1 osteotomy. (*Illustration by Robert Brown.*)

◆ Complications of Maxillary Procedures

LeFort I Osteotomy

The LeFort I osteotomy (**Fig. 16.5**) has an impressive list of complications, all of which underscore the technical challenges encountered with maxillary surgery (**Table 16.6**).

Malpositioning

Proper preoperative planning is the only way to ensure accurate positioning of the maxilla. To achieve an ideal outcome, the surgeon must obtain mounted models with accurate centric relation and an accurate midline assessment. Concomitant mandibular surgery may be considered. Intraoperative swelling, bleeding, and the nasotracheal tube location all confuse the picture. The most common cause of malpositioning after a LeFort I osteotomy is an inability to seat the mandibular condyles properly. The surgeon must be certain that the condyles are seated first; then the maxillomandibular complex may be rotated superiorly into position until the first contact is felt (Dawson's technique).[74] After fixation of the maxilla, the jaws should be unwired, and

a critical assessment of the occlusion should then be made. If the occlusion is not ideal at this stage, adjustments to the osteotomy should be made.

Bleeding

Maxillary osteotomies, especially LeFort I and II osteotomies, have the potential for the most serious bleeding sequelae in orthognathic surgery. These complications may present as immediate intraoperative bleeding or as postoperative swelling or epistaxis. For two-jaw surgeries, the authors recommend preoperative type and screen for at least 2 units of packed red blood cells. Intraoperative hypotensive anesthesia is also suggested. The most common sources of hemorrhage are the terminal branches of the internal maxillary artery, especially the descending palatine or sphenopalatine artery. Bleeding from these may be caused by an improper or overly aggressive use of osteotomies, drilling, an oscillating saw, or downfracture of the maxilla. The downfracture may even damage the internal carotid artery if a basal skull fracture ensues that involves areas such as the foramen lacerum and the carotid canal. Even arteriovenous fistulas are possible.[75,76] The anterior and posterior superior alveolar and nasopalatine arteries are often intention-

Table 16.6

LeFort I Osteotomy Complications

- Malpositioning[107]

- Bleeding[108]

- Infraorbital nerve traction injury

- Vascular compromise[109]

- Periodontal defects[110]

- Devitalized teeth[110]

- Nerve injury[78]

- Ophthalmic artery injury[111]

- Nasolacrimal injury[112]

- Oronasal and oroantral fistulas[89]

- Nasal septal deviations

- Maxillary sinusitis

- Poor aesthetic soft-tissue changes

- Injury to the parotid duct

- Unfavorable fractures (pterygoid plate, sphenoid bone, middle cranial fossa)

- Nonunion

- Eustachian tube dysfunction

- Velopharyngeal incompetence

- Arteriovenous fistulas (carotid cavernous sinus)

- Dysphagia

- Transverse relapse

ally severed during maxillary surgery. Thrombogenic substances (e.g., microfibrillar collagen, topical thrombin) are often used to assist in hemostasis. Direct ligation of the descending palatine artery is recommended and is easily accomplished if dissection in a subperiosteal plane is performed.[77]

If bleeding occurs posterior to the pterygomaxillary osteotomy, packing is the best solution. Absorbable packing may be necessary. Hemorrhage from the internal maxillary artery may require direct ligation or even an external approach to the external carotid artery.[77]

Postoperatively, epistaxis should be treated with nasal packing, head elevation, and control of hypertension. If bleeding remains uncontrolled after anterior or poste-

rior nasal packing, then an arteriogram with possible embolization may be indicated before a return trip to the operating room. Certainly, removal of MMF and a tracheostomy may be necessary if bleeding is affecting the patient's airway.

Vascular Insufficiency

Patients with previous palatal surgery (cleft palate) or previous LeFort I osteotomy and maxillary downfracture should be evaluated preoperatively for compromise in their blood supply. Significant palatal scarring is an indication to preserve one labial artery pedicle. In the case of a previous LeFort osteotomy, evaluation of the gingiva may reveal edematous gingiva, which indicates poor venous return. This knowledge will guide the surgeon intraoperatively.

Intraoperative laser Doppler studies can confirm that anterior maxillary perfusion decreases gradually during downfracture and mobilization. It is recommended that the surgeon maintain constant vigilance during the operation to assess anterior perfusion. Intermittent relaxation will allow the maxilla to reperfuse. Segmental osteotomies will also compromise blood supply.[78] If severe perfusion deficiencies are noted during the operation, the surgeon may need to fix the maxilla rigidly into its original position and abort the procedure. Severe, prolonged disturbances in blood circulation may lead to avascular tissue necrosis, which may cause tooth devitalization, periodontal defects, or even loss of major bone segments. Because of the dense network of anastomoses in the face, this is a rare event, but it may manifest both in the maxilla and in the mandible, especially in association with segmental osteotomies. The anterior part of the maxilla is a zone of special risk.[77–80] Preservation of the descending palatine artery was not found to be critical for maintaining blood flow to the downfractured maxilla in animal studies,[80–82] but it has been recommended that the artery should be preserved whenever possible and segmentalization of the maxilla should be minimized. A wide, intact soft-tissue pedicle is important for the circulation of the downfractured maxilla. In the mandible, avascular necrosis can usually be avoided by minimal stripping of the periosteum and muscle attachments.[83] If frank necrosis occurs, then the wound should be managed conservatively with local wound care. Aggressive debridement is not indicated and may worsen the situation.

Periodontal Defects

Preoperative assessment of planned maxillary movement should alert the surgeon to future forces on the gingiva. Maintaining a healthy cuff of gingiva attached to the teeth during the horizontal vestibular incision will prevent necrosis. Tooth root disruption is avoided with a carefully planned osteotomy. Following maxillary advancement, grafting with bone or an alloplast is often helpful. Postoperative periodontal disease may be prevented with standard hygiene and good nutrition; however referral to a periodontist is an option.

Nerve Injury

Nerve injuries in maxillary downfracture can be divided into sensory, motor, secretory motor, and special sensory (optic nerve) injuries. Mastery of local anatomy is essential. During the procedure, sensory changes that are secondary to retraction injury are expected. The infraorbital, anterior, middle, and posterior superior alveolar, nasopalatine, and descending palatine nerves are all at risk. Despite a direct cut to the nerve, neurosensory innervation returns to the palate, gingiva, and teeth in nearly all cases. Approximately 25% of cases will have persistent hypesthesia.[84] Careful monitoring of fracture planes will typically prevent motor nerve injury. However, the optic nerve, nasociliary nerve, and cranial nerves III and VI may be at risk due to postoperative hematoma or seroma collection. Injury to these nerves is rarely recognized at the time of surgery.

Postoperatively, reassurance is recommended if neurosensory deficits present themselves. Cases of abducens nerve (VI) palsy have been reported, and all spontaneously resolved.[85] Oculomotor nerve (CN III) injury has also occurred and resolved in the postoperative period.[86] Blindness has also been reported.[78] In one case, multiple sphenoid and middle cranial fossa fractures were seen on postoperative CT scans. Retrobulbar hematoma was blamed for the other two cases.[78] Blindness persisted in one patient with a hematoma and in the patient with multiple sphenoid fractures. Finally, xerophthalmia has been seen secondary to injury of the secretory fibers of the abducens nerve.[78] Supportive therapy is recommended in this situation.

Ophthalmic and Nasolacrimal Injuries

Ophthalmic complications are rare sequelae of maxillary osteotomies. They include decreased visual acuity, extraocular muscle dysfunction, neuroparalytic keratitis, and nasolacrimal problems.[78] These injuries appear to be caused by indirect trauma to the neurovascular structures during the pterygomaxillary fractures that extend to the base of the skull. Use of topical sympathomimetics and injectible vasoconstrictive agents can result in pupil dilation and confuse the postoperative eye examination. Visual acuity testing should be performed, and ophthalmologic consultation to assess globe pressures must be obtained without hesitation. In the extreme case of frank proptosis, lateral canthotomy and high-dose steroids must be instituted.

Most patients undergoing maxillary downfracture experience some measure of epiphora that resolves spontaneously. Persistent epiphora seems to be more common with high LeFort osteotomies.[87] Disruption of the nasolacrimal duct[88] and nasal septal deviations[78] are the primary causes. Treatment of these complications is cause-specific.

Oronasal and Oroantral Fistulas

Large (greater than 8 mm) maxillary advancements increase the risk of relapse and soft-tissue breakdown. Oronasal fistulas are slightly more common than oroantral. Perhaps the cause of this is the greater tension placed on the palatal mucosa as the maxilla is widened.[89] The key to prevention of these fistulas is protection of the nasal mucosa. Excessive tension at closure or mucosal tears increase the risk of fistula. Postoperatively, patients should be careful to avoid nose blowing to prevent subcutaneous emphysema. Proper oral hygiene and use of a loose obturator are often recommended as initial treatment of a fistula. Decongestants, nasal sprays, and antibiotics may all assist with patient comfort and maxillary sinus health. Fistulas that persist after six months may be treated with surgical procedures, including a buccal fat pad, a tongue flap, or a facial artery musculomucosal flap.[90]

Nasal Septal Deviation

Preoperative evaluation of the symmetry, function, and appearance of the nose will help guide the postoperative management of it. Deviation of the nasal septum secondary to maxillary osteotomy has been associated with increased airway resistance and aesthetic complaints.[89] The anterior edge of the nasal spine rises superiorly as it progresses toward the nasopalatine foramen. It then arcs and falls posteriorly. If the maxilla is repositioned anteriorly, this arc will create buckling in the caudal nasal septum that may be addressed with a slight trim of the septum inferiorly. During advancement, both the inferior surface caudal septum and the superior surface of the ANS should be contoured to prevent deviation.[91] A 2-0 permanent suture may be used to reaffix the caudal septum in the midline by drilling a small hole in the nasal spine or appropriate midline. Postoperative deviation may need to be corrected during a separate operation. If deviation is noted in the immediate postoperative period, gentle manipulation or nasal packing may guide healing, but this is notoriously unreliable compared with good intraoperative technique.

Unacceptable Soft-Tissue Changes

A preoperative discussion of the changes of the nasal appearance with maxillary advancement is imperative to prepare the patient for possible secondary procedures. At least three to six months of healing following orthognathic surgery are advocated before septorhinoplasty with alar base reductions. Excessive maxillary movements will affect lip position, amount of incisor tooth showing at rest, fullness of the upper lip, and alar base support.

Unfavorable Fractures

Unusual fractures have been noted, including complete vomer avulsion,[92] pterygoid plate fracture,[93] sphenoid bone fracture,[94] and middle cranial fossa fracture.[95] Good surgical exposure and completion of all planned osteotomy cuts are paramount to prevent non-ideal fracture planes.

Nonunion (Delayed Union)

Nonunion and delayed union were far more common before rigid fixation.[96] Mobility or poor bony contact can incite a fibrous union or delayed union. Likewise, if maxillary mobility persists, vertical bone resorption may occur, causing foreshortening of the maxillary height with unplanned and untoward aesthetic results.

Transverse Relapse

Transverse relapse is a phenomenon associated with multiple-piece maxillary osteotomy.[97] When transverse relapse occurs, we get a constriction of segments toward the midline with occlusal prematurities that result in an open bite clinically. If a multiple-piece LeFort osteotomy is done, the segments need to be adequately mobilized or grafted to keep them apart. Surgically assisted rapid palatal expansion has been shown to be effective as a separate procedure before a LeFort I osteotomy.[98]

Associated Functional Complications

Eustachian tube dysfunction is possible after any palatal procedure, because the levator veli palatini and the tensor veli palatini have been repositioned. Therefore, many patients complain of fullness in the ears, decreased hearing, and pain. Postoperative decongestants, nasal sprays, and reassurance are essential. Routine microscopic evaluation is mandatory to rule out serous otitis media and the need for tympanostomy tube management of the middle ear space.

Velopharyngeal dysfunction has been shown to occur to a minor degree after every maxillary osteotomy.[99] However, it is much more common following advancement in patients with a cleft palate.[100] Preoperative evaluation by a speech pathologist is essential to document the degree of insufficiency, and the surgeon must have a thorough discussion with the patient and the family about its possible worsening following advancement. Also, further consultation is required to discuss adjunctive procedures that can be performed postoperatively to correct the issue. Other complications present in the literature are rare instances of arteriovenous fistulas (including cavernous sinus fistulas),[101] dysphagia,[102] and condylar resorption.[103] These complications may be related to surgical technique or to other unknown factors.

Anterior Maxillary Segmental Osteotomy

Complications of anterior maxillary segmental osteotomy include vascular complications and hemorrhage in the maxilla.

Bleeding

Severe hemorrhage has been previously documented with both maxillary and mandibular surgery. Massive hemorrhage is rare, but it is possible during the osteotomy of the posterior maxilla or if the cut is incomplete and one attempts to force the maxilla to downfracture and produces a fracture at the base of the skull. Bleeding may also occur from careless use of chisels or saws in the posterior maxilla. This can result in direct or indirect vascular injury to the major vessels in the neck or skull base, including the internal carotid artery and internal jugular vein. Efforts should be made to direct osteotomies properly in the pterygoid plates and to downfracture the maxilla without excessive force. This principle becomes paramount in revision procedures involving a maxillary osteotomy, as previous procedures could have easily created unusual fusion lines. Other vessels at risk include the internal maxillary artery, the posterior superior alveolar artery, and the greater palatine artery.

Stretch injury of the internal carotid artery is also possible secondary to positioning. During neck extension, the carotid is compressed upon the vertebral column. Adding a rotational component to the neck for exposure places the vessel at risk for postoperative thrombosis. Mortality associated with thrombosis of the internal carotid has been estimated at 40%, with an additional 52% of the patients being left with a serious neurological deficit.

Following a LeFort I osteotomy, delayed bleeding may occur immediately after surgery or as late as nine days postoperatively. The vessels most frequently involved are the greater palatine artery, the internal maxillary, and the pterygoid plexus of veins.

◆ Conclusion

Orthognathic surgery requires astute preoperative assessment, careful preoperative planning and surgical modeling, and accurate surgical management to prevent common complications. When choosing the procedures with the patient, the orthognathic surgeon must weigh the risks with the ultimate goals by considering the patient's global health, tobacco use, and previous surgical procedures. Intraoperative vigilance is imperative to prevent alar necrosis from nasotracheal or nasogastric tubes, external scars, cautery burns, nerve or vascular injury, or excessive vascular compromise of the bony segments. When complications arise, the surgeon must address the concerns of the patient as well as act promptly to prevent negative long-term sequelae.

PEARLS OF WISDOM

Meticulous preoperative planning and model surgery will help to limit bony segment malposition.

Prevention of an unfavorable split depends on proper cortical bone cuts that extend through the inferior mandibular border.

The most common sensory nerve injury in the bilateral sagittal-split osteotomy is to the inferior alveolar nerve.

In the vertical ramus osteotomy, an improperly seated condyle in the glenoid fossa (condylar sag) can result in a postoperative open bite deformity.

A common cause of poor maxillary positioning in LeFort I osteotomy is inadequate seating of the condyles.

Severe proximal segment rotation in the vertical ramus osteotomy can be prevented by direct visualization of the planned cuts and by identification of the antilingula on the buccal (lateral) surface of the mandible for orientation of the lingula.

References

1. Spaey YJ, Bettens RM, Mommaerts MY, et al. A prospective study on infectious complications in orthognathic surgery. J Craniomaxillofac Surg 2005;33(1):24–29
2. Martis C, Karabouta I. Infection after orthognathic surgery, with and without preventive antibiotics. Int J Oral Surg 1984;13(6):490–494
3. Perko M. Maxillary sinus and surgical movement of maxilla. Int J Oral Surg 1972;1(4):177–184
4. Zijderveld SA, Smeele LE, Kostense PJ, Tuinzing DB. Preoperative antibiotic prophylaxis in orthognathic surgery: a randomized, double-blind, and placebo-controlled clinical study. J Oral Maxillofac Surg 1999;57(12):1403–1406, discussion 1406–1407
5. Peterson LJ. Antibiotic prophylaxis against wound infections in oral and maxillofacial surgery. J Oral Maxillofac Surg 1990;48(6):617–620
6. Van Sickels JE, Richardson DA. Stability of orthognathic surgery: a review of rigid fixation. Br J Oral Maxillofac Surg 1996;34(4):279–285
7. Dolce C, Hatch JP, Van Sickels JE, Rugh JD. Rigid versus wire fixation for mandibular advancement: skeletal and dental changes after 5 years. Am J Orthod Dentofacial Orthop 2002;121(6):610–619
8. Keeling SD, Dolce C, Van Sickels JE, Bays RA, Clark GM, Rugh JD. A comparative study of skeletal and dental stability between rigid and wire fixation for mandibular advancement. Am J Orthod Dentofacial Orthop 2000;117(6):638–649
9. Lee DY, Bailey LJ, Proffit WR. Soft tissue changes after superior repositioning of the maxilla with Le Fort I osteotomy: 5-year follow-up. Int J Adult Orthodon Orthognath Surg 1996;11(4):301–311
10. Smith GC, Moloney FB, West RA. Mandibular advancement surgery. A study of the lower border wiring technique for osteosynthesis. Oral Surg Oral Med Oral Pathol 1985;60(5):467–475
11. Baker DL, Stoelinga PJ, Blijdorp PA, Brouns JJ. Long-term stability after inferior maxillary repositioning by miniplate fixation. Int J Oral Maxillofac Surg 1992;21(6):320–326
12. Louis PJ, Waite PD, Austin RB. Long-term skeletal stability after rigid fixation of Le Fort I osteotomies with advancements. Int J Oral Maxillofac Surg 1993;22(2):82–86
13. van Merkesteyn JP, Groot RH, van Leeuwaarden R, Kroon FH. Intra-operative complications in sagittal and vertical ramus osteotomies. Int J Oral Maxillofac Surg 1987;16(6):665–670
14. Ylikontiola L, Moberg K, Huumonen S, Soikkonen K, Oikarinen K. Comparison of three radiographic methods used to locate the mandibular canal in the buccolingual direction before bilateral sagittal split osteotomy. Oral Surg Oral Med Oral Pathol Oral Radiol Endod 2002;93(6):736–742
15. O'Ryan F. Complications of orthognathic surgery. Oral Maxillofac Surg Clin North Am 1990;2:593
16. Hunsuck EE. A modified intraoral sagittal splitting technic for correction of mandibular prognathism. J Oral Surg 1968;26(4):250–253
17. Hunsuck EE. A method of intraoral open reduction of fractured mandibles. J Oral Surg 1967;25(6):533–541
18. Epker BN. Modifications in the sagittal osteotomy of the mandible. J Oral Surg 1977;35(2):157–159
19. Wolford LM, Bennett MA, Rafferty CG. Modification of the mandibular ramus sagittal split osteotomy. Oral Surg Oral Med Oral Pathol 1987;64(2):146–155
20. Dal Pont G. Retromolar osteotomy for the correction of prognathism. J Oral Surg Anesth Hosp Dent Serv 1961;19:42–47
21. Bays RA. Arthrotomy and Orthognathic Surgery for TMD. In: Kraus SL, ed. Temporomandibular Disorders, 2 ed. New York: Churchhill Livingstone; 1994:237
22. Wolford LM, Davis WM Jr. The mandibular inferior border split: a modification in the sagittal split osteotomy. J Oral Maxillofac Surg 1990;48(1):92–94
23. Epkcr BN, Wolford LM. Modified Sagittal Ramus Osteotomy. In: Epker BN, Wolford LM, eds. Dentofacial Deformities: Surgical Orthodontic Correction. St. Louis: CV Mosby; 1980:66
24. Turvey TA. Intraoperative complications of sagittal osteotomy of the mandibular ramus: incidence and management. J Oral Maxillofac Surg 1985;43(7):504–509
25. Panula K, Finne K, Oikarinen K. Incidence of complications and problems related to orthognathic surgery: a review of 655 patients. J Oral Maxillofac Surg 2001;59(10):1128–1136, discussion 1137
26. Lindquist CC, Obeid G. Complications of genioplasty done alone or in combination with sagittal split-ramus osteotomy. Oral Surg Oral Med Oral Pathol 1988;66(1):13–16
27. Walter JM Jr, Gregg JM. Analysis of postsurgical neurologic alteration in the trigeminal nerve. J Oral Surg 1979;37(6):410–414
28. Westermark A, Bystedt H, von Konow L. Inferior alveolar nerve function after sagittal split osteotomy of the mandible: correlation with degree of intraoperative nerve encounter

and other variables in 496 operations. Br J Oral Maxillofac Surg 1998;36(6):429–433

29. Van Sickels JE, Hatch JP, Dolce C, Bays RA, Rugh JD. Effects of age, amount of advancement, and genioplasty on neurosensory disturbance after a bilateral sagittal split osteotomy. J Oral Maxillofac Surg 2002;60(9):1012–1017

30. Jones DL, Wolford LM, Hartog JM. Comparison of methods to assess neurosensory alterations following orthognathic surgery. Int J Adult Orthodon Orthognath Surg 1990;5(1):35–42

31. Jääskeläinen SK, Peltola JK, Forssell K, Vähätalo K. Evaluating function of the inferior alveolar nerve with repeated nerve conduction tests during mandibular sagittal split osteotomy. J Oral Maxillofac Surg 1995;53(3):269–279

32. Westermark A, Englesson L, Bongenhielm U. Neurosensory function after sagittal split osteotomy of the mandible: a comparison between subjective evaluation and objective assessment. Int J Adult Orthodon Orthognath Surg 1999; 14(4):268–275

33. Cunningham LL, Tiner BD, Clark GM, Bays RA, Keeling SD, Rugh JD. Surgeon's assessment of nerve damage vs. patients' report of neurosensory deficit. J Dent Res 1995;74(Special Issue):156

34. Schendel SA, Epker BN. Results after mandibular advancement surgery: an analysis of 87 cases. J Oral Surg 1980;38(4): 265–282

35. Jacks SC, Zuniga JR, Turvey TA, Schalit C. A retrospective analysis of lingual nerve sensory changes after mandibular bilateral sagittal split osteotomy. J Oral Maxillofac Surg 1998; 56(6):700–704, discussion 705

36. de Vries K, Devriese PP, Hovinga J, van den Akker HP. Facial palsy after sagittal split osteotomies. A survey of 1747 sagittal split osteotomies. J Craniomaxillofac Surg 1993;21(2): 50–53

37. Van Sickels JE, Tucker MR. Prevention and Management of Complications in Orthognathic Surgery. In: Peterson LJ, ed. Principles of Oral and Maxillofacial Surgery. Philadelphia: JB Lippincott; 1992:1465

38. Jones JK, Van Sickels JE. Facial nerve injuries associated with orthognathic surgery: a review of incidence and management. J Oral Maxillofac Surg 1991;49(7):740–744 Review

39. Blumenthal F, May M. Electrodiagnosis. In: May M, ed. The Facial Nerve. New York: Thieme; 1986:1

40. Christiansen RL, Soudah HP. Disseminated intravascular coagulation following orthognathic surgery. Int J Adult Orthodon Orthognath Surg 1993;8(3):217–224

41. Lanigan DT, Hey JH, West RA. Major vascular complications of orthognathic surgery: hemorrhage associated with Le Fort I osteotomies. J Oral Maxillofac Surg 1990;48(6):561–573

42. Neuwirth BR, White RP Jr, Collins ML, Phillips C. Recovery following orthognathic surgery and autologous blood transfusion. Int J Adult Orthodon Orthognath Surg 1992;7(4): 221–228

43. Ellis E III, Hinton RJ. Histologic examination of the temporomandibular joint after mandibular advancement with and without rigid fixation: an experimental investigation in adult *Macaca mulatta.* J Oral Maxillofac Surg 1991;49(12): 1316–1327

44. Nitzan DW, Dolwick MF. Temporomandibular joint fibrous ankylosis following orthognathic surgery: report of eight cases. Int J Adult Orthodon Orthognath Surg 1989;4(1):7–11

45. Gallagher DM, Bell WH, Storum KA. Soft tissue changes associated with advancement genioplasty performed con-

comitantly with superior repositioning of the maxilla. J Oral Maxillofac Surg 1984;42(4):238–242

46. Kerstens HC, Tuinzing DB, Golding RP, van der Kwast WA. Condylar atrophy and osteoarthrosis after bimaxillary surgery. Oral Surg Oral Med Oral Pathol 1990;69(3):274–280

47. Moore KE, Gooris PJ, Stoelinga PJ. The contributing role of condylar resorption to skeletal relapse following mandibular advancement surgery: report of five cases. J Oral Maxillofac Surg 1991;49(5):448–460

48. Merkx MA, Van Damme PA. Condylar resorption after orthognathic surgery. Evaluation of treatment in 8 patients. J Craniomaxillofac Surg 1994;22(1):53–58

49. Bouwman JP, Kerstens HC, Tuinzing DB. Condylar resorption in orthognathic surgery. The role of intermaxillary fixation. Oral Surg Oral Med Oral Pathol 1994;78(2):138–141

50. Arnett GW, Milam SB, Gottesman L. Progressive mandibular retrusion—idiopathic condylar resorption. Part I. Am J Orthod Dentofacial Orthop 1996;110(1):8–15 Review

51. Hoppenreijs TJ, Freihofer HP, Stoelinga PJ, Tuinzing DB, van't Hof MA. Condylar remodelling and resorption after Le Fort I and bimaxillary osteotomies in patients with anterior open bite. A clinical and radiological study. Int J Oral Maxillofac Surg 1998;27(2):81–91

52. Hwang SJ, Haers PE, Zimmermann A, Oechslin C, Seifert B, Sailer HF. Surgical risk factors for condylar resorption after orthognathic surgery. Oral Surg Oral Med Oral Pathol Oral Radiol Endod 2000;89(5):542–552

53. Schellhas KP, Wilkes CH, Fritts HM, Omlie MR, Lagrotteria LB. MR of osteochondritis dissecans and avascular necrosis of the mandibular condyle. AJR Am J Roentgenol 1989;152(3): 551–560

54. Moore KE, Gooris PJ, Stoelinga PJ. The contributing role of condylar resorption to skeletal relapse following mandibular advancement surgery: report of five cases. J Oral Maxillofac Surg 1991;49(5):448–460

55. Cutbirth M, Van Sickels JE, Thrash WJ. Condylar resorption after bicortical screw fixation of mandibular advancement. J Oral Maxillofac Surg 1998;56(2):178–182, discussion 183

56. Kerstens HC, Tuinzing DB, Golding RP, van der Kwast WA. Condylar atrophy and osteoarthrosis after bimaxillary surgery. Oral Surg Oral Med Oral Pathol 1990;69(3):274–280

57. Moore KE, Gooris PJ, Stoelinga PJ. The contributing role of condylar resorption to skeletal relapse following mandibular advancement surgery: report of five cases. J Oral Maxillofac Surg 1991;49(5):448–460

58. De Clercq CA, Neyt LF, Mommaerts MY, Abeloos JV, De Mot BM. Condylar resorption in orthognathic surgery: a retrospective study. Int J Adult Orthodon Orthognath Surg 1994;9(3):233–240

59. Bays RA, Fisher KL. Evaluation of condylar position and rigid fixation of sagittal split osteotomies. American Association of Oral and Maxillofacial Surgeons, Anaheim, CA 1987. Abstract.

60. Singer RS, Bays RA. A comparison between superior and inferior border wiring techniques in sagittal split ramus osteotomy. J Oral Maxillofac Surg 1985;43(6):444–449

61. Tuinzing DB, Greebe RB. Complications related to the intraoral vertical ramus osteotomy. Int J Oral Surg 1985;14(4): 319–324

62. Zaytoun HS Jr, Phillips C, Terry BC. Long-term neurosensory deficits following transoral vertical ramus and sagittal split osteotomies for mandibular prognathism. J Oral Maxillofac Surg 1986;44(3):193–196

63. Egyedi P, Houwing M, Juten E. The oblique subcondylar osteotomy: report of results of 100 cases. J Oral Surg 1981;39(11):871–873

64. Guralnick W, Kelly JP. Palsy of the facial nerve after intraoral oblique osteotomies of the mandible. J Oral Surg 1979;37(10):743

65. Van Sickels JE, Tucker MR. Prevention and Management of Complications in Orthognathic Surgery. In: Peterson LJ, ed. Principles of Oral and Maxillofacial Surgery. Philadelphia: JB Lippincott; 1992:1465

66. Eckerdal O, Sund G, Astrand P. Skeletal remodeling in the TMJ after oblique sliding osteotomy of the mandibular rami. Int J Oral Maxillofac Surg 1986;15:233-239

67. Hall HD, Chase DC, Payor LG. Evaluation and refinement of the intraoral vertical subcondylar osteotomy. J Oral Surg 1975;33(5):333–341

68. Boyer CC, Williams TW, Stevens FH. Blood supply of the temporomandibular joint. J Dent Res 1964;43:224–228

69. Hale RG, Timmis DP, Bays RA. A new mandibulotomy technique for the dentate patient. Plast Reconstr Surg 1991;87(2):362–364

70. Dorfman HS, Turvey TA. Alterations in osseous crestal height following interdental osteotomies. Oral Surg Oral Med Oral Pathol 1979;48(2):120–125

71. Karras SC, Wolford LM. Augmentation genioplasty with hard tissue replacement implants. J Oral Maxillofac Surg 1998;56(5):549–552

72. Papel ID, Capone RB. Botulinum toxin A for mentalis muscle dysfunction. Arch Facial Plast Surg 2001;3(4):268–269

73. Zide BM, McCarthy J. The mentalis muscle: an essential component of chin and lower lip position. Plast Reconstr Surg 1989;83(3):413–420

74. Dawson PE. Centric relation. Its effect on occluso-muscle harmony. Dent Clin North Am 1979;23(2):169–180

75. Lanigan DT, Hey JH, West RA. Major vascular complications of orthognathic surgery: hemorrhage associated with Le Fort I osteotomies. J Oral Maxillofac Surg 1990;48(6):561–573

76. Mehra P, Cottrell DA, Caiazzo A, Lincoln R. Life-threatening, delayed epistaxis after surgically assisted rapid palatal expansion: a case report. J Oral Maxillofac Surg 1999;57(2):201–204

77. Lanigan DT, West RA. Management of postoperative hemorrhage following the Le Fort I maxillary osteotomy. J Oral Maxillofac Surg 1984;42(6):367–375

78. Lanigan D, Hey J, West RA. Aseptic necrosis of the maxilla: report of 36 cases. J Oral Maxillofac Surg 1990;48(2):142–156 Review

79. Epker BN. Vascular considerations in orthognathic surgery. I. Mandibular osteotomies. Oral Surg Oral Med Oral Pathol 1984;57(5):467–472

80. Lanigan DT, Loewy J. Postoperative computed tomography scan study of the pterygomaxillary separation during the Le Fort I osteotomy using a micro-oscillating saw. J Oral Maxillofac Surg 1995;53(10):1161–1166

81. Bell WH, Fonseca RJ, Kenneky JW, Levy BM. Bone healing and revascularization after total maxillary osteotomy. J Oral Surg 1975;33(4):253–260

82. Bell WH, You ZH, Finn RA, Fields RT. Wound healing after multisegmental Le Fort I osteotomy and transection of the descending palatine vessels. J Oral Maxillofac Surg 1995;53(12):1425–1433, discussion 1433–1434

83. Bell WH, Schendel SA. Biologic basis for modification of the sagittal ramus split operation. J Oral Surg 1977;35(5):362–369

84. de Jongh M, Barnard D, Birnie D. Sensory nerve morbidity following Le Fort I osteotomy. J Maxillofac Surg 1986;14(1):10–13

85. Watts PG. Unilateral abducent nerve palsy: a rare complication following a Le Fort I maxillary osteotomy. Br J Oral Maxillofac Surg 1984;22(3):212–215

86. Carr RJ, Gilbert P. Isolated partial third nerve palsy following Le Fort I maxillary osteotomy in a patient with cleft lip and palate. Br J Oral Maxillofac Surg 1986;24(3):206–211

87. Keller EE, Sather AH. Quadrangular Le Fort I osteotomy: surgical technique and review of 54 patients. J Oral Maxillofac Surg 1990;48(1):2–11, discussion 12–13

88. Tomasetti BJ, Broutsas M, Gormley M, Jarrett W. Lack of tearing after Le Fort I osteotomy. J Oral Surg 1976;34(12):1095–1097

89. Sher MR. Treatment of oro-antral-nasal fistula after anterior maxillary osteotomy. J Oral Surg 1980;38(3):212–214

90. Pribaz J, Stephens W, Crespo L, Gifford G. A new intraoral flap: facial artery musculomucosal (FAMM) flap. Plast Reconstr Surg 1992;90(3):421–429

91. Bays RA, Timmis DP. Techniques for Maxillary Orthognathic Surgery. In: Peterson L, ed. Principles of Oral and Maxillofacial Surgery. Philadelphia: JB Lippincott; 1991:1349

92. Smith KS, Heggie AA. Vomero-sphenoidal disarticulation during the Le Fort I maxillary osteotomy: report of case. J Oral Maxillofac Surg 1995;53(4):465–467

93. Robinson PP, Hendy CW. Pterygoid plate fractures caused by the Le Fort I osteotomy. Br J Oral Maxillofac Surg 1986;24(3):198–202

94. Lanigan DT, Romanchuk K, Olson CK. Ophthalmic complications associated with orthognathic surgery. J Oral Maxillofac Surg 1993;51(5):480–494 Review

95. Precious DS, Goodday RH, Bourget L, Skulsky FG. Pterygoid plate fracture in Le Fort I osteotomy with and without pterygoid chisel: a computed tomography scan evaluation of 58 patients. J Oral Maxillofac Surg 1993;51(2):151–153

96. Schendel SA, Eisenfeld JH, Bell WH, Epker BN. Superior repositioning of the maxilla: stability and soft tissue osseous relations. Am J Orthod 1976;70(6):663–674

97. Bell WH, Jacobs JD, Quejada JG. Simultaneous repositioning of the maxilla, mandible, and chin. Treatment planning and analysis of soft tissues. Am J Orthod 1986;89(1):28–50

98. Kuo PC, Will LA. Surgical-orthodontic treatment of maxillary constriction. Oral Maxillofac Surg Clin North Am 1990;2:751–759

99. Kummer AW, Strife JL, Grau WH, Creaghead NA, Lee L. The effects of Le Fort I osteotomy with maxillary movement on articulation, resonance, and velopharyngeal function. Cleft Palate J 1989;26(3):193–199, discussion 199–200

100. Schwarz C, Gruner E. Logopaedic findings following advancement of the maxilla. J Maxillofac Surg 1976;4(1):40–55

101. Habal MB. A carotid cavernous sinus fistula after maxillary osteotomy. Plast Reconstr Surg 1986;77(6):981–987

102. Gaukroger MC. Dysphagia following bimaxillary osteotomy. Br J Oral Maxillofac Surg 1993;31(3):189–190

103. de Mol van Otterloo JJ, Dorenbos J, Tuinzing DB, van der Kwast WA. TMJ performance and behaviour in patients more than 6 years after Le Fort I osteotomy. Br J Oral Maxillofac Surg 1993;31(2):83–86

104. Lindquist CC, Obeid G. Complications of genioplasty done alone or in combination with sagittal split-ramus osteotomy. Oral Surg Oral Med Oral Pathol 1988;66(1):13–16

105. O'Ryan F. Complications of orthognathic surgery. Oral Maxillofac Surg Clin North Am 1990;2:593

106. Park HS, Ellis E III, Fonseca RJ, Reynolds ST, Mayo KH. A retrospective study of advancement genioplasty. Oral Surg Oral Med Oral Pathol 1989;67(5):481–489

107. Frost DE, Koutnik AW. Alternative stabilization of the maxilla during simultaneous jaw-mobilization procedures. Oral Surg Oral Med Oral Pathol 1983;56(2):125–127

108. Lanigan DT, Hey JH, West RA. Major vascular complications of orthognathic surgery: hemorrhage associated with Le Fort I osteotomies. J Oral Maxillofac Surg 1990;48(6):561–573

109. Parnes EI, Becker ML. Necrosis of the anterior maxilla following osteotomy. Oral Surg Oral Med Oral Pathol 1972; 33(3):326–330

110. Vedtofte P, Nattestad A. Pulp sensibility and pulp necrosis after Le Fort I osteotomy. J Craniomaxillofac Surg 1989;17(4): 167–171

111. Reiner S, Willoughby JH. Transient abducens nerve palsy following a Le Fort I maxillary osteotomy: report of a case. J Oral Maxillofac Surg 1988;46(8):699–701

112. Shoshani Y, Samet N, Ardekian L, Taicher S. Nasolacrimal duct injury after LeFort I osteotomy. J Oral Maxillofac Surg 1994;52(4):406–407

17

Overcoming Adversities in Hair Restoration

John E. Frank

Even though the scalp possesses less anatomic and physiologic complexity than other areas of the head and neck, microscopic hair transplantation is a highly technical procedure, with results that are highly visible. As such, there is always the potential for troublesome events. Any adverse outcome in a modern hair restoration practice may create temporal and economic burdens for surgeons, but unfulfilled expectations may be psychologically devastating for patients.

Hair restoration techniques have evolved, and the types of complications and the manner in which they occur have changed accordingly. Before 1990, scalp reductions, flaps, and plug grafting were the procedures of choice. Common problems included flap death, wide scalp scars, misdirected hair, and conspicuous unsightly pluggy hair grafts. Today, most hair restoration complications occur with microfollicular grafting and the attendant challenge of producing thick, natural looking hairlines without accompanying donor site morbidity.

The incidence of hair transplant complications has declined as knowledge, training, and practitioner skills have increased, and the majority of cases proceed without adversity.[1] However, because many transplants are performed in procedure rooms rather than accredited operating rooms, complications undoubtedly are underreported. In addition, the presence of sensational marketing campaigns may lead prospective patients to arrive with fantastic and often unrealistic expectations. Because these hopes cannot be always met with current methods, failure to meet patient expectations will be considered.

This chapter is divided into three sections covering preventative strategies, intraoperative complications, and postoperative complications. Complications involving donor and recipient areas will be discussed separately, and because we still rely upon scalp reductions for targeted cases, the challenges associated with flaps and reductions and ways to conquer them will also be discussed.[2,3]

◆ Prevention Strategies

Patient Expectations and Transplant Design

It cannot be overstated that the transplant surgeon should personally and diligently inform each candidate of the realistic expectations for the procedure as well as any potential adverse outcomes. Patients must be informed that maximum hair density may be achieved only by undergoing more than a single procedure. Many other intangibles contribute to the complexity of results, and hair color, curl, scalp complexion and future hair loss are all important factors influencing the outcome. Therefore, even with lengthy preoperative discussions and comprehensive consent forms, it is still idealistic to believe that each patient will develop a true appreciation of the anticipated results. Any patient who cannot clearly comprehend the limitations of microscopic hair transplantation should not be considered an appropriate candidate. Because hair loss is usually progressive with age, many advanced transplant surgeons are apprehensive about transplanting patients under the age of 25 years. In some instances, hair loss prevention is a far more important strategy than hair restoration. Convincing an emotionally distraught 20-year-old of this approach can be very difficult. It is perfectly appropriate to insist a relative or close friend be present during the initial consultation (or series of consultations). Although a hair restoration complication may not manifest until balding has progressed, it is the responsibility of the initial surgeon to use the utmost discretion. With regard to hairline design, it is imperative to stress the importance of the temporal recession instead of a straight line. In addition, transplanting aggressively low in the forehead will ultimately result in extremely unfavorable results.

An additional challenge occurs with women, for they commonly suffer from postoperative anagen and telogen effluvium (shock loss). Regrowth may not occur for over one year's time, leading to a very uncomfortable waiting period for both the patient and the surgeon. Hair and scalp surgery may exacerbate any telogen effluvium occurring preoperatively. Shock loss may be limited by use of some preventative strategies, such as administering preoperative minoxidil, limiting the amount of intraoperative epinephrine, and gentle tissue handling with minimization of damage to surrounding follicles.[4] Unfortunately, there is no proven preventative remedy, and this fact must be communicated to all patients at risk. Assessment of the prevailing hair cell cycles via preoperative hair pull tests and microscopic hair pluck root exams helps to differentiate between the typical miniaturization associated with male- and female-pattern hair loss and effluvium, as well as to determine other dermatologic conditions of the hair and scalp[5]. This knowledge is important and may identify some patients as poor hair transplant candidates. A sound understanding of these tests and dermatologic conditions is incumbent upon any hair transplant surgeon.

Another concern should be individuals requesting vertex or crown transplants. Although many advances have been made with regard to the design of the crown, such as the whorl pattern, it is still very difficult to achieve thick, natural coverage in this area.[6] Patients must be clearly informed of this challenge and the necessity of multiple procedures. The potential for progressive hair loss is also very high in this area, so surgeons are forewarned to proceed carefully. It is possible that the entire donor supply may be usurped after several transplant sessions, leaving no reserves for the anterior scalp. The vertex is also more difficult to cover because of the illusion of less hair when the crown is observed from above. A basic tenet of microscopic hair transplant is that valuable donor hair should be allocated in a front-to-back pattern. In contrast, frontal hair tends to cover balder areas posteriorly, especially when viewed anteriorly. In all cases, it is recommended to reiterate the patient's requests preoperatively, and it may also be helpful to depict the plan with a simple line drawing.

Anesthesia

A major advantage of microfollicular hair transplantation is that the entire procedure may be completed using local anesthesia only. However, substantial risk is present when large dosages of anesthetics are applied. As with any cosmetic procedure, the surgeon's tolerance for withholding an operation on a medically fragile patient should be low. For individuals who may have low amounts of coagulants, whether from aspirin, ibuprofen, coumadin, clopidogrel (Plavix), other NSAIDS, vitamins, or natural supplements, a test procedure using a small number of grafts may furnish clues as to what to expect from the definitive larger procedure.

Despite the high dosages of lidocaine administered in hair transplantation, toxicity is surprisingly rare. However, the surgeon must be aware of the standard dosages (lidocaine without epinephrine is 5 mg/kg, or up to 7 mg/kg if given with epinephrine) and the signs and symptoms of toxicity—the progression of tongue paresthesia, light-headedness, and changes in vision leading to unconsciousness and possible seizure. Should this occur, the patient should be immediately moved to an acute care center where serum lidocaine levels can be drawn (toxicities may be observed at 6 mcg/ml but more commonly occur once levels exceed 10 mcg/ml)[7] and where the patient's cardiopulmonary status can be secured.

Preoperatively, patients should be also screened for prior episodes of fainting. Vasovagal syncope may occur, most commonly during the application of local anesthesia. The high frequency of this event during hair transplantation may be related to the fact that middle-aged males constitute the largest demographic for patients undergoing this procedure. Systemic, nonspecific β-blockers can potentiate the injected epinephrine and cause toxic hypertension. Although this complication is unusual, no surgeon should ever hesitate to postpone a procedure until the patient is converted to a cardiac-specific β-blocker.[8]

◆ Identification and Management of Intraoperative Complications

Anesthesia

One of the earliest problems encountered in hair transplantation is an anxious patient intolerant of the administration of local anesthesia. Depending upon the facility and the resources available, sedation may be useful. A small preoperative dose of a benzodiazepine is optimal. Other options include lorazepam or diazepam, both which have an onset of less than 30 minutes and a duration of several hours. Proven techniques for decreasing the pain of the administration of local anesthetic include buffering with sodium bicarbonate, warming, and hypnosis.[9,10] A one part in ten bicarbonate dilution and temperatures may be titrated to find the most gentle and least irritating solution possible. What may appear as a trivial matter for the highly skilled surgeon is actually an invaluable opportunity to set the tone for the entire procedure and further the relationship with the patient. Different techniques and devices are available for delivering local anesthesia. Nothing, however, can substitute for the slow, gentle, and relaxed delivery by the surgeon or his delegate.

The epinephrine component of the local anesthetic frequently precipitates episodes of anxiety and tachycardia. Premixed and commercially available packaged local anesthetics with epinephrine are rarely problematic; however, surgeons may encounter side effects when mixing greater than 1 mg of epinephrine in 30 cc of saline. In addition, paradoxical rebound vasodilation may also occur, causing graft popping and oozing so that many surgeons commonly avoid these "super juice" solutions.

Antihypertensive medications should be available, but they are rarely required. Sedatives may be more useful in calming a patient and subsequently decreasing blood pressure and heart rate. Local maneuvers such as Valsalva and deep breathing are helpful. In the absence of a bruit or history of cardiovascular disease, a carotid massage may also be used. Patients with a history of anxiety or difficulty with local anesthesia may benefit from a benzodiazepine or even a 0.1 mg oral dose of clonidine if they are tachycardic or hypertensive.

Donor Morbidity

Bleeding or other intraoperative complications of the donor area are rare. Many surgeons limit the amount of cautery to prevent damage to the surrounding hair follicles. Intraoperative hematomas are unusual, but if they are suspected, they should be explored and any bleeding vessel ligated.

Wound closure and edge approximation may be problematic if the width of the harvest is excessive, since the scalp is relatively inelastic. This is especially true in repeat procedures. Typically, elliptical incisions will close when the width of excision remains less than 1.2 cm. It may also be helpful to measure the elasticity of the donor area before excision.[11-13] In the event of difficult wound approximation, wide undermining should mobilize the edges sufficiently to allow closure. Pulling the edges together with a penetrating towel clamp may also be helpful. Interestingly, it has been postulated that the scar resulting from an unclosed wound that heals by secondary intention will ultimately be no wider than the scar of a wound closed with excessive tension. The postauricular area is typically the most difficult area to close and usually heals with the most scarring (**Fig. 17.1**). Narrowly tapering the elliptical incision toward the mastoid may be helpful. Paradoxically, scalps that have the greatest elasticity and are easiest to close may ultimately lead to the widest scarring. This may be a manifestation of the Ehlers-Danlos syndrome.[14]

Finally, despite careful calculation and measurement of the donor strip, it is common for the calculated number of harvested micro grafts not to match exactly the anticipated number of promised recipient sites. This may require opening the already-sutured donor site and harvesting additional tissue. The surgeon should carefully consider the extra trauma that additional tissue harvesting creates, as this will invariably increase the tension across the wound. Should the surgeon choose

to harvest extra tissue, then it becomes prudent to avoid the postauricular area entirely. Also, prior to re-incising, it may be helpful to leave the closure sutures intact as they will act as tissue retractors.

Hair Graft Handling

Surgical assistants have a very important role in hair transplantation. Following removal of the donor strip by the surgeon, assistants must use special care while transferring, dissecting, storing, and placing the grafts. Once removed from the body, hair follicles are extremely sensitive to insults from crushing and desiccation.[15,16] A small amount of subdermal fatty tissue should be retained around each follicular unit, as this will serve to protect the fragile follicle; binocular microscopy will aid in this process.[17] Each graft must be sized appropriately to fit snugly into the recipient openings. Grafts that are too large will be traumatized during placement, and grafts that are too small will not adequately fill the recipient site. Optimally, the graft cutting stations should physically reside in the procedure room so patient-to-patient crossover is avoided.

Recipient Sites

The surgeon may encounter technical complications while creating recipient incisions or while placing the grafts. One of the first challenges is initiating and sustaining profound anesthesia. Patients who experience pain throughout the procedure are likely be hypertensive, with subsequent oozing and graft popping. This will ultimately affect the final outcome. Oral, intramuscular, and intravenous analgesics may mitigate these

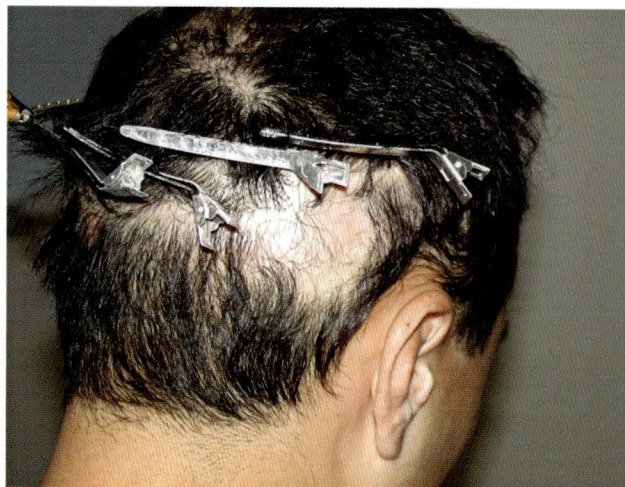

Fig. 17.1 The retroauricular area is most prone to develop wide donor scarring, especially after multiple procedures.

circumstances. The effects of lidocaine will diminish with time, and frequent reapplication or stacking of injections will prevent the lidocaine from wearing off and disrupting the placement process. As the sensory nerves run most superficially in the dermis, deeper infiltration of anesthesia will miss the intended nerves and will also dissipate more easily through the deeper dermis and subcutaneous fat. Therefore, the thin subcutaneous administration of local anesthesia is mandatory.

Matching the size and the depth of the recipient incisions will minimize problems with graft placement. The grafts must fit easily yet snugly into each opening. Excessively skinny grafts will yield poorer survival.[18] At some point, however, every surgeon will be faced with grafts that tend to pop during the placement period. The cause of this problem may be hypertension or vascular oozing. Additionally, graft popping occurs secondary to inherent skin properties. Increasing the concentration of the "super juice" (dilute epinephrine in normal saline) may ameliorate this condition. However a balance must be struck; excessive volumes and concentrations of epinephrine may cause transient tachycardia or potentially diminish blood flow and hamper healing. In addition, rebound hyperemia should be expected following liberal use of concentrated epinephrine solutions. Excessive graft popping may be also technique- and operator-dependent. Surgeons should familiarize themselves with the various techniques for graft placement.[19]

Intraoperative headache may be treated with analgesics; however, the pain may also be alleviated by simply removing the circumferential dressing. Ketorolac 15 to 30 mg IM or IV may be helpful. Regardless of the patient's blood pressure or coagulation status, the transplanted grafts may continue to elevate or pop. This is probably more related to dermal elasticity, and a gentle pressure dressing may be applied. Alternatively, a salon hair dryer set to low heat should serve to limit popping until the openings coagulate and dry. At home, patients should be instructed to use direct pressure if oozing occurs. Optimally, patients should keep the grafted area as moist as possible by using a misting spray bottle. This will prevent excessive crusting during the postoperative phase.

◆ Diagnosis and Management of Postoperative Complications

General

During postoperative days 2–6, edema migrates from the top of the scalp to the forehead and throughout the soft tissues of the face. This commonly results in periorbital ecchymosis and facial edema. The edema may be limited by mixing triamcinolone 40 mg with the local anesthesia of the recipient area.[20] Nonetheless, even when the surgeon is diligent about notifying the patient

of this complication preoperatively, the sight of postoperative facial edema may be unsettling to patients. Besides the use of corticosteroids, it is helpful to reassure the patient calmly that this is common and that it will simply resolve with time. After several days, very few patients experience any pain in the recipient area.

Donor Site

Donor site complications may arise in the immediate postoperative period, over several weeks, or over months as the wound remodels. During the first two weeks, it is not uncommon for patients to complain about donor site discomfort. This usually resolves with suture removal. Although staples are easier to place, they are more uncomfortable than traditional sutures.[21] During the weeks to months following suture removal, localized areas of thickening may arise. These are typically caused by retained suture remnants or dermal elements. It may be difficult to distinguish suture material from hair keratin fibers. Localized wound irritations may be treated with widely available commercial 1–2% topical triamcinolone cream.

Total wound dehiscence may also occur. This is more likely to occur in patients undergoing repeat procedures where scar tissue is present and the tension across the wound is high. If this occurs, local wound hygiene is important while the wound granulates and heals by secondary intention. Once the wound has completely epithelialized, a sizable scar will be evident, because most of the follicles will have been destroyed. This can truly be a problematic issue for patients and hair restoration surgeons. Unfortunately, most scar revision techniques fail, ultimately resulting in a persistent, lifelong occipital scar that can, practically speaking, only be camoflauged by hair styling techniques in the back of the scalp. Because local flaps in this area have not proven successful in eliminating donor scars, surgeons have been left with few options, such as actually transplanting hair from the temporal area into the occipital scar or tattooing the scarred dermis with permanent ink as a way to conceal the bare scar.

Other localized wound complications confounding hair surgeons are hypertrophic scarring, pyogenic granuloma, and arteriovenous fistula formation. Hypertrophic scarring may be treated with serial Kenalog (Bristol-Myers Squibb, Princeton, NJ) injections; however, overuse of concentrated Kenalog injections may cause skin depressions secondary to atrophy of the subdermal fat. Pyogenic granulomas should be treated with local wound care and silver nitrate cauterization (**Fig. 17.2**). An arteriovenous (AV) fistula may present anywhere from several days to several weeks postoperatively. This will typically be perceived as a slightly painful swelling in the area of the donor excision. On examination, a pulsating mass confirms the diagnosis. Some operators choose to allow this to resolve sponta-

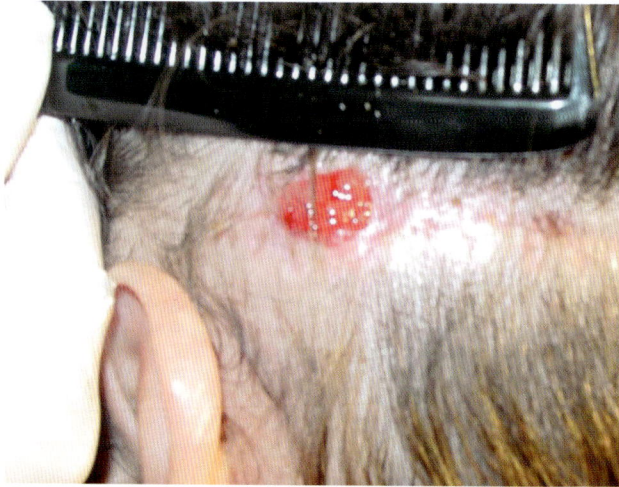

Fig. 17.2 A pyogenic granuloma is noted in the left side of a patient's donor area. This was treated with serial silver nitrate cauterization.

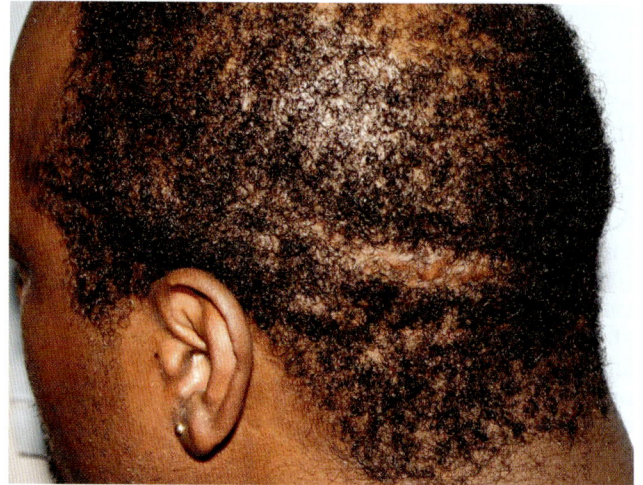

Fig. 17.3 Keloid formation is rare, and this formation developed after an attempted scar revision.

neously; however, the most effective treatment for an uncomfortable AV fistula is a local excision and ligation of the feeding vessel.[22]

Patients may inquire about the potential for keloid formation (**Fig. 17.3**). Fortunately, the occurrence of keloids is extremely rare. More commonly, a donor area may undergo significant telogen effluvium or shock loss. Although the donor area is less noticeable, any amount of shock loss can be extremely unnerving (**Fig. 17.4**). The surgeon at this point is obligated to offer gentle reassurance that the hair will in fact grow back.

Following any donor wound complications, a wider scar may form. In fact, even in uncomplicated surgeries patients will have a range in the size of the donor scar. A larger scar is often seen after repeat procedures; therefore, some surgeons will choose to harvest in a completely separate area, either above or below the original scar. It may be easier to camouflage several fine lines as opposed to a single wide scar (**Fig. 17.5**). Although several scar-reduction techniques are available, converting a widened scar to an invisible line is extremely difficult, as previously mentioned. Simple scar excision

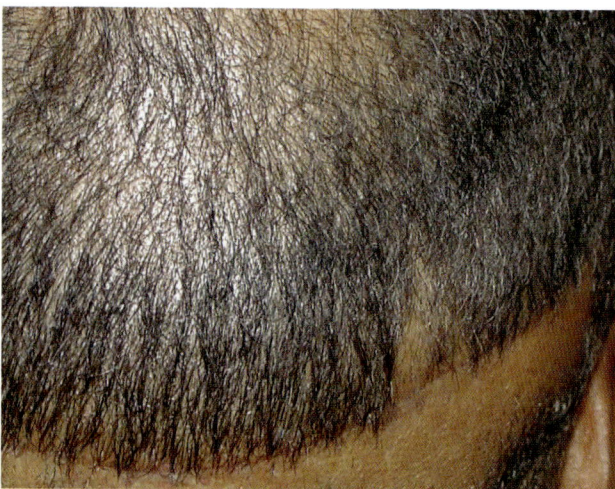

Fig. 17.4 Telogen and anagen effluvium developed in the donor area. It is more difficult to conceal in this patient with short hair.

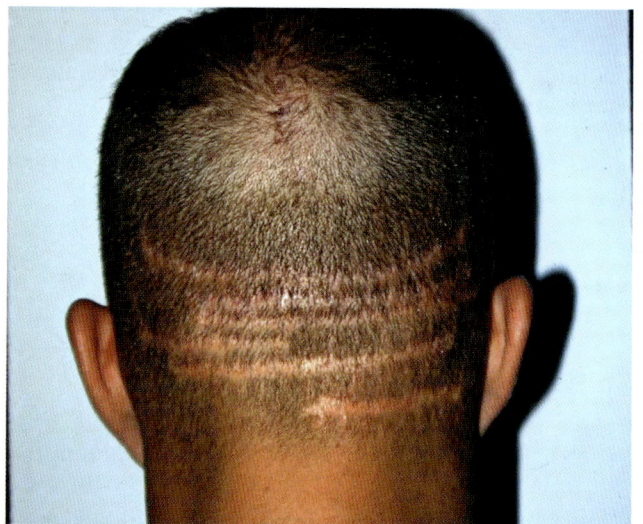

Fig. 17.5 Stacked donor scars may be more cosmetically appealing than one large scar.

may be tempting; however, donor scar revisions have a low aesthetic yield. Despite the will of a surgeon determined to do big cases, conservative donor excision minimizes donor scarring by limiting the tension across the wound. Once again, the retroauricular area tends to have the widest scarring, and careful preoperative planning will minimize this problem. Prepare for a widened scar when harvesting below the external occipital protuberance, as tension from the extensor muscles of the neck may contribute to widening. Deep fixation sutures may serve to decrease tension across the wound and theoretically prevent the scar from widening.[23,24] A small series of running 30°, 45°, or 60° Z-plasties or M-plasties may serve to break the line as well as to convert the angle of the tension across the wound from horizontal to vertical. In patients with ample donor supply, hair may be transplanted into the scar to help camouflage the donor scar.[3] Other methods of repair, such as using tissue expansion or trichophytic excisions, have been infrequently described.[25-27]

Recipient

Complications in the recipient area are rare in the first two postoperative days. Some patients may report bleeding from some of the incision sites. They should be instructed to apply gentle pressure. Oozing beyond 48 hours is unusual and should raise concern for a bleeding abnormality. Scabbing is to be expected. However, if the grafted areas are kept moist with either a saline-based spray or an ointment, then the crusts and scabs resolve by day 7. Crusts and scabs may be gently removed, but prolonged crusting should not be confused with the development of seborrheic plaques. In this event, treatment is targeted at the proliferating *Malassezia* yeast (formerly *Pityrospirum ovale*) and may include an antifungal shampoo, pyrithione zinc, topical corticosteroid, or 20% salicylic acid.[28,29]

Crusting may also conceal recipient wound healing abnormalities. One such problem is frontal central necrosis (**Fig. 17.6**). Although it is considered a rare complication, its true incidence is unknown, for many cases may go unreported.[30] The exact cause is also unclear. Rousso postulates that prolonged numbness may lead to itching and self-excoriation, while Seager feels that necrosis is the result of a compromised blood supply from exceedingly dense packing.[31,32] A necrotic area should be treated with local wound care and antibiotics, culturing any evidence of purulence. The objective of the oral antibiotic is to minimize the bacterial load of normal skin flora in the infected area while granulation tissue forms. However, one is advised to inspect the wound routinely for evidence of advancing cellulitis, particularly in any patient with compromised blood flow, such as a patient with type 1 diabetes. Should cellulitis occur, the antibiotics should be carefully adjusted based upon cultures and sensitivities, with IV antibiotics used if necessary.

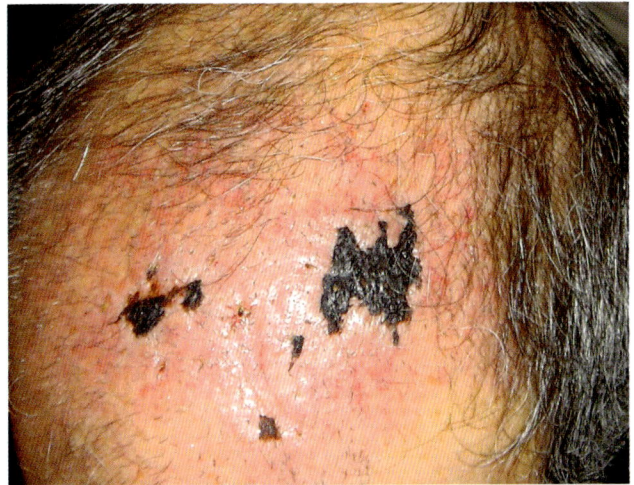

Fig. 17.6 Frontal central necrosis.

The eschar may be left intact as a biologic dressing until granulation tissue forms. If the wound is small, the edges may contract to cover the area completely; otherwise, the wound will heal by secondary intention. Tissue expansion may be used to create enough tissue for primary closure. Several weeks should elapse before a conservative attempt to add additional grafts.

During the months following the procedure, epidermal inclusion cysts occur in at least 10% of all follicular unit transplant cases.[33] Ironically, the occurrence of cysts may herald the growth of the new grafts. Patients should be instructed on procedures for home hygiene using topical rubbing alcohol and warm compresses.[34] Most cysts will be self-limiting; however, larger cysts may require incision and drainage. Persistent cysts occasionally progress to scalp infections requiring oral antibiotics. Rarely will this lead to loss of grafts.

Unfortunately, there is not yet a proven way to predict the occurrence of anagen and telogen effluvium (shock loss) nor a way to limit its severity. Parsely recommends minimizing the packing in already dense areas, and Kassimir has tried using minoxidil.[4,30] Because of the unpredictability of this possible temporary outcome and its potential for emotional distress, all patients should be carefully counseled regarding it.

Patients should expect new hair growth between the second and fifth month; however, individual deviations may occur (**Table 17.1**). Growth may be delayed beyond six months. Simple reassurance is helpful during follow-up exams, and demonstration of early growth with a microscopic device may be helpful. If the ultimate growth is less than expected, then several causes should be investigated. Poor handling may have created crush injury or desiccation. The quality of the donor hair may also have been poor. The surrounding hair may be

Table 17.1

Growth Problems	
Poor growth	Handling errors, weak donor, continued hair loss, count error, ergonomics, hairpiece
Poor planning	Asymmetry, too low, too straight, wrong area
Individual graft problem	Pitting, cobblestoning, wrong angles, kinky

experiencing continued hair loss, making it very difficult to determine the final results. On occasion, despite meticulous technique, the graft counts may have been tallied incorrectly. In any event, it may be very difficult to quantify the final outcome. Practically speaking, this final step of graft placement requires the highest level of skill and technical acumen. To enable the greatest graft survival, the surgeon must ensure patient comfort and safety as well as facilitating a perfect environment for the technicians, including brilliant lighting, magnification, precision instruments, and logistics. Hairpiece wearers have notoriously poor or delayed growth. Several reasons have been postulated; however, current dogma is to limit the amount of time the patient wears the hairpiece postoperatively, and the hair should be fixed to the scalp only with clips—hair adhesives should be avoided. Anecdotal evidence supports the notion that artificial hair should not be worn in the immediate postoperative period (during the first 3–5 days); however, this often presents social limits for patients, and they have been known to place hairpieces directly on the healing grafts. The same is true preoperatively, when patients are encouraged to maximize the health and natural state of the scalp follicle environment by limiting the time they wear their hairpiece. More scientific work needs to be completed that studies the effect of scalp hygiene on hair growth. As the tools for measuring postoperative results for hair transplant and other aesthetic surgeries evolve, patients should be encouraged to maintain meticulous scalp hygiene and to avoid any unnecessary traction on the grafts.

Even with robust growth, surgical errors may still occur in the planning and design. Poor outcomes include asymmetry or perhaps the placement of grafts in areas that were not acceptable to the patient. Patients also have been known to change their minds. It may be helpful to ask patients to sign a copy of the preoperative design, either on a drawing or a marked photograph. Obviously, this should be done before any sedation is administered. Finally, despite excellent growth and execution of a well-designed transplant, each individual graft may still appear cosmetically unsatisfactory. Some

known problems include pitting, ridging, cobblestoning, improper hair/scalp angling, and excessively curly or kinky hair growth. Hair styling may camouflage some problems, but ultimately the surgeon always has the option to excise unwanted hair or to add additional grafts to create blending. The same concepts are true for repairing older techniques, such as the hairline with unsightly multifollicular plugs. Experienced transplant surgeons have developed several elegant techniques for repairing undesirable results from prior procedures by either completely or partially excising standard grafts (hair plugs) and transplanting smaller, microscopic grafts in the immediate area.[14,35–37] The basic idea is to break up all or parts of the older hair plug (standard graft) using a small dermatologic circular biopsy punch, reprocess the grafts, and reinsert smaller, follicular unit grafts and thereby create a new, blended hairline.

◆ Flaps and Scalp Reduction

Fairly recent surveys conducted by the International Society of Hair Restoration Surgery revealed that only 1.2% of all surgical hair restoration procedures involve alopecia reductions or flaps.[38] Many current hair surgeons may not even be familiar with the techniques. By way of review, the classic temporoparietal flap (Juri flap or Fleming-Mayer flap) is a pedicled flap using a terminal branch of the superficial temporal artery. Hair-bearing scalp is transferred to the frontal hairline, and several separate flaps may allow the transfer of large amounts of thick hair. Although the transferred hair yields complete density, the flap delivers far from satisfactory aesthetic results by today's standards. Complications associated with the Juri flap, such as necrosis, asymmetry, and faulty hair direction, spawned techniques designed to correct them.[39] Because of their marginal aesthetics and elevated risk of complications, as well as the advancement of micrografting, Juri flaps have become relatively obsolete except in rare instances associated with trauma or burn scars.

On the other hand, alopecia reductions may still be useful in selected cases of alopecia. Different designs excise unwanted bald scalp while advancing hair-bearing tissue. Serial excisions as well as tissue expansion will maximize the size of the reduction. The techniques are useful for revising scars and reconstructing scalp defects.[40,41] Infection, hematoma, and implant exposure are all possible complications when tissue expanders are used. In addition, the complications of any scalp reduction procedure include diminished density of the surrounding hair and a visible scar. Perhaps the most troubling cosmetic deformity is the development of a "slot defect," with hair falling unnaturally away from the scar (**Fig. 17.7**). Frechet describes using a triple transposition flaps to deal with the slot formation (**Fig. 17.8**).[2]

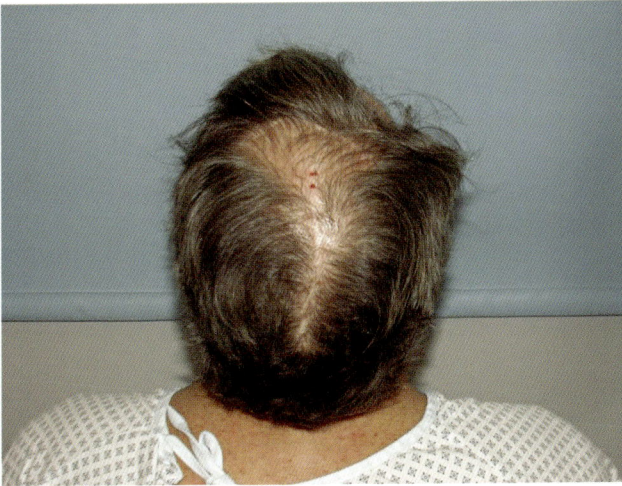

Fig. 17.7 This photograph shows the slot defect that may occur after a reduction performed to alleviate vertex alopecia.

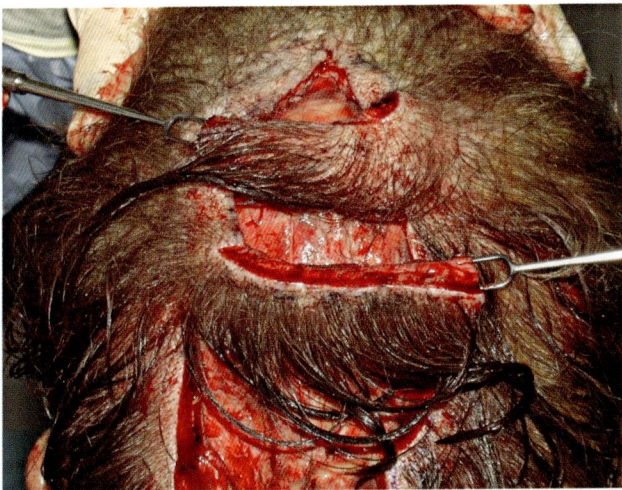

Fig. 17.8 The slot defect may be repaired with the transposition of three hair-bearing flaps, allowing both coverage of the slot as well as a natural direction of the hair falling inferiorly.

◆ Conclusion

This chapter has described the complications of hair restoration and techniques for their prevention and mitigation. Despite proper planning and execution, experienced transplant surgeons will still encounter patients whose expectations have not been met. Maintaining close follow-up and good communications should limit the problems when unexpected results or complications occur. As always, avoidance of complications is the best practice.

PEARLS OF WISDOM

Preparing hair restoration patients to have realistic expectations will help tremendously with patient satisfaction.

Patients must understand that hair loss is progressive and that most hair restoration patients will require more than one procedure.

It is always easier to add additional hair than to attempt correcting poorly placed grafts.

The best hair results occur when patients are relaxed and at ease.

When there is doubt, a preliminary test procedure using approximately 100 grafts may allay the fears of both the surgeon and patient.

Promising new techniques using Follicular Unit Extraction (FUE) and automation devices will undoubtedly be associated with newer, but hopefully less serious, complications.

References

1. Adler SC, Rousso D. Evaluation of past and present hair replacement techniques. Aesthetic improvement, effectiveness, postoperative pain, and complications. Arch Facial Plast Surg 1999;1(4):266–271
2. Frechet P. A new method for correction of the vertical scar observed following scalp reduction for extensive alopecia. J Dermatol Surg Oncol 1990;16(7):640–644
3. Epstein JS. Hair transplantation in women: treating female pattern baldness and repairing distortion and scarring from prior cosmetic surgery. Arch Facial Plast Surg 2003;5(1):121–126
4. Kassimir JJ. Use of topical minoxidil as a possible adjunct to hair transplant surgery. A pilot study. J Am Acad Dermatol 1987;16(3 Pt 2):685–687
5. Olsen E. In: Disorders of Hair Growth: Diagnosis and Treatment. New York: McGraw-Hill; 2004:77–81
6. Ziering C, Krenitsky G. The Ziering whorl classification of scalp hair. Dermatol Surg 2003;29(8):817–821, discussion 821
7. Klein J. Cytochrome P450 3A4 and Lidocaine Metabolism. In: Klein JP, ed. Tumescent Techniques. St. Louis: Mosby; 2000:131–140
8. Zhang CBD, Banting DW, Gelb AW, Hamilton JT. Effect of beta-adrenoreceptor blockade with nadolol on the duration of local anesthesia. J Am Dent Assoc 1999;130(12):1773–1780
9. Nusbaum BP. Techniques to reduce pain associated with hair transplantation: optimizing anesthesia and analgesia. Am J Clin Dermatol 2004;5(1):9–15
10. Hammond D. Hypnotic Inductions. In: Hammond DC, ed. Hypnotic Induction and Suggestion. Chicago: American Society of Hypnosis; 1998:20–44
11. Feldman C. Tissue laxity based on donor tissue ballooning. Hair Trans Forum Intl 2001;11(4):119

12. Mayer ML. P.T., Scalp Elasticity Scale. Hair Trans Forum Intl 2005;15(4):122–123

13. Bosley LL, Hope CR, Montroy RE, Straub PM. Reduction of male pattern baldness in multiple stages: a retrospective study. J Dermatol Surg Oncol 1980;6(6):498–503

14. Bernstein RM, Rassman WR, Rashid N, Shiell RC. The art of repair in surgical hair restoration part I: basic repair strategies. Dermatol Surg 2002;28(9):783–794

15. Kim J, Hwang S. The Effects of Dehydration, Preservation Temperature and Time, and Hydrogen Peroxide on Hair Grafts. In: Unger WP, ed. Hair Transplantation. New York: Marcel Dekker; 1995:285–286

16. Greco JF, Kramer RD, Reynolds GD. A "crush study" review of micrograft survival. Dermatol Surg 1997;23(9):752–755

17. Cooley JE, Vogel JE. Follicle trauma and the role of the dissecting microscope in hair transplantation: A multicenter study. Dermatol Clin 1999;17(2):307–312, viii; discussion 312–313

18. Seager DJ. Micrograft size and subsequent survival. Dermatol Surg 1997;23(9):757–761, discussion 762

19. Whitworth JM, Stough DB, Limmer B, et al. A comparison of graft implantation techniques for hair transplantation. Semin Cutan Med Surg 1999;18(2):177–183

20. Gholamali A, Sepideh P, Susan E. Hair transplantation without post-operative edema. Hair Trans Forum Int 2005;15(5):149, 158

21. Bernstein RM, Rassman WR, Rashid N. A new suture for hair transplantation: poliglecaprone 25. Dermatol Surg 2001; 27(1):5–11

22. Davis AJ, Nelson PK. Arteriovenous fistula of the scalp secondary to punch autograft hair transplantation: angioarchitecture, histopathology, and endovascular and surgical therapy. Plast Reconstr Surg 1997;100(1):242–249

23. Seery GE. Hair transplantation: management of donor area. Dermatol Surg 2002;28(2):136–142

24. Bernstein RM, Rassman WR, Rashid N, Shiell RC. The art of repair in surgical hair restoration—part II: the tactics of repair. Dermatol Surg 2002;28(10):873–893

25. Brandy DA. Intricacies of the single-scar technique for donor harvesting in hair transplantation surgery. Dermatol Surg 2004;30(6):837–844, discussion 844–845

26. Seery GE. Improved scalp surgery results by controlling tension vector forces in the tissues by galea to pericranium fixation sutures. Dermatol Surg 2001;27(6):569–574

27. Seyhan A, Yoleri L, Barutçu A. Immediate hair transplantation into a newly closed wound to conceal the final scar on the hair-bearing skin. Plast Reconstr Surg 2000 Apr;105(5):1866–1870, discussion 1871

28. Cotterill P. Seborrheic dermatitis. Hair Trans Forum Intl 1997;7(6):13

29. DeAngelis YMG, Gemmer CM, Kaczvinsky JR, Kenneally DC, Schwartz JR, Dawson TL Jr. Three etiologic facets of dandruff and seborrheic dermatitis: fungi, sebaceous lipids, and individual sensitivity. J Investig Dermatol Symp Proc 2005;10(3):295–297

30. Parsley W. Management of the Postoperative Period. In: Unger WP, ed. Hair Transplantation. New York: Marcel Dekker; 2004:562

31. Rousso DE. Repostoperative frontal central necrosis. Hair Trans Forum Intl. 1999;9(5):158

32. Seager DJ. Pitfalls of Follicular Unit Hair Transplantation and How to Avoid Them In: Unger WP, ed. Hair Transplantation. New York: Marcel Dekker; 2004:409–410

33. Whiting DA, Stough DB. Posttransplant epidermoid cysts secondary to small graft hair transplantation. Dermatol Surg 1995;21(10):863–866

34. Barrera A. Micrograft and minigraft megasession hair transplantation results after a single session. Plast Reconstr Surg 1997;100(6):1524–1530

35. Epstein JS. Revision surgical hair restoration: repair of undesirable results. Plast Reconstr Surg 1999;104(1):222–232, discussion 233–236

36. Vogel JE. Correcting problems in hair restoration surgery: an update. Facial Plast Surg Clin North Am 2004;12(2):263–278

37. Swinehart JM. Hair repair surgery. Corrective measures for improvement of older large-graft procedures and scalp scars. Dermatol Surg 1999;25(7):523–528, discussion 529

38. International Society of Hair Restoration Surgery. Hair Restoration Surgical Procedures by Type of Procedure. Practice Census Statistics, 2005:18

39. Brandy DA. Corrective hair restoration techniques for the aesthetic problems of temperoparietal flaps. Dermatol Surg 2003;29(3):230–234, discussion 234

40. Epstein JS. The role of tissue expansion in hair transplant surgery: presentation of two unique cases. Hair Trans Forum Intl 2002;12(3):108–109

41. Ramirez A, Kabaker SS. Reducing the female forehead without hair transplantation. Hair Trans Forum Intl 2004;14(2):93–94

Index

Note: Page numbers followed by *f* and *t* indicate figures and tables, respectively.